Immunology: Overview and Laboratory Manual

Tobili Y. Sam-Yellowe

Immunology: Overview and Laboratory Manual

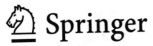 Springer

Tobili Y. Sam-Yellowe
Cleveland State University
Cleveland, OH, USA

ISBN 978-3-030-64688-2   ISBN 978-3-030-64686-8   (eBook)
https://doi.org/10.1007/978-3-030-64686-8

This Springer imprint is published by the registered company Springer Nature Switzerland AG
The registered company address is: Gewerbestrasse 11, 6330 Cham, Switzerland

To Samuel Itode and Tobili Ann Idiowa Hatcher

Preface

Immunology is an exciting and fascinating subject. New discoveries and a deeper understanding of cellular and molecular interactions continue to result in a proliferation of publications in the literature. The use of traditional as well as new laboratory techniques for investigating immunological processes and detecting antibodies and antigens continue to provide new information and expand our knowledge of immunology and its contributions to other areas such as oncology, parasitology and virology. Increased understanding of regulatory pathways during cell activation in innate and adaptive immunity along with the identification of disease markers is providing improved ways to approach clinical therapies for cancer, autoimmune diseases and allergies using bioinformatics and immunological systems. An increased understanding of the human immune system has ushered in a reality for vaccines against parasitic diseases using novel vaccine delivery systems. Due to the highly experimental nature of immunology and the importance of being able to refer to the theory underlying a particular laboratory exercise, I wanted to write a book that combines the laboratory exercises with the theory in one book to give students a fuller appreciation of immunology. Illustrations are provided in the laboratory manual to aid understanding of the flow of the protocols described. Exercises progress from basic protocols introducing students to the microscope, pipetting, performing dilutions in the laboratory, counting and differentiating leukocytes to more complex exercises involving immunoassays and tissue culture. Exercises employing molecular biology techniques are included to round out the laboratory exercises. Each exercise can be performed alone or combined with others to provide a more detailed understanding of concepts. The experiments are suitable for students beginning immunology as well as those that already have a background in immunology at the undergraduate or graduate level. Questions are provided at the end of to aid review of the material covered in the overview and laboratory exercises. The overview portion of the book describes the organization of innate and adaptive immunity with an explanation of lymphoid organs, cell organization and function, properties of antigens, development and activation of B and T lymphocytes and the process of lymphocyte migration and apoptosis. Sections are included for hypersensitivities, parasite immunity, vaccines, transplantation, immune regulation and autoimmunity, immunodeficiencies and cancer. Study guides and questions to aid review of the topics are included at the end of the overview. A list of vendors where reagents can be obtained for the laboratory and a list of immunology websites is provided. I am grateful for the reviewers who provided feedback on the book proposal and for their helpful suggestions. I look forward to receiving questions, comments and suggestions regarding the book.

Cleveland, OH, USA

Tobili Y. Sam-Yellowe

Acknowledgements

I thank all my students of immunology from the past 30 years. I have appreciated their many comments, probing questions, and their help in keeping immunology fresh and always fascinating. I thank my immunology professors who first sparked my interest in the subject of immunology with their vivid illustrations and explanations of cellular interactions and the genuine enthusiasm with which they taught the subject of immunology. They made immunology exercises exciting and helped to strengthen understanding of concepts in immunology. These exercises continue to help students understand immunological concepts and increase their desire to continue the study of immunology. I am grateful to the editorial team at Springer Nature for all their help with this book. I thank my children Samuel and Tobili Ann for their understanding, patience and continued support. I am extremely grateful to Aidan M. Walsh for preparing the illustrations used in the cover, overview and lab manual.

Contents

Part I
Immunology Overview

Chapter 1
Immunity

Organization of the Immune System

The human immune system is essential for survival. The human host is exposed to a myriad of organisms with potential to cause infections. Some organisms are opportunistic and will cause infections in immunocompromised and some immunocompetent individuals, while other organisms are pathogenic and will cause infections in immunocompetent individuals. Entry of infectious agents into the host through the skin, or through breaches in the mucosal barriers of the body can elicit immune responses that can ultimately eliminate the pathogen. Elimination can occur through the innate immune system or through the combined efforts of both innate and adaptive immune responses. The way in which host cells detect pathogens and their antigens, leading to signal transduction within cells resulting in cytokine secretion and the events bridging innate immunity to activation of the adaptive immune response, will be the subject of the overview section of this book. The laboratory protocols used to identify antigens, antibodies, cytokines and their cellular interactions will be the subject of the laboratory exercises in the lab manual. The first task of the overview section is to define the organization of the immune system. What is the immune system? Where is it located in the body? These are questions that we will answer as we discuss how the immune system works. Among different vertebrate and invertebrate organisms, mechanisms of immunity are present ranging from the presence of phagocytic cells and humoral substances to the activity of effector cells utilizing variable lymphoid receptors to respond in "adaptive" responses in ways similar to the variable receptors on human cells generated from the variable, diversity and joining (VDJ) gene recombination events resulting in the expression of variable B and T lymphocyte antigen binding receptors. Pathogenic agents comprise prokaryotes (bacteria, archaea), eukaryotes (protozoans, helminths, and fungi), viruses and prions. The human immune system is designed and equipped to meet the challenges of exposure to and encounter with pathogenic agents. In addition to infectious agents, the immune system is also equipped to respond to

© Springer Nature Switzerland AG 2021
T. Y. Sam-Yellowe, *Immunology: Overview and Laboratory Manual*,
https://doi.org/10.1007/978-3-030-64686-8_1

chemical antigens, natural or synthetic. A competent immune system copes effectively with most of these agents, generating immune responses that lead to the production of memory B and T lymphocytes. An immunologically incompetent (immunosuppressed) immune system is deficient in many responses, tolerized or anergic and cannot cope with antigenic agents by mounting an effective immune response. The emphasis of this overview text will be on the vertebrate immune system, mainly the human immune system. The overview will serve as ready reference for the exercises contained in the laboratory manual section of the text. In the chapters that follow, we will use examples from results of mouse and human studies to explain various immunological concepts in innate and adaptive immunity. The mouse is the most commonly used animal model in experimental immunology. Another important animal model frequently used, particularly for antibody production is the rabbit. We will also use examples from experiments performed using cell lines in tissue culture to discuss, illustrate and explain various immunological concepts.

Within the host, the immune system is organized as a network of interacting cells, soluble factors, **intracellular** and **intercellular** signals all cooperating to mount the most effective and efficient immune response. The immune response is highly coordinated and regulated, with cells in continuous communication using cytokines and chemokines as the medium for coordination. This vast network also in coordination with the neuroendocrine system and gut microbiome is aimed at protecting the host and maintaining immune homeostasis. The major barriers protecting the body from extracellular agents include the skin and mucosal epithelium. These barriers contain immune cells capable of sensing, detecting, and phagocytosing pathogens for eventual elimination. How do host cells "know" that barriers have been breached? We will discuss the sentinel cells that "sound the alarm" announcing the presence of invaders in the body. The barriers also contain antimicrobial peptides and proteins secreted by cells of the epithelium. The fundamental approach of the immune system in providing protection is to eliminate foreign agents **(antigens)** by the use of cells and soluble factors in innate immunity, binding and eliminating antigens in response to soluble factors such as cytokines from **T helper cells** and **antibodies (immunoglobulins)** from **B cells** in humoral immunity or attacking target cells directly using cell mediated immunity by the use of **cytotoxic T lymphocytes (CTLs) or natural killer (NK) cells**. T helper and cytotoxic T lymphocytes recognize antigen associated with **major histocompatibility complex (MHC)** proteins. Activation of the T cells generates effector and memory cell populations. Both humoral and cell-mediated immunity are branches of specific or adaptive (also known as acquired or induced) immunity that together can recognize extracellular and intracellular antigens. Cytokines produced by cells in innate and adaptive immune responses, enhance cell activation and result in cell recruitment and migration.

We will also discuss **tolerance**, a specific non response to antigens by B and T lymphocytes, which can occur upon exposure to pathogens and in chronic diseases such as autoimmune disease and cancers and in some parasitic infections. The role of central and peripheral tolerance in the function of regulatory T cells (TREG) will be discussed. During development of the host, the immune system develops in a manner that allows cells to recognize foreign antigens on pathogens and **alloantigens** on **histoincompatible** tissue. The process of readiness i.e. cell preparation involves recognition of antigen by host cells using specific antigen binding receptors followed by cell activation. Cells that cannot enter the activation pathway become **anergic** or die by **programmed cell death** (PCD) also known as **apoptosis**. While most activity of the immune system in its protective capacity is beneficial, the immune system can also "malfunction" or breakdown, allowing the immune system to attack host tissue. This **autoreactivity** is known as an autoimmune response (autoimmunity). The immune response can also become highly exaggerated leading to extensive tissue damage and inflammation. These exaggerated responses are known as **hypersensitive** responses or **hypersensitivities**. An example is an allergic response made to allergen exposure. The regulation provided by the commensal organisms of the gut microbiome will be discussed with reference to the "Old friends" or "Hygiene hypothesis" to provide an understanding of the interdependence that exists between the gut microbiome and immune homeostasis. Parts of the immune system may be nonfunctional through **immunodeficiencies** (both congenital and acquired) leaving the host highly vulnerable to infectious disease agents, neoplastic or abnormal cell growth such as tumors and cancers. Tissue transplants may be vigorously attacked following transplantation leading to tissue rejection. Figure 1.1 presents an overview of the immune system as it responds to pathogens.

The major system responsible for transportation of components of the immune system is the **lymphatic system**. This is the second circulatory system in the body. The components are transported mainly as lymph, which consists of proteinaceous fluid collected from intercellular spaces, during blood circulation, as well as lymphocytes. The lymph circulates through lymphatic vessels, regional lymph nodes and eventually through the **thoracic duct** (also known as the left lymphatic duct, the largest lymphatic vessel) and subclavian veins which empty into the heart through the vena cava. The lymph is filtered through regional lymph nodes where foreign substances are trapped for antigen processing and degradation. Every tissue in the body is sampled for pathogens. On the basis of this circulation, immune cells are located in regional lymph nodes strategically located in the body and immune cells are also found in the peripheral blood circulation. The discipline of immunology is highly experimental and accompanied by prolific publications of new findings and advances in the field of immunology. The discipline is highly integrated with molecular biology, cell biology, genetics, evolutionary biology, clinical medicine and the fields of infectious diseases and parasitology. The following overall objectives will guide a course utilizing this book:

- Students will develop an excellent working knowledge of how the immune system develops and works under normal circumstances, and under conditions where portions of the system are "dysfunctional".
- Students completing the course will have an excellent working knowledge of the various cellular components, cellular and signaling networks and regulatory features that permit effective and efficient function of the immune system.

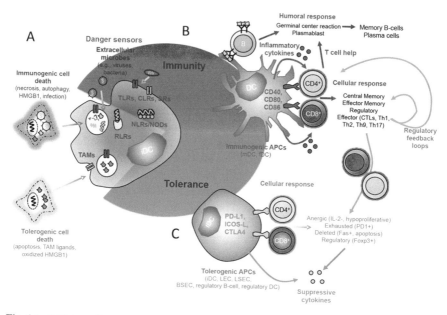

Fig. 1.1 Bridging of innate and adaptive immune responses. (**a**) Dendritic cells (DCs) are major sentinel cells responsible for detecting and responding to molecules released from damaged and dying cells and from pathogen invasion of tissues. Immature DCs (iDCs) expressing pattern recognition receptors (PRRs) such as TLRs, CLRs, NLRs, RLRs and SRs on the cell surface and within the cytoplasm bind to pathogen associated molecular patterns (PAMPs) and damage associated molecular patterns (DAMPs) from damaged tissue and initiate innate immune responses. Signals received by iDCs may lead to T lymphocyte activation for the production of effector T cells or signals may induce anergy or tolerance. (**b**) Cytokines released by iDCs polarize T helper subsets (TH1, TH2, TH9, TH17) and enhance T cell recognition of antigen and effector cell and memory cell development. Cytokines secreted enhance B and T cell cooperation in adaptive immune responses. Cross presentation of antigens to cytotoxic T cells (Tc) also leads to activation and induction of apoptosis in targets cells. (**c**) Inhibitory signals and lack of coreceptor expression or engagement can lead to anergy and tolerance. The Tyro-3, Ax1 and Mer (TAM) family receptor tyrosine kinases become activated, inhibiting DC activation and maturation. [*Republished with permission of SpringerNature publishing from Irvine, D. J., et al., "Engineering synthetic vaccines using cues from natural immunity." Nat Mater 2013 November; 12(11):978-990, Figure 1. Conveyed through STM permission guidelines 2014*]

- Students completing the course will be able to identify specific immune diseases and understand the mechanism of disease development and the contribution of specific immune mechanisms to the development of disease.
- Students will be able to identify the molecules and features that characterize antigens/immunogens (proteins, carbohydrates, lipids and nucleic acid) with potential as strong vaccine molecules.

Based on our discussions in the chapters of this overview, students will learn the different ways in which immune responses are evaluated in the host using serological, immunological and molecular assays. We will examine the organization of the immune system, and cells and organs of the immune system including hematopoiesis and regulation. We will then examine properties of antigens, antigen processing and presentation on major histocompatibility complex (MHC) proteins, the development of B and T lymphocytes and cell signaling following antigen binding by B and T cell receptors. Applications of immune mechanisms to apoptosis, hypersensitivities, parasite immunity, autoimmunity, rejection of transplanted tissue, immunodeficiencies and cancer will be discussed.

Selected References

Irvine DJ, Swartz MA, Szeto GL (2013) Engineering synthetic vaccines using cues from natural immunity. Nat Mater 12:978–990

Murphy K, Weaver C (2017) Janeway's immunobiology, 9th edn. Garland Press, New York

Parkin J, Cohen B (2001) An overview of the immune system. Lancet 357:1777–1789

Punt J, Stranford SA, Jones PP, Owen JA (2019) Kuby immunology, 8th edn. W.H. Freeman and Company, New York. Chapter 20, Antigen-Antibody Interactions.

Shanker A, Marincola FM (2011) Cooperativity of adaptive and innate immunity: implications for cancer therapy. Cancer Immunol Immunother 60:1061–1074

Simon AK, Hollander GA, McMichael A (2015) Evolution of the immune system in humans from infancy to old age. Proc R Soc B 282:20143085

Yatim KM, Lakkis FG (2015) A brief journey through the immune system. Clin J Am Soc Nephrol 10:1274–1281

Chapter 2
Components of Immunity

The first area that we will address regarding immunity is how to identify the components of the immune system which will allow us to know those components that function in the innate and adaptive immune systems. How is the immune system organized? How does the immune system work? In our discussions we will provide answers to these questions. The immune system comprises a coordinated, closed as well as open network of cells, molecules, fluid and compartmentalized organs or domains within the body. Each organ or domain and each cell and molecule has a distinct function for defense. Blood and lymphatic vessels combine to transport cells and molecules into and out of organs to facilitate antigen recognition by B and T cells, cell activation and access of effector molecules and cells with pathogens and their products. Cell adhesion molecules (CAMs) enable cells to interact and communicate, thereby facilitating coordinated responses and movement of cells out of blood vessels and across compartments into tissues, through diapedesis. The various organs, cells, molecules and interconnected network of lymphatic and blood vessels responsible for immunity constitute the immune system. The immune response generated is strengthened by interactions of immune cells with products of the gut microbiome such as the short chain fatty acids (SCFAs), butyrate, propionate and acetate. The cumulative and coordinated response to antigens (foreign and self antigen) resulting in effector function and memory cell development is the immune response. The major components of the immune system include leukocytes for defense. Leukocytes comprise granulocytes which include neutrophils, eosinophils, basophils, mast cells and agranulocytes such as monocytes (including tissue macrophages), lymphocytes and dendritic cells. For example, B lymphocytes secrete antibodies and cytokines, T lymphocytes secrete cytokines and some T cells mediate cytotoxicity. Plasma and lymph is used for transportation of cells and molecules throughout the body. Erythrocytes facilitate the survival of leukocytes by ensuring availability of oxygen for cell respiration and metabolism through gas exchange.

The second area will focus on an understanding of what the immune system is. This leads us to ask where the immune system is located. Where are the effector cells and lymphoid organs located in the body? Cells that function in the immune

© Springer Nature Switzerland AG 2021
T. Y. Sam-Yellowe, *Immunology: Overview and Laboratory Manual*,
https://doi.org/10.1007/978-3-030-64686-8_2

system are dispersed throughout the body in association with a network of lymphatic vessels, lymphoid organs and mucosal surfaces lining body cavities. A major factor in coordinating the immune system is the closed circulatory system through the heart as well as the open lymphatic system consisting of lymphatic vessels, whose contents pass through lymph nodes, continue unidirectionally through lymphatic vessels and enter the subclavian veins as they make their way to the heart through the vena cava. Lymph moves through the body by muscular action as it transports cells and cell products.

The third area will examine the definition of immunity and will be helpful as we begin our discussions of how immune cells "sense" and encounter pathogens that breach the skin and mucosal barriers of the body resulting in the initiation of an immune response. What is immunity? A simple and generalized definition would be, protection from infectious disease. Other definitions include the body's reaction to foreign substances and host molecules collectively known as antigens, the components of pathogens such as bacteria, fungi, parasites and viruses. The various macromolecules which include proteins, polysaccharides, lipids, nucleic acids which are components of the secretory and excretory products of pathogens along with membrane and cytoplasmic contents of the pathogens are known as antigens. Other antigen sources include autoantigens, transplanted tissue, tumors, secreted products from microorganisms and synthetic antigens. Immunity can be innate (native, natural, non-specific) or it can be adaptive (acquired, specific, induced). The immune response can be humoral or cellular. Historically, the study of immunology was focused on interactions between antibodies and antigens, known as serology. Modern immunology comprises the study of specific **biochemical, physiological, histological, cellular, molecular, genetic and epigenetic** events that occur within a host following an encounter with, and recognition of foreign substances (antigens) such as microbes, parasites, macromolecules, transplanted tissue, or tumors, including tumor associated and tumor specific antigens. The study of immunology also comprises an understanding of the gut microbiome and the gut-brain axis as well as the role of SCFAs in modulating immune cell function. Immune mechanisms while protective can also cause injury (allergies and other hypersensitivity conditions) and disease (autoimmune diseases) under certain conditions. The mammalian antigen specific immune system increases the efficiency of host defense by selectively targeting foreign invaders using powerful effector mechanisms. The immune system consists of the cells and the molecules responsible for immunity such that the cumulative and coordinated response to the foreign substance is the immune response. The immune response is a result of specific recognition of **foreign substances**, collectively known as **antigens** and the host response to the antigens. Generally there is a coordination of both humoral and cellular responses as a result of exposure to or contact with antigen. This results in immunity. In general the interrelationships are established among the pathogen or infectious agent, the host, the infection or disease that results and the resulting immunity. The basic unit of the immune system is the antigen specific lymphocyte clone, but successful host defense requires clonal activity and regulated coordinated activities to ensure consistent and efficacious response to antigen regardless of entry site. For cutaneous and mucosal sites, the response is primarily innate immunity. However, cells from adaptive immunity are also activated following antigen presentation. For entry through the blood circulation and at the systemic level, adaptive immunity is the primary response with assistance from innate immune responses. A major requirement of immunity is a micro-environment to support production, maturation and differentiation of leukocytes and erythrocytes from pluripotent, non-functional precursors in primary lymphoid organs.

A fourth area we will address is the effector function of immunity. What features are required for the development of immunity? Following the maturity of lymphocytes, for example B and T lymphocytes in primary lymphoid organs, antigen contact will be made using the proper antigen receptors in specialized micro-environments in secondary and tertiary lymphoid organs. Contact with antigen will include communication with accessory cells to support and regulate the resulting antigen driven clonal expansion and differentiation of the responding lymphocytes. In this environment, pathogens are filtered through lymph nodes, the immune response is initiated following antigen contact and lymphocytes traverse the general circulation entering and leaving the lymph nodes until antigen contact is made. Cells failing to contact antigen die by apoptosis. Following lymphocyte proliferation, cells must have the correct environment to differentiate into effector and memory cells. The effector and memory lymphocyte populations must be dispersed to sites in the body for elimination of the invaders and for surveillance of host tissues for future antigen contact and elimination of neoplastic growth. To ensure that the immune system functions efficiently the mammalian immune system is compartmentalized into distinct organs and tissues. The compartments are unified, functionally, through a large network of targeted lymphocytes that circulate through both tissues and organs. An induced and sustained immune response is a result of specific recognition of an antigen by the host immune system, and the resulting cellular activity, which leads to secretion of antibodies, cytokines or activation of cells into cytotoxic effector cells. The central premise of immunity is Recognition versus Response. Membrane receptors on lymphocytes and other cells such as neutrophils, macrophages, epithelial cells lining the mucosa recognize and bind ligands from pathogens, antigens expressed on host cell surfaces or molecules exposed following tissue damage. For example:

Diverse molecular patterns on pathogens vs Innate responses; Antigens vs Humoral responses; Antigens vs Cellular responses.

Summary of the adaptive immune response: Cells participating in the immune system include lymphocytes and antigen presenting cells with cytokines and chemokines coordinating responses.

Lymphocytes

Bone marrow -> Thymus

B lymphocytes   Antigenically committed T lymphocytes

Effector cells plus memory cells   •Antigen contact   Effector cells plus
                                                             APCs   memory cells
2×10^3 antibody molecules secreted   Cytokines
                                                                                          CD4$^+$ cells: TH1, TH2,
                                                      • MHC proteins   TH17, Treg
                                                                                          CD8$^+$ cells Tc
Isotypes: lgM, IgG, IgA, IgD, IgE   Alpha/beta TCR
                                                                                          Gamma/delta TCR

Maturation and activation states of the lymphocyte influences the migration pattern of the cells due to the types of cell adhesion molecules expressed by the cells and endothelial cells of blood vessels. Cell activation is as a result of antigen contact. Naïve resting cells migrate to the secondary lymphoid tissue, activated cells migrate to inflammatory sites or home to specific sites within the secondary and tertiary tissues. Memory cells recirculate into the secondary lymphoid organs and the bone marrow. Memory cells cross the vascular endothelium at the high endothelial venules (HEVs) when they enter lymph nodes. The following features interact and lead to antigen recognition, cell activation followed by cytokine and antibody secretion and generation of cytotoxic killer cells:

- Pathogen
- Host
- Infection
- Disease
- Immunity
- Memory

In order to generate an immune response, recognition molecules need to be assembled in the **afferent branch** (also known as the **input branch**) of the immune system. The secretion of effector molecules such as antibodies and the activation of cells for effector function for target destruction constitute the **efferent branch** (also known as the **output branch**) of the immune system. Both afferent and efferent branches function cooperatively with the major histocompatibility complex (MHC) proteins and are regulated by cytokines, to generate a successful immune response. Although responses are not linear, cellular interactions lead to sequential events within networks that lead to effective responses that result in elimination of antigens and production of memory cells.

Selected References

Antonioli L, Blandizzi C, Pacher P, Guilliams M, Hasko G (2019) Rethinking communication in the immune system: The quorum sensing concept. Trends Immunol 40:88–97

Muraille E, Goriely S (2017) The nonspecific face of adaptive immunity. Curr Opin Immunol 48:38–43

Murphy K, Weaver C (2017) Janeway's immunobiology, 9th edn. Garland Press, New York

Punt J, Stranford SA, Jones PP (2019) In: Owen JA (ed) Kuby immunology, 8th edn. W.H. Freeman and Company, New York. Chapter 20, Antigen-antibody interactions

Chapter 3
Hematopoiesis

In order to recognize antigens and mount an immune response, different cell types are required to perform immunosurveillance, sense and detect pathogens and continuously survey the landscape of host tissues for breaches and host cell alterations. Each cell bears surface receptors that facilitate specific functions. Where do the cells come from? How can each cell type be differentiated? The various cells of the immune system develop from a common pluripotent stem cell known as the **hematopoietic stem cell (HSC)** which makes up 0.05% of all bone marrow cells. This is a cell type maintained at homeostatic levels and low frequency. The process of blood cell formation and differentiation in the bone marrow is known as **hematopoiesis**. The HSC is highly regulated, self-renewing and highly proliferative on demand. From these cells, myeloid and lymphoid progenitors arise that are capable of giving rise to granulocytic, erythroid and myeloid lineages (megakaryocytic, monocytic-dendritic), and into B lymphocytes, T lymphocytes and innate lymphoid cells (ILCs), respectively. The HSC responds to cytokines such as IL-1, IL-3, IL-7, GM-CSFs and examples of surface antigens identifying HSC are stem cell antigen (Sca-1), CD34 and CD38. Lineage specific markers are absent on HSCs. The cells most commonly associated with immunity include the leukocytes; lymphocytes (B, T and Natural killer), neutrophils, eosinophils, basophils, mast cells, monocytes, macrophages, dendritic cells and innate lymphoid cells. Erythrocytes (red blood cells) and leukocytes (white blood cells) develop in the bone marrow, within the medullary cavity, from pluripotent HSCs. CD34-biotin can be used to affinity purify stem cells for clinical use. In the presence of the appropriate cytokines, these cells in vitro can give rise to all the major leukocytes. Surface antigens expressed by cells during development and differentiation identify the phenotype of embryonic and maturation stages of the cells. Cluster of differentiation (CD) markers identified by specific monoclonal and polyclonal antibodies are used to identify specific cell types. Following hematopoiesis, lymphocytes exist in a resting state as naive or unprimed cells in G phase. Following antigen contact lymphocytes progress from $G_0 \rightarrow G_1 \rightarrow S \rightarrow G_2 \rightarrow M$. Cytokine microenvironments further polarize subsets of effector cells such as in T helper subsets to aid specific effector functions of the cells in antigen clearance.

© Springer Nature Switzerland AG 2021
T. Y. Sam-Yellowe, *Immunology: Overview and Laboratory Manual*,
https://doi.org/10.1007/978-3-030-64686-8_3

Cell Lineage Development from HSCs

The HSCs are in direct contact with stromal cells in the bone marrow and receive nutrients and signals required for cell proliferation, differentiation and trafficking within the bone marrow and migration to the periphery. Homing receptors consisting of cell adhesion molecules and chemokine receptors expressed by cells facilitates cell migration and trafficking to peripheral tissues. Several cell populations make up the stroma that supports HSC growth and differentiation in the bone marrow. These include endothelial cells lining blood vessels, perivascular cells interacting with the endothelia, bone forming osteoblasts that influence lymphoid cell development, macrophages and sympathetic nerves. The latter two support other cells within the stroma. During gestation, hematopoietic activity occurs in the placenta, fetal liver, yolk sac, aorta-gonad-mesonephros (AGM) and shifts to the bone marrow before birth. Long term (LT) and short term (ST) HSCs give rise to multipotent progenitor (MPP) cells. Common myeloid (CMP) and lymphoid-primed multipotent progenitor (LMPP) cells differentiate from MPP. Early lymphoid progenitor (ELP) cells differentiated from LMPP further differentiate into common lymphoid progenitor (CLP) cells from which T and B lymphocytes, natural killer (NK) cells and dendritic cells (DCs) differentiate. Each progenitor cell expresses cell surface markers and transcription factors that influence lineage commitment toward myeloid or lymphoid cell development.

Hematopoietic stem cells are self-renewing, capable of responding to growth factors and cytokines and differentiate into progenitor cells in response to specific growth factors. Two major progenitors differentiate from HSCs, responsible for myeloid and lymphoid cells. The common myeloid progenitor (CMP) gives rise to myeloid cells and the common lymphoid progenitor (CLP) differentiates into lymphoid cells. Cells of myeloid origin include the granulocytes; neutrophils, eosinophils and basophils. Additionally, monocytes, dendritic cells, mast cells, erythrocytes and platelets which are derived from megakaryocytes, also differentiate from CMP. Monocytes differentiate into macrophages as well as dendritic cells in tissues. Lymphoid cells include T and B lymphocytes, innate lymphoid cells (ILCs) and dendritic cells. The natural killer (NK) cell is the most well studied cell among the ILCs. The process of hematopoiesis is highly regulated through processes dependent on receptor down regulation and apoptosis. T lymphocytes migrate from the bone marrow to the thymus as thymocytes and complete maturation as cytotoxic, helper or regulatory T cells. Lymphocytes are not easily distinguished by staining of blood cells with Giemsa stain. They are very similar morphologically. However, lymphocytes can be distinguished by cluster of differentiation (CD) molecules. The use of techniques such as flow cytometry where monoclonal antibodies specific to CD molecules were used to identify cells expressing CD molecules was instrumental in identifying various cells, at different developmental stages of lymphoid and myeloid cell lineages.

Cell Lineage Markers

Flow cytometry continues to be an essential technique used for immunophenotyping of leukocytes. For example, expression of CD3 identifies T cells. Additional expression of CD4 and CD8 along with CD3, identifies TH cells and CTLs, respectively. Expression of CD19, CD20 and CD21 identifies B cells and CD16 identifies NK cells. The molecules c-kit and Sca-1 identify lineage negative (Lin⁻) HSC and early progenitors such as MPP also express CD34. Progenitor cells can express the same markers. The progenitor cells LMPP, ELP and CLP express flt-3. As progenitor cells for lymphoid cells begin to differentiate toward B and T cell lineages, the recombinase enzymes RAG1/RAG2 and the enzyme Tdt become active. Both enzymes are required for recombination of the variable regions of the immunoglobulin and T cell receptor genes. Transcription factors also influence lineage commitment. Ikaros is required for lymphoid cell development and not myeloid cells. PU.1 at high levels commits cells towards myeloid cells. Within the thymus, commitment to single positive CD4⁺ T cells is influenced by Th-POK while expression of CD8 on T cells (CD8⁺) is activated by Runx3. Hematopoiesis is highly regulated, and decreased expression of cell surface antigens and induction of apoptosis are examples of mechanisms that decrease cell number and control cell proliferation. Activation of cells leading to differentiation is also regulated by epigenetic processes. Bivalent histone modification has been shown to influence gene activation in the production of cell lineages.

Cluster of Differentiation (CD) Antigens

These are leukocyte surface antigens identified and characterized by monoclonal antibodies. Monoclonal antibodies reacting with a particular membrane molecule are grouped together as a cluster of differentiation. Identification of specific patterns of leukocyte surface antigen expression (CD antigen expression) is essential in understanding the differentiation of leukocyte subpopulations and functions of the cells. These markers are crucial molecules that allow differentiation of leukocyte subpopulations using cell sorting or flow cytometry methods. Different developmental stages or cell lineages can be distinguished by the type of cell surface molecule expressed. Cells developing from the bone marrow and thymus will become involved in innate and adaptive immune responses. Adaptive immune responses include humoral and cell-mediated immune responses. In the following chapters we will examine the features of both branches of immunity. A short summary of the humoral and cellular immune responses is provided below.

Humoral immunity is also known as B cell or antibody-mediated immunity. The B cell receptor complex recognizes antigen. Following crosslinking and B cell activation, a specific antibody is synthesized by differentiated B cells known as plasma cells. Different isotypes or classes of antibodies can be secreted by plasma cells.

These include IgM, IgG, IgA, IgE and IgD. Specific antibody synthesis is mediated by CD4+ T helper cells in association with MHC class II antigens. Antibodies synthesized, function in the following different ways to eliminate pathogens: neutralization, precipitation, agglutination, opsonization and complement fixation.

Cell-mediated immunity (CMI) known as T cell or cytokine-mediated immunity involves cytotoxic T (Tc) lymphocytes. The T cell receptor complex on CD8+ cytotoxic T cells, and T helper 1 cells in association with MHC class I and MHC class II antigens respectively, mediates direct killing activity on pathogen infected cells. Tc cells differentiate into cytotoxic T lymphocytes (CTLs) which recognize altered self-cells intracellularly infected by pathogens or undergoing neoplastic transformation. Other cells participating in cell mediated responses include macrophages.

Selected References

Abraham BJ, Cui K, Tang Q, Zhao K (2013) Dynamic regulation of epigenomic landcsapesduring hematopoiesis. BMC Genomics 14:193

Antoniani C, Romano D, Miccio A (2017) Epigenetic regulation of hematopoiesis: Biological insights and0020therapeutic applications. Stem Cells Transl Med 6:2106–2114

Engel P, Boumsell L, Balderas R et al (2015) CD nomenclature 2015 :Human leukocyte differentiation antigen workshops as a driving force in immunology. J Immunol 195:4555–4563

Murphy K, Weaver C (2017) Janeway's immunobiology, 9th edn. Garland Press, New York

Punt J, Stranford SA, Jones PP, Owen JA (2019) Kuby immunology, 8th edn. W.H. Freeman and Company, New York. Chapter 20, Antigen-antibody interactions

Chapter 4
The Immune System: Pathogen Sensing and Detection

When the immune system is functioning optimally, it is responsible for detecting and eliminating pathogens that enter the body, and for maintaining homeostasis with our microbiome. The immune system consists primarily of two branches, each specialized in the types of responses that will be mounted, but working cooperatively to detect and eliminate pathogens. These branches are known as **innate** and **adaptive** branches. Macromolecules associated with pathogens on cell surfaces, or secreted by pathogens within the host are known as **antigens**. In response to the antigens, the infected host mounts an immune response aimed at eliminating the pathogen by the use of cellular attack by **phagocytosis** or by the use of antimicrobial molecules present in the blood and mucosal environments. The host can also mount a specific response that involves the secretion of **antibodies** or the activation of **cytotoxic T cells (killer)** cells. The first branch of the immune system concerned with surveillance and surveying the "landscape" of our tissues for breaches, aberrant receptor topology on host cells, and rapid response to defend the host is known as the **innate** system. The second branch of the immune system specialized to recognize specific molecules from pathogens and deliver selective attack to destroy and eliminate pathogens is known as the **adaptive** (acquired or induced) immune response. In the first branch, cells of the innate immune system bearing receptors on their surfaces act as sentinels to raise the alarm regarding the breach of the host's defenses. These receptors are collectively called **pattern recognition receptors (PRRs)** and are found on cell surfaces as well as within the cytoplasm and in endosome-lysosomes. The ligands for the receptors are various molecules on the surface of pathogens, including molecules secreted by the pathogens known as **pathogen associated molecular patterns (PAMPs)**. Viral genomes (RNA and DNA) are also recognized by PRRs located within the host cell cytoplasm and within the endosomal system within cells. Other danger signals; **damage associated molecular patterns (DAMPs)**, resulting from damaged tissue due to the invading pathogens are detected by the sentinels and signals conveyed to effector cells of the innate immune system resulting in the production of molecules that help to protect tissues from further damage and contribute to the destruction of the pathogens. Ligation of

© Springer Nature Switzerland AG 2021
T. Y. Sam-Yellowe, *Immunology: Overview and Laboratory Manual*,
https://doi.org/10.1007/978-3-030-64686-8_4

PAMPs with PRRs activates cell signaling cascades that lead to the production of transcription factors that will influence the transcription of genes encoding pro-inflammatory cytokines. A combination of molecules, cells, tissues, organs, blood and lymphatic vessels form the framework that is organized to form the immune system. A brief description of the characteristics of cells of the innate system are provided below. Effector functions of each cell will be addressed in later chapters. A more detailed discussion of dendritic cells and macrophages is given in this chapter to facilitate later discussions about T lymphocytes.

Cells of the Immune System

The cells of the immune system are comprised of leukocytes (white blood cells), categorized as **granulocytes** and **agranulocytes**. The former includes neutrophils (polymorphonuclear cells), eosinophils, basophils and mast cells. The latter includes monocytes, lymphocytes and dendritic cells. Monocytes differentiate into macrophages in the tissues. Within tissues, the macrophages consist of a network known as the reticuloendothelial system (RES) or mononuclear phagocytic system (MPS). Leukocytes, erythrocytes and thrombocytes (platelets) are derived from HSCs in the bone marrow. Myeloid progenitors (producing myeloid cells) arising from the HSCs differentiate into neutrophils, eosinophils, basophils, mast cells, monocytes and some dendritic cells. Lymphoid progenitors producing lymphoid cells from HSCs differentiate into B and T lymphocytes, innate lymphoid cells (ILCs) such as natural killer (NK) cells, ILC1, ILC2, ILC17, ILC22, LTi cells and dendritic cells. The ILCs are grouped according to the types of cytokines secreted. Group1 ILCs include NK and ILC1 cells, group 2 ILC include ILC2 cells and group 3 ILCs include ILC17, ILC22 and LTi cells. The NK cells are the most widely studied of the ILCs. Cells develop, differentiate and mature within microenvironments that provide tissue support as well as growth factors and other molecules required for development. Dendritic cells and macrophages digest antigens associated with pathogens and then present them on their cell surfaces in association with major histocompatibility complex (MHC) proteins, to naïve T cells known as helper T (Th) cells. The digestion of antigens is known as **antigen processing** and the cells such as dendritic cells, macrophages and B lymphocytes that process (digest) antigen are known as **antigen presenting cells (APCs)**. In addition to cytokines, cells of the immune system can be distinguished by markers known as CD antigens. Monoclonal antibodies made against the markers are used in various immunoassays, including flow cytometry to determine the distribution of the cells in tissue following identification of the markers by antibodies. The presence of the T cell receptor (TCR) and CD3 identifies T cells. The presence of CD4 or CD8 along with $TCR^+/CD3^+$ identifies the T cell as a T helper and cytotoxic T cell, respectively. B lymphocytes also express the cell surface molecules CD19, CD20, CD21 along with the B cell receptor (immunoglobulin, Ig) and Igα/Igβ (CD79α/CD79β). Natural killer cells express CD16 and CD56 (human), different populations of macrophages can be identified using CD14 and CD16, and different populations of dendritic cells can be identified using CD11c, CD11b and CD103. Individually each cell type plays a significant role in orchestrating pathogen sensing, recognition, processing or delivering antigen to secondary and tertiary lymphoid organs. A summary of characteristics and functions of cells of the immune system are discussed below.

Neutrophils are professional phagocytes that represent the most numerous leukocytes in blood. Over 70% of leukocytes recirculate approximately every 48 h and enter tissue in response to chemotactic stimuli.

Neutrophils opsonize antigen using antibody and complement receptors. Neutrophils are recruited to sites of inflammation. They produce toxic oxidizing molecules (H_2O_2, OH^-, hypochlorite) and nicotinamide adenine dinucleotide phosphate (NADPH) oxidative burst that can kill pathogens. Neutrophils have been shown to release nucleic acids associated with histones that function as extracellular traps to capture bacteria. The traps are known as neutrophil extracellular traps (NETs).

Eosinophils comprise 2–5% of leukocytes. They possess numerous cytoplasmic granules that contain basic protein which causes damage to parasites especially in helminth (worm) infections. Secretion of major basic protein (MBP), MBP2, eosinophil cationic protein (ECP), and eosinophil peroxidase (EPO) characterize the effector function of eosinophils. Granules also contain histaminase and aryl sulphatase which down regulate inflammatory responses. Eosinophils produce autocrine cytokines like IL-3 and GM-CSF which enhance cytotoxic killing activity of eosinophils. Human eosinophils secrete IL-4 which is associated with the TH2 immune responses and inflammation. Eosinophils perform the role of APCs in draining lymph nodes, presenting antigen to TH2 cells.

Basophils are functionally similar to mast cells with numerous large cytoplasmic granules. The granules contain inflammatory mediators such as histamine. Basophils comprise approximately 0.5% of leukocytes. However, in worm infections, basophils play important roles through degranulation and cytokine secretion which aids in the recruitment of cells such as lymphocytes.

Mast cells are present in most tissue adjoining blood vessels, contain numerous granules and upon stimulation by cross linked IgE-antigen, degranulation takes place releasing inflammatory mediators such as histamine and platelet activating factor (PAF). Mast cells guide the process of inflammation. There are two types of mast cells; (a) Connective tissue mast cells-CTMCs and (b) Mucosal mast cells -MMCS. The former is the main tissue mast cell, the latter is found in the gut and lungs and is dependent on IL-3 and IL4 for proliferation. The MMCs increase during parasitic infection. Appropriate inflammation brings relevant immune cells to the desired site whereas inappropriate inflammation destroys host tissue and can cause illness e.g. asthma, hay fever.

Lymphocytes are the major immune cell of adaptive immunity. There are approximately 10^{12} lymphocytes in humans, roughly the cellular mass of the brain or liver. Lymphocytes constitute 25% of the leukocyte population and 99% of the nucleated cells in the lymph. Three major types of lymphocytes are produced during lymphopoiesis. B and T lymphocytes and innate lymphoid cells of which the natural killer cell is the most widely studied.

B lymphocytes contain several subsets. Two of the subsets will be discussed here and in the chapter examining B cell development, additional subsets will be discussed. **B1 cells** (CD5$^+$ CD23$^-$) are a minor population of cells that appear to be self-renewing. They develop early and respond to a number of common microbial antigens and T independent antigens. They also generate autoantibodies, mostly IgM. **B2 cells** (CD5$^-$ CD23 $^+$) constitute the majority of B cells. They interact with antigens, develop a greater diversity of antigen receptors, differentiate into plasma cells responsible for secreting antibodies and function in humoral immunity. B lymphocytes are located in the bone marrow, spleen, lymph nodes and peripheral blood. B cells differentiate into effector cells called plasma cells and memory cells. Plasma cells are terminal cells (end cells) which synthesize and secrete antibodies (immunoglobulin) of five **isotypes** known as **Immunoglobulin (Ig) M, IgD, IgG, IgA and IgE**. These are major components of humoral immunity. Plasma cells lack membrane bound antibody. Surface markers used to identify B cells include; **mIg, class** II **MHC antigens, CD220/CD45, CD19, CD20, CD21, CD22, CD32, CD35, CD40, CD80 (B7-1), CD86 (B7-2), Leukocyte functional antigen (LFA) and ICAM.**

A B cell receptor complex is formed on the surface of B cells and includes mIg on the surface of B cells associated with an Igα/Igβ non-antigen specific heterodimer.

T lymphocytes consist of T helper (TH) cells (CD3$^+$CD4$^+$) and cytotoxic T cells (Tc) (CD3$^+$CD8$^+$). T helper cells possess several subsets defined by the type of cytokines polarizing their differentiation and the types of cytokines they secrete. Additional types of T cells including regulatory T cells (Treg), the natural killer T cell (NKT) cell and intraepithelial T cells (IELs) will be discussed in the chapter on T cell development. The NKT cell possesses a T cell receptor restricted not by the classical MHC class I or II antigens but by a molecule known as CD1. T helper cells develop from a TH0 precursor, and under cytokine influence differentiate into various subsets. For example **TH1** cells secrete TNFα and IFNγ and enhance cell-mediated immunity. TH1 cells also help with antibody production by B cells. **TH2** cells secrete IL-4, IL-5 and IL13, and provides B cell help for antibody production. Tc also secrete cytokines but they also express FasL (CD95L) which binds to Fas (CD95) on host target cells leading to apoptosis in target cells, through the secretion of perforin and granzymes which facilitate the activation of the apoptotic pathway. T lymphocytes interact with antigens in association with products of the major histocompatibility (MHC) gene complexes for class I and II genes. **This is known as MHC restriction.** T helper cells also interact with B cells to aid in the generation of antibodies and in the affinity maturation and isotype switching of antibodies. T lymphocytes synthesize and secrete cytokines and upon activation differentiate into effector and memory cells. They express membrane bound T cell receptor (TCR) of either α/β or γ/δ type. **Other T cell surface markers include CD3, Thy-1, CD2, CD4, CD5, CD8, CD28, CD40L, LFA and ICAM.** T lymphocytes function in both cellular and humoral immunity and are located in the thymus, spleen, lymph nodes, and in peripheral blood.

Innate lymphoid cells (ILCs) interact with antigen directly, in antibody mediated killing and function in cell-mediated immunity. The most well known ILC are NK cells which mediate killing of virus infected cells and transformed host cells.

Cell surface markers include; **CD2, CD16 (Fcγ III receptor), NKR-PL and CD69**. They are located in the spleen, lymph nodes and peripheral blood. Due to the presence of the Fc receptor on the surface of NK cells, they can carry out antibody dependent cellular cytotoxicity (ADCC) reactions. The different types of lymphocytes function in the two branches of adaptive immunity known as **humoral (HI)** and **cell-mediated immunity (CMI)** as well as in innate immunity, for NK cells. We discuss the role of ILCs in different aspects of immunity below.

Natural killer cells are a heterogeneous population of ILCs that do not express recombined antigen binding receptors. Like T and B lymphocytes, NK cells are differentiated from the CLP. NK cells express activating and inhibitory receptors that once activated can lead to cell killing or survival, respectively. The initial discovery of NK cells showed they could kill tumor cells without previous encounter with the tumor cells, suggesting a different killing mechanism from other cytotoxic cells. NK activating receptors induce signals through intracellular immunoreceptor tyrosine-based activation motif (ITAM) sequences that result in NK killing of target host cells in the absence of "sufficient" inhibitory signals. NK inhibitory receptors prevent host cell killing by NK cells. Engagement of inhibitory receptors with MHC class I proteins prevents NK proliferation and cytokine release, such that transduced signals inhibit NK killing of the host cell through intracellular immunoreceptor tyrosine-based inhibitory motif (ITIM) sequences. Natural killer cells participate in both innate and adaptive immune responses. NK cells active in innate immunity respond to IL-12 and type 1 interferons. They also secrete IFNγ which is important for TH1 cell effector function and they express IL-2Rβ (CD122). They have phenotypic differences with respect to the surface molecules expressed in mice and humans. Both human and mouse NK cells express CD16 the Fc receptor for IgG (FcγIII), CD2 and IL-2Rβ. Human NK cells express CD56, a cell adhesion molecule and mouse NK cells express CD49b and NK1.1 family of receptor molecules. NK cells recognize alterations of MHC class I proteins on host cell surfaces and can become activated to kill cells by apoptosis. Human NK cells express killer-cell immunoglobulin like receptors (KIRs) which contain both activating and inhibitory types of receptors. KIRs are diverse and polymorphic and can bind both HLA-B and HLA-C class I MHC allelic variants at polymorphic sites. Another receptor family expressed by NK cells is the NKG2 family which also contains activating and inhibitory receptors and is found in human and mouse NK cells. NKG2A is an inhibitory receptor which can bind to HLA-E bound to peptides derived from HLA-A, B or C proteins. Other NKG2 receptor family members are activating receptors. The NKG2D receptors found on mouse and human NK cells is an important activating receptor. NKG2D binds to non-polymorphic MHCI-like molecules on cells undergoing DNA damage, infected host cells and other cells undergoing stress. The MHCI-like molecules lack β2-microglobulin. In mice, the activating receptor Ly49H binds to an MHCI-like protein produced by murine cytomegalovirus (MCMV). A group of receptors known as natural cytotoxicity receptors (NCRs) in humans are activating receptors that bind antigens on tumor cells and virus-infected host cells.

Antigen presenting cells (APCs) play a prominent role in initiating adaptive immunity. Pathogens endocytosed or phagocytosed are digested to obtain peptides which combine with MHC proteins and become displayed on the surface of the APC for recognition by T cells. There are three professional APCs, dendritic cells (DCs), macrophages and B lymphocytes. What features distinguish each cell type? In the next section we will examine the defining features of macrophages and DCs.

Monocytes are phagocytic cells derived from myeloid progenitors that differentiate into macrophages and dendritic cells in tissues. Monocytes constitute a heterogenous population of cells. However, subsets of monocytes can be identified based on the expression of CD14, a coreceptor for the PRR toll-like receptor 4 (TLR4) and CD16 the Fc receptor for IgG. Following recruitment and migration of monocytes into tissues, they encounter cytokine microenvironments that shape their response and differentiation to macrophages or dendritic cells. Monocytes perform patrolling and sensing functions, and they detect PAMPs and DAMPs. Inflammatory and patrolling subsets of monocytes function in immune responses. Inflammatory monocytes are recruited into tissues rapidly where they differentiate into macrophages while patrolling subsets are involved in blood vessel repair. Encounter with specific pathogens or inflammatory mediators influences monocyte differentiation to macrophages that can mediate innate immune effector function as well as perform antigen presentation to T lymphocytes in adaptive immune responses. Monocytes detect PAMPs and DAMPS through TLRs like TLR4 and TLR7.

Macrophages are also involved in adaptive immune responses as major antigen processing and presenting cells (APCs). They are large phagocytic cells present in most tissues. Resident tissue macrophages can remain in tissue for years. Others function as APCs and recirculate through secondary lymphoid tissue.

Macrophages function in phagocytosis, antigen processing, antigen presentation and they also carry out cytotoxic activity. Macrophages also secrete a variety of cytokines, enzymes, and other soluble proteins including some complement proteins, defensins and they generate free oxygen and nitrogen radicals. Macrophages carry out cytotoxic activity by oxygen dependent killing and oxygen independent killing. In oxygen dependent killing also known as respiratory burst, reactive oxygen and nitrogen intermediates such as superoxide anion and nitric oxide, respectively are produced. Both of these substances have antibacterial activity. In oxygen independent killing, defensins are produced by macrophages. This substance forms ion-permeable pores in cell membranes. Other antigen presenting cells include dendritic cells, follicular dendritic cells found in B cell rich areas, non-lymphoid or "veiled" dendritic cells and interdigitating dendritic cells found in T cell rich areas of secondary lymphoid organs.

Types of macrophages:

Kupffer cells in the liver

Mesangial phagocytes in the glomerular endothelium/capillaries enter Bowman's capsule.

Microglial cells in the brain

Alveolar macrophages in the lungs

Osteoclasts in the bones

Synovial A cells are phagocytes which lie on the synovium in contact with synovial fluid.

Macrophages maintain homeostasis through host defense, wound healing and immune regulation. The various macrophage subsets reflect each of these functions. Macrophages are derived from monocytes. However, there is evidence demonstrating that some macrophages are self-renewing and populate tissues from early hematopoioetic precursors. Monocyte cell populations are heterogeneous, and are identified by expression of the cell surface molecules CD16$^+$ or CD14$^+$. In mice where monocyte subset distinctions are better understood, recruitment of monocytes into various tissues is dependent on acute or chronic inflammation in affected tissues. Expression of chemokine receptors influences the migration of monocytes into tissue sites. Classical monocyte subset utilizes CCR2 and non-classical monocyte subset utilizes CXCR1. Macrophages are heterogeneous cells with a plastic phenotype. Macrophages form the mononuclear phagocytic system in the body (the RES) and are therefore widely distributed in lymphoid and non-lymphoid tissue (liver, lungs, brain, kidneys, bone). Differentiation of macrophages depends on colony stimulating factors (CSFs) and cytokine signals in particular tissue microenvironments leading to the development of macrophage subsets that are pro-inflammatory (M1 subset) or anti-inflammatory (M2 subset).

Macrophages become activated in response to cytokines. Ligation of cytokines to cytokine receptors on macrophages leads to cytokine signaling, specific signal transducer and activation of transcription (STAT) proteins and transcription factors that determine the differentiation pathway of macrophages. STAT-1 and NF-κB promote M1 differentiation while STAT-3, STAT-6 and interferon regulatory factor 3 (IRF-3) promote M2 differentiation. TH1 derived cytokines IFNγ and TNFα influence the development of M1 macrophages with resultant secretion of the proinflammatory cytokines, IL-1α, IL-1β, TNFα, IL-6, IL-12, IL-23 and low levels of IL-10. Anti-inflammatory M2 macrophages can also develop as a result of the cytokines IL-4 and IL-13 secreted by TH2, as well as IL-21 and IL-33 leading to the secretion of the effector cytokines, IL-10 and TGFβ and low levels of IL-12 by M2 macrophage subsets. Although M1 and M2 polarizations has been observed in vitro, it is unclear whether the subsets are distinct in vivo. The M2 subset is further categorized into M2a, M2b, M2c and M2d subsets, each polarized by specific cytokines, TLRs, glucocorticoids and TLR agonists. M2a (induced by IL-4, IL-13), M2b (induced by immune complexes, TLRs, FcγR), M2c (induced by IL-10, TGFβ, glucocorticoids) and M2d (induced by TLR agonists).

Dendritic cells are a heterogeneous group of cells derived from myeloid and lymphoid precursors during hematopoiesis. They possess diverse phenotypes and are distributed in different tissues and organs of the body (Fig. 4.1). DCs function in innate immunity as important sentinel cells "sensing" the presence of pathogens in the body and binding to ligands on pathogens using pathogen recognition receptors (PRRs), such as Toll-like receptors. DCs also respond to signals from damaged tissue. The DC occupies a central position in the events that initiate innate immunity and in the events that bridge innate and adaptive immunity. DCs are strategic bridges between innate and adaptive immune responses, where they present processed antigen to naive T helper cells in secondary lymphoid organs. Development and differentiation of DCs during hematopoiesis is dependent on colony stimulating factors

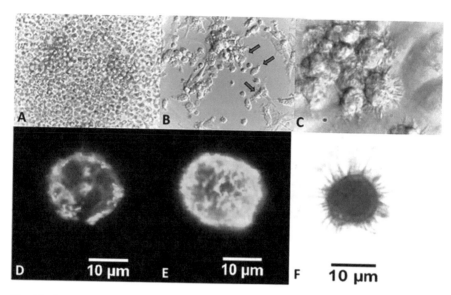

Fig. 4.1 Dendritic cells cultured from bone marrow precursors with GM-CSF (**a**) cultures at 24 h, (**b, c**) cultures at 6 days, red arrows (**b**) showing long and thin extensions (dendrites). (**d**) Positive immunofluorescent label of MHC class II on iDC at 6 day culture. (**e**) Positive immunofluorescent label of MHC class II on iDC after 2 h culture with LPS. (**e**) Toluidine blue stained DC showing extensions (dendrites). [*Republished with permission of IntechOpen publishing from Castell-Rodriguez et al., "Dendritic cells: Location, Function, and Clinical Implications." Biology of Myelomonocytic Cells.* https://doi.org/10.5772/intechopen.68352, *2017, Figure 2. Conveyed through STM permission guidelines 2014*]

(CSFs), cytokines and transcription factors which determine the effector function of the DCs. Monocyte colony stimulating factor (MCS-F), granulocyte-monocyte CSF (GM-CSF), TGFβ and Flt3L drive differentiation of DCs under non-inflammatory and inflammatory conditions. The transcription factors PU.1, Ikaros, Gfi-1, E2–2 and IRF8 participate in DC development and differentiation. The microenvironment of the developing DC will determine whether activation or tolerance occurs. DCs possess a characteristic morphology with dendrites, elongated membrane used for the capture of antigen. Dendritic cells are distributed in primary and secondary lymphoid organs, circulating in blood and located in tissue sites within the gastrointestinal tract, skin, liver, lungs, kidneys and muscle. Dendritic cells capture and process antigen for presentation to naïve T helper cells. Along with macrophages and B lymphocytes, DCs constitute the professional antigen presenting cells in the body. Antigen is presented on MHC class II proteins to T helper cells in secondary and tertiary lymphoid organs. However, DCs are potent in their role as APCs due to the ability of immature DCs to capture antigen and process the antigen as they mature. DCs also function to polarize naïve T helper cells into effector T cell subsets. DCs also promote tolerance in T cells.

DCs express MHC class II proteins (Fig. 4.1) and CD11c. DCs are categorized as conventional DCs (cDCs), (also known as myeloid DCs), plasmacytoid DCs (pDC) (also known as lymphoid DCs, Langerhans cells localized in the epidermis of the skin and monocyte- derived DCs (Blood DCs). Conventional DCs are the major APC, possessing varying function which include antigen presentation to naïve T helper cells and cross presentation of exogenous antigen to $CD8^+$ cytotoxic T lymphocytes (CTLs). Expression of CD1c and CD141 defines chemokine secreting and cross presenting cDCs, respectively. cDCs possess subsets that define migratory and tissue resident populations denoted as mDC1 and mDC2, respectively. The former express the chemokine receptor XCR1 and CD103 (E-cadherin receptor). The latter express, CD8 and CD11b (integrin). High levels of MHC class II and CD11c expression define migratory cDCs. Conventional DCs express TLR2 and TLR4 and release the cytokines IL-6, IL-12, TNF and chemokines following receptor signaling. Migratory DCs are located in the dermis (dermal DCs), skin and mucosa. The presence of the markers CD4, $CD8\alpha$, CD11b and CD103, identify dendritic cells important for different aspects of immunity and tolerance induction. DCs mediating antiviral immunity with antigen presentation to CTLs express $MHCII^+CD8\alpha^+CD103^+$. Plasmacytoid DCs are also important in viral immunity and secrete type 1 interferons, e. g. $IFN\alpha$ in response to viral infection. pDCs bind to virus genomes using cytoplasmic PRRs such as TLR7 and TLR9. Expression of the surface molecules, $CD11c^{low}$, MHC class II^{low}, blood DC antigen-2 (BDCA-2), CD45RA, Siglec-H^+ and bone marrow stromal antigen-2 (BST2) (tetherin) distinguish pDCs from cDCs. pDC function as APCs for naïve TH cells but can also tolerize T cells resulting in anergy instead of activation. Expression of IRF8 and E2-2 is required for pDC development.

Langerhans cells are located in the epidermis of the skin where they come into contact with pathogens and their associated antigens when they invade through the skin. Langerhans cells migrate through the dermis to deliver captured antigen to lymph nodes draining the skin. Langerhans cells are characterized by the presence of Birbeck granules which contain langerin. They also express MHC class II proteins used for antigen presentation to naïve T helper cells.

Under non-inflammatory conditions, peripheral blood monocytes ($CD11b^+$ $CD11c^-MHCII^-$) can differentiate into dendritic cells in response to monocyte-colony stimulating factor (MCSF) binding to MCSF receptors (MCSF-R). Monocyte-derived DCs represent immature DCs (iDCs/veiled cells) in blood. Monocyte-derived DCs can activate antigen processing and presentation pathways under inflammatory conditions leading to antigen presentation to naïve T helper cells and cross presentation of exogenous antigen to $CD8^+$ cytotoxic T cells. Upregulation of coreceptor molecules such as CD40, CD80/B7.1, CD86/B7.2 and CCR7 facilitates migration of cells into lymph nodes for engagement with naïve T helper cells for polarization and activation. iDCs express the blood dendritic cells antigens, BDCA-2, BDCA-3 and BDCA-4.

Categories of Immune Responses

Similarities have been observed in the cytokine profiles of ILCs and T helper cells and in the types of immune responses the cells engage in. Based on these differences, three categories of immune responses are recognized as follows: Types 1, 2 and 3 immunity. Type 1 immunity is induced against intracellular pathogens such as viruses, intracellular bacteria and parasites. Inflammatory responses and autoimmune responses are also categorized as type 1 immunity. Immunity to helminths, venoms and allergens is known as type 2 immunity. Immune responses to extracellular pathogens that induces inflammation and autoimmune reactions is a type 3 immunity. Innate lymphoid cells and T cells originate from a common lymphoid progenitor and have a cytokine profile similar to that found in T helper cells. ILC1 cells secrete type 1 cytokines, ILC2 cells secrete type 2 cytokines and ILC3 cells including lymphoid tissue inducer cells secrete type 17 cytokines. ILCs function in innate and adaptive immunity and can license other innate cells by the cytokines that they secrete. ILCs share transcription factors with TH and Tc cells.

In **type 1 immunity** the major group1 ILC, NK cells is activated along with TH1 and Tc1 cells. Cytotoxic activity of NK and CTLs targets intracellularly infected cells. IgG1 and IgG2 isotypes interact with Fc receptors on NK cells for ADCC reactions. IFNγ produced by ILC1 cells is important for TH1 cell polarization and for NK cell activity early in innate immunity. As adaptive immunity develops, CTLs respond to specific antigen and mediate clearance by induction of apoptosis in target cells and phagocytosis by macrophages. Macrophages secrete IL-12 and IL-18.

Type 2 immunity is mediated by group 2 ILCs, TH2 and Tc2 cells and directed towards multicellular helminth parasites. Additional cells important in type 2 immune responses include basophils and mast cells. IgE bound to Fc receptors on mast cells and basophils characterizes responses in type 2 immunity. Cytokines important for activating cells include thymic stromal lymphopoietin (TSLP) which activates ILC2 cells within mucosal environments. Additional cytokines produced within the mucosal environment are IL-33 and IL-25. The cytokines IL-5 and IL-13 are also produced by ILC2 cells and act on eosinophils to kill worms and induce goblet cell secretion of mucus, respectively. Dendritic cell polarization of TH2 cells is also mediated by IL-13.

Type 3 immunity is characterized by group 3 ILCs, TH17 and Tc17 cells. Activation of different subsets of ILCs early in innate responses induces the polarization of type 1, 2, and 3 immune responses. The immune responses to extracellular bacteria and fungi include the secretion of IL-17A, IL-17F, IL-22 and IL-26 from TH17 cells. ILC3 cells are present before birth and are known as lymphoid tissue inducer cells. These cells respond to IL-23 and IL-1β and promote the secretion of the proinflammatory cytokine IL-17 and IL-22. These cells promote the development of lymph nodes and Peyers patches during fetal development. Unlike TH cells, no polarization, priming or differentiation is needed for ILC effector function. ILCs respond rapidly and amplify responses of innate effector cells. Interleukin 17 acts on stromal cells, epithelial cells and myeloid cells and stimulates secretion of IL-6, IL-1β, G-CSF and GM-CSF. Chemokine production leads to recruitment of neutrophils and monocytes. The cytokine IL-22 targets epithelial cells in the mucosa leading to the secretion of antimicrobial peptides, IL-6, IL-1β and strengthening of the mucosal barrier. TH17 cells in the mucosal lymphoid tissue undergo differentiation in the presence of increased levels of IL-6, IL-1β and IL-23.

Mucosal Immunity

The mucosal epithelium and the skin present large barriers to the entry of pathogens into the body. Both barriers are important parts of the innate immune system. Commensal organisms making up the human microbiome are most abundant in the mucosal environment especially in the gastrointestinal (GI) tract. Interaction of metabolic products like short chain fatty acids (SCFAs) secreted from the commensal organisms with cells of the immune system helps to maintain immune homeostasis and tolerance to the commensals. The presence of the commensal organisms in the right proportions helps to prevent colonization of the mucosal environment by pathogens. The mucosal associated lymphoid tissue (MALT) consists of cells that produce antimicrobial agents and have phagocytic activity as well as molecules that have cellular activity for the elimination of various pathogens including bacteria, viruses, parasites and fungi. Mucosal epithelial cells in the GI tract also known as enterocytes express PRRs that bind to PAMPs. They also secrete antimicrobial peptides. Macrophages and dendritic cells found in the lamina propria below the epithelial lining also express PRRs that bind to PAMPs and facilitate phagocytosis of pathogens from the lumen of the GI tract. Innate lymphoid cells play important roles in mucosal immunity through the cytokines they secrete. Type 1 immune responses mounted against pathogens involve TH1, TH17, ILC1, ILC3 and NK cells. Cytotoxic T cells, CD8$^+$ intraepithelial lymphocytes (IELs) expressing either γδ or αβ TCR, iNKT and mucosal associated invariant T (MAIT) cells also provide effector functions protecting the mucosa. Cytokines secreted by cells in type I responses include IFNγ from TH1 and ILC1 cells, IL-17, IL-22 and IL-21 from TFH (follicular helper T) cells. Worm infections elicit type II immune responses and activation of TH2 cells which secrete IL-4, IL-5, IL-13 and IL-9 from TH9 cells. ILC2 and TH9 cells also function in type 2 responses. B cell activation in response to antigen and interaction with TH cells leads to production of IgG, IgE and IgA. The presence of secretory IgA in the mucosal environment promotes a tolerogenic response and effector function of FoxP3$^+$ TREG cells, through the production of IL-10 and TGFβ. Epithelial cells interacting with the gut microbiome through PRRs secrete retinoic acid (RA), TGFβ and thymic stromal lymphopoietin (TSLP) which together sustain the tolerogenic environment within the gut. Proinflammatory cytokines such as TNFα and IL-17 result in inflammatory responses which can contribute to damaged tissue, recruitment of cells and release of DAMPs. CX$_3$CR1$^+$macrophages and migrating CD103$^+$dendritic cells interact with TH and B cells. The macrophages and dendritic cells can retrieve antigens from the gut lumen, for processing and presentation. Similar to TREG, they secrete IL-10 contributing to gut homeostasis and generating persistent peripheral TREG. B cell activating factor (BAFF), a proliferation-inducing ligand (APRIL) secreted by epithelial cells and APCs and IL-10, aid IgA production by B cells in the lamina propria in a T-independent and T-dependent manner. Dimerized secretory IgA held together by a J-chain, bind to polyIgRs in the basal face of the epithelial cells and become transcytosed across the epithelium to the gut lumen, where it binds to microbes preventing breaches of the gut epithelium. IgA secreting plasma cells express the mucosal homing molecules, integrin $\alpha_4\beta_7$ (LPAM-1) and the chemokine receptor CCR7, which directs their extravasation into the mucosal environment. Additional cells important in mucosal immunity include Paneth cells which are found in the small intestine, goblet cells which are also present in the small intestine but are abundant in the large intestine where they produce a thick layer of mucus that coats the epithelium (Fig. 4.2). Goblet cells also secrete antimicrobial peptides.

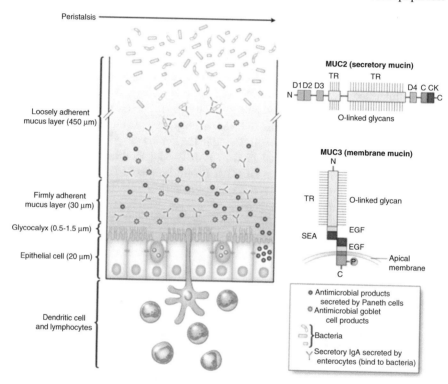

Fig. 4.2 Gut mucosal barrier. The illustration depicts two mucus layers overlaying the gut epithelium (left) and domain structures of secretory (*MUC2*) and membrane-bound (*MUC3*) mucins on the right. *MUC3* and *MUC17* are part of the glycocalyx, which makes up membrane-bound mucins covering the epithelium and loosely adherent mucin layer composed of *MUC2* secreted by goblet cells, paneth cells and enterocytes. Microbes are associated with the loose mucin layer. The domain structure of *MUC2* monomer shows central tandem repeat (TR) regions rich in proline, threonine, and serine (PTS domain) to which many oligosaccharide side chains (O-linked glycan) are linked, and four von Willebrand factor D domains flanking the tandem repeat (PTS) domains and C-terminal knot (CK) domain, which is involved in initial *MUC2* dimerization. The domain structure of *MUC3* mucin shows that it consists of two subunits, one extracellular and one membrane-bound. The extracellular subunit consists of a glycosylated tandem repeat (PTS) domain and two epidermal growth factor (EGF)-like domains separated by sperm protein, enterokinase, and agrin (SEA) motif (a proteolytic cleavage site during biosynthesis) a membrane-bound subunit that consists of membrane-spanning domain and a cytoplasmic tail with potential phosphorylation (P) sites. [*Republished with permission of SpringerNature publishing from Kim, Y. S. and Ho, S. B. (2010), "Intestinal goblet cells and mucins in health and disease: Recent insights and progress." Curr Gastroenterol Rep; 12:319-330, Figure 1. Conveyed through STM permission guidelines 2014*]

Peyer's patches located in the small intestine in the ileum conatin lymphoid follicles and germinal centers indicating active adaptive immune response following antigen delivery by Paneth cells. Microfold (M) cells like Paneth cells also capture antigen from the GI lumen and deliver the antigens to dendritic cells in the Peyer's patches. Along with epithelial cells, they secrete defensins, AMPs and regenerating islet-derived protein (REG3) family members which target bacterial membranes. REG3 proteins target gram-positive bacterial cells. Tuft cells secrete molecules that aid worm expulsion in the GI. Isolated lymphoid follicles (ILFs) containing B lymphocytes also provide gut immunity. ILC3 cells, TH17, TREG, TFH, IELs and IgA secreting B cells are important in maintaining gut homeostasis. The lumenal sequesteration of commensal gut microbiota within the GI tract from the immune system provides a level of "immunological ignorance" that leads to gut and immune homeostasis. The effect of the cytokines secreted by lymphocytes increases the effector activity of granulocytes such as eosinophils that can also participate in type 2 responses.

Selected References

Castell-Rodriguez A, Pinon-Zarate G, Herrera-Enriquez M, Jarquin-Yanez K, Medina-Solares I (2017) Dendritic cells: location, function, and clinical implications. Chapter 2. IntechOpen biology of myelomonocytic cells

Italiani P, Boraschi D (2014) From monocytes to M1/M2 macrophages: phenotypical vs. functional differentiation. Frontiers in Immunology 5:514

Kim YS, Ho SB (2010) Intestinal goblet cells and mucins in health and disease: Recent insights and progress. Curr Gastroenterol Rep 12:319–330

Kita H (2011) Eosinophils: multifaceted biologic properties and roles in health and disease. Immunol Rev 242:161–177

Kotas ME, Locksley RM (2018) Why ILC's? Immunity 48:1081–1090

Murphy K, Weaver C (2017) Janeway's immunobiology, 9th edn. Garland Press, New York

Neill DR, Flynn RJ (2018) Origins and evolution of innate lymphoid cells: Wardens of barrier immunity. Parasite immunology 40:e12436

Punt J, Stranford SA, Jones PP, Owen JA (2019) Kuby immunology, 8th edn. W.H. Freeman and Company, New York. Chapter 20, Antigen-antibody interactions

Shapouri-Mpghaddam A, Mohammadian S, Vazini H, Taghadosi M, Esmaaelli S, Mardani F, Seifi B, Mohammadi A, Afshari JT, Sahebkar A (2018) Macrophage plasticity, polarization, and function in health and disease. J Cell Physiol. 233:6425–6440

Walsh KP, Mills KHG (2013) Dendritic celss and othe innate determinants of T helper cell polarization. Trends Immunol 34(11):521–530

Wojno EDT, Artis D (2016) Emerging concepts and future challenges in innate lymphoid cell biology. J. Exp. Med. 213:2229–2248

Yipp BG, Kubes P (2013) NETosis: how vital is it? Blood 122:2784–2794

Chapter 5
Lymphoid Organs

Unlike other major organ locations in the body such as the heart, lungs and kidneys that define specific systems, the immune system like the endocrine system has organs and tissues that are distributed strategically all over the body. For the immune system, blood and lymphatic vessels maintain connections among the organs and tissues. The immune system consists of structurally and functionally diverse organs and tissues dispersed throughout the body. The organs are classified as primary, secondary and tertiary lymphoid organs. Lymphocytes and other blood cells are produced in the bone marrow from a hematopoietic pluripotent stem cell. Following production, lymphocytes migrate and accumulate within compartments in specialized lymphoid organs.

Lymphoid Organs and Tissue

These consist of areas rich in reticular fibers produced by reticular cells and areas where lymphocytes "home" to within the organs. Lymphoid organs contain stromal and parenchymal tissue. There are B lymphocyte rich zones and T lymphocyte rich zones within the organs and areas rich in B and T lymphocytes. Lymphocytes leaving the bone marrow and thymus enter secondary and tertiary lymphoid organs and tissue in response to cytokines (chemokines) and using cell adhesion molecules expressed on the cell surfaces and on the endothelial cell surfaces. If antigen is not encountered, cells recirculate and reenter the lymphoid organs and tissues. Types of lymphoid tissue include dense lymphoid tissue (cells held together, fixed), loose lymphoid tissue (cells free, enter and exit tissue) and follicular tissue (lymphoid nodules).

Primary lymphoid organs contain a microenvironment for the formation and maturation of blood cells. The bone marrow and thymus are **primary lymphoid organs**. The bone marrow is the Bursal equivalent, and major hematopoietic organ that constantly monitors the need for differentiated erythrocytes and leukocytes in

© Springer Nature Switzerland AG 2021
T. Y. Sam-Yellowe, *Immunology: Overview and Laboratory Manual*,
https://doi.org/10.1007/978-3-030-64686-8_5

the body. Hematopoiesis occurs in different tissues during fetal development, including the yolk sac, placenta, fetal liver and the aorta-gonad-mesonephros (AGM) region. After birth and throughout adult life, hematopoiesis occurs in the bone marrow. Hematopoietic stem cells reside within the bone marrow and also circulate in the blood. The **bone marrow** consists of red and yellow marrow. Hematopoiesis occurs within the **red marrow** of the long bones, in the medullary cavity of the femur and in the humerus (Fig. 5.1). Different cell lineages develop during hematopoiesis (Fig. 5.2). Bones of the vertebrae, skull, ribs, sternum and pelvis support blood cell development mostly before puberty. The bone marrow is organized into two compartments, the **endosteal** (**endosteum**) niche and **perivascular** niche. The endosteal niche lines the inner cavity of the long bones and the perivascular niche lines the blood vessels found in the center of the bone. Sinusoids containing blood cells are also found with the marrow. The endothelial cells lining the blood vessels interact with the perivascular cells to maintain HSCs and the hematopoietic cells differentiated from the HSCs. Osteoblasts from the bone matrix contribute to the regulation of lymphoid cell differentiation. Macrophages contribute to the development of hematopoietic cells within the bone marrow niches and sympathetic nerves provide signals to the cells within the microenvironments within the medullary cavity. Stromal tissue containing reticular fibers consisting of types I and III collagen provide support for hematopoietic cells distributed as cords within the marrow. Adipose tissue is found within the adult marrow. Fibroblastic stromal cells, provide a support network for hematopoietic cells as they undergo mitosis,

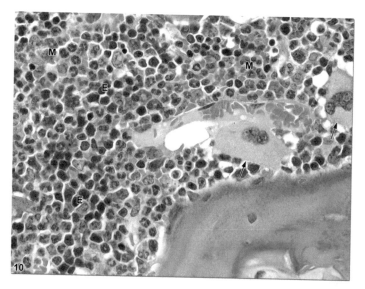

Fig. 5.1 Mouse (6 month old 129 mouse) bone marrow showing hematopoiesis. *M* Myeloid, *E* Erythroid regions and megakaryocytes (arrows). [*Republished with permission of SAGE publishing from Travlos, G. S., "Normal structure, function, and histology of the bone marrow." Toxicologic Pathology, 34:548-565, 2006, Figure 10. Conveyed through STM permission guidelines 2014*]

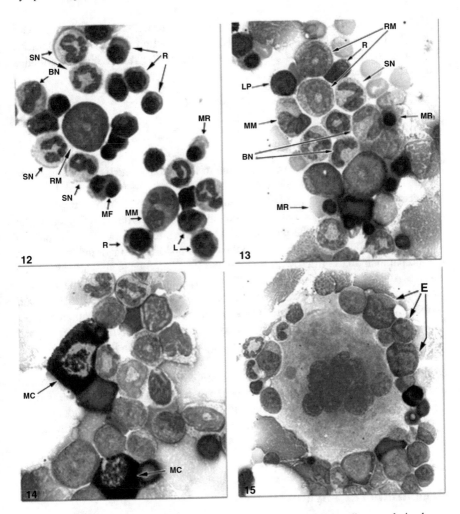

Fig. 5.2 Bone marrow smear from a normal rat showing cells of different lineages during hematopoiesis. *BN* Band neutrophil, *L* Lymphocyte, *MF* Mitotic figure, *MM* Metamyelocyte, *MR* Metarubricyte, *R* Rubricyte, *RM* Ring form myelocyte, *SN* Segmented neutrophil. [*Republished with permission of SAGE publishing from Travlos, G. S., "Normal structure, function, and histology of the bone marrow." Toxicologic Pathology, 34:548-565, 2006, Figure 12. Conveyed through STM permission guidelines 2014*]

proliferate, differentiate and mature. Stromal cells provide sites for adherence, nutrients, cytokines, chemokines, colony stimulating factors and growth factors. Transcription factors expressed by hematopoietic cells in response to signals from the stroma drive lineage differentiation. HSCs become nonself-renewing multipotent progenitors (MMPs) capable of producing lymphoid and myeloid cells. MMPs express the cytokine receptor FLT3 (CD135), a surface receptor tyrosine kinase which binds to the cytokine FLT3 ligand (FLT3L) on the surface of stromal cells.

Additional molecules expressed on the surface of stromal cells include stem cell factor (SCF) and the chemokine CXCL12 which function in B cell development. SCF binds to the receptor tyrosine kinase Kit (CD117). Yellow marrow contains more adipose than the red marrow.

Thymus

Thymocytes from the bone marrow migrate to the thymus where they mature. The thymus is important both for cell-mediated immune responses and humoral responses. The thymus is a lobulated lymphoid organ covered by a capsule and divided into two major compartments, the cortex and medulla. Histologically, the cortex stains darker than the pale medulla. The thymus does not filter blood and lacks reticular fibers like those found in the lymph node. In younger individuals, the thymic paranchyma is filled with lymphocytes. As individuals age, adipose tissue replaces the lymphocyte population. This is due to involution of the thymus. However, reticulo-epithelial cells form the blood-thymic barrier. Pericytes are found at the capillary basal lamina and the basal lamina of reticulo-endothelial cells. Thymocytes mature in the thymus before distribution to other lymphoid organs and the peripheral circulation. Blood vessels enter and exit through the thymic capsule. The capsular artery transporting thymocytes branches in the septa and enters the corticomedullary arterioles, continues into the cortical capillaries and enters the medulla. T lymphocytes leave the thymus through the venules to enter the periphery. The absence of a thymus results in DiGeorge syndrome. Individuals may develop mild to severe immunodeficiencies as a result of having a small thymus or completely lacking a thymus, respectively.

Organization of Thymus

The capsule covering the thymus is composed of connective tissue. Septa subdivide the lobes of the thymus into lobules. Blood vessels enter through the septa. The cortex is the outer edge of the thymus. Large numbers of thymocytes, macrophages, reticular cells (secrete thymic hormones) and thymic epithelial cells are located in the cortex. The medulla is the inner portion of the thymus where differentiated T lymphocytes, reticular cells, macrophages and Hassal's corpuscles (thymic corpuscles) are located. Hassal's corpuscles are composed of flat keratinized epithelial cells in a concentric organization. These are concentric arrangements of flat keratinized epithelial cells. There are no afferent lymphatics, lymphoid nodules, B cells or antibody production in the thymus (Fig. 5.3). **Positive** and **Negative selection** of thymocytes occurs within the thymus to ensure maturing T cells are not self-reactive, and that cells exiting the thymus react with processed peptides presented by MHC proteins of host background, respectively.

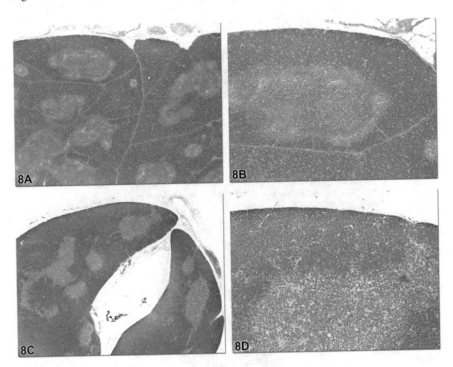

Fig. 5.3 Rat and mouse thymus. (**a**) Rat (3-month old female Wistar rat) thymus showing cortex and medulla and thymic lobules. (**b**) Higher magnification of (**a**). (**c**) Mouse (3-month old B6C3F1 mouse) thymus showing absence of thymic lobules. (**d**) Higher magnification of C. [*Republished with permission of SAGE publishing from Pearse, G. "Normal structure, function, and histology of the thymus." Toxicologic Pathology, 504-514, 2006, Figure 8. Conveyed through STM permission guidelines 2014*]

Secondary lymphoid organs are sites for cell differentiation. Secondary lymphoid organs contain an optimum microenvironment for effective cellular interaction, T and B lymphocyte activation and differentiation and germinal center development. In addition to possessing discrete sites for B and T cell residence, the architecture of the organs maximizes antigen trapping and lymphocyte interaction. The spleen and lymph nodes make up the secondary lymphoid organs. The spleen filters the blood while the lymph nodes filter extracellular fluid. Regional lymph nodes are clustered in strategic locations throughout the body especially at junctions of lymphatic vessels where they filter lymph. Most antigens make their initial contact with macrophages and lymphocytes in regional lymph nodes. The lymph nodes are secondary lymphoid organs. They contain high endothelial venules (HEVs) used by lymphocytes for entry into the nodes.

Lymph nodes are encapsulated bean-shaped structures found along lymphatic vessels. B and T lymphocytes are distributed in different compartments within the node. A capsule surrounds the lymph nodes and branches into the matrix of the node forming trabeculae. Both capsule and trabeculae are composed of connective tissue.

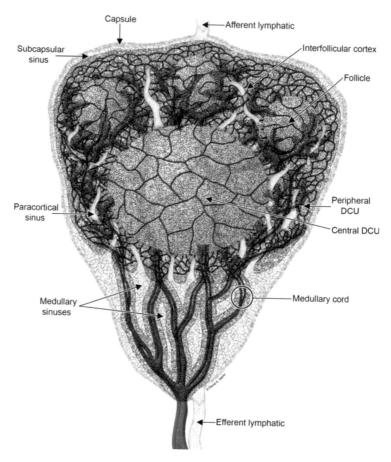

Capsule

Afferent lymphatic

Subcapsular
sinus

Interfollicular cortex

Follicle

Paracortical
sinus

Peripheral
DCU

Central DCU

Medullary
sinuses

Medullary cord

Efferent lymphatic

Fig. 5.4 Illustration of a single lymph node lobule showing afferent and efferent lymphatic vessels, subcapsular sinus, follicles, medullary sinuses, medullary cord and deep cortical unit (DCU) containing paracortex. [*Republished with permission of SAGE publishing from Willard-Mack, C. L., "Normal structure, function, and histology of lymph nodes." Toxicologic Pathology, 34:409-424, 2006, Figure 1. Conveyed through STM permission guidelines 2014*]

Afferent lymphatic vessels enter the node at the capsule, transporting lymph and cells, and continues into the subcapsular space where the subcapsular sinus is also located (Fig. 5.4). The subcapsular sinus is lined by a layer of endothelial cells, below which are macrophages that function to capture antigen from lymph in the lumen of the sinus. The lymph node is divided into three main compartments, the **cortex**, **paracortex** and **medulla**. Cortical and medullary sinuses are present. Macrophages are found mostly in the paracortex and medulla and reticular cells are also found in the nodes. Reticular fibers formed by the reticular cells form part of the lymph node stroma. The paracortex is a *thymic dependent* zone of the lymph nodes and is T cell rich. Lymphoid follicles and germinal centers are located in the cortex, and represent B cell rich areas of the lymph node. Aggregates of lymphoid tissue known as medullary cords are found in the medulla. Medullary sinuses are also located within the compartment of the medulla. Blood vessels enter and exit the lymph nodes at the hilus. Post capillary venules lined with cuboidal epithelium and known as high endothelial venules (HEVs) are used by lymphocytes to migrate into the lymph nodes and are located deep within the cortex. Lymphocytes and endothelial cells express cell adhesion molecules such as selectins and integrins to facilitate diapedesis (also known as extravasation or transendothelial migration) of cells into the lymph node. Larger venules and arteriolar branches exit the lymph nodes. Medullary sinuses merge at the hilus to form efferent lymphatic vessels that exit the lymph node. A summary of the direction of lymph flow into the lymph node is shown below.

Direction of flow of lymph entering and exiting lymph node: afferent lymphatic vessels → capsule → subcapsular space (subcapsular sinus) → trabeculae → paracortex → medullary sinus → efferent lymphatic vessel

Lymphatic vessels travel with veins. They arise near capillary beds in the connective tissue matrix and move towards lymphatic ducts. Lymphatic vessels have large lumens with irregular diameter. Large lymphatic vessels possess valves. The lymphatic vessels are lined with endothelial cells and contain sparse connective tissue. They transport interstitial fluid, within the capillaries known as lymph, to secondary lymphoid organs. The lymph contains few lymphocytes but no erythrocytes. A decrease in hydrostatic pressure and increase in osomotic pressure at the venous end of the capillary beds forces water into the capillaries. Lymph from the body enters the thoracic duct, and moves towards the left subclavian vein in the neck. In the right arm and right side of the head, lymphatic vessels converge to form the right lymphatic duct that enters the right subclavian vein thereby ensuring that steady-state levels of fluid is maintained in the blood circulation. Infections within the lymphatic system can lead to inflammation of the lymphatic vessels known as lymphangitis, a condition in which red streaks are visible under the skin. Swelling of lymph nodes, lymphadenitis (also known as bubos), occurs due to inflammation.

The **spleen** is a secondary lymphoid organ located below the diaphragm, under the rib cage on the left side of the body. The spleen filters blood, traps blood borne pathogens and removes damaged or senescent blood cells from blood circulation. There are no high endothelial venules (HEVs) in the spleen.

Organization of the Spleen

The spleen is surrounded by a capsule composed of dense connective tissue. Trabeculae branch and extend from the capsule into the parenchyma (functional areas) of the spleen (Fig. 5.5). The parenchymal area is known as the pulp. The pulp is divided into **red pulp** and **white pulp.** The red pulp contains splenic sinusoids (thin-walled blood vessels), splenic cords of Billroth (parenchymal tissue), reticular connective tissue and venous sinuses. The white pulp makes up round, whitish areas

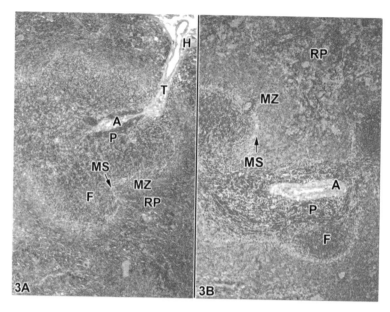

Fig. 5.5 Mouse (20 week old female B6C3F1 mouse) spleen, (left) and rat (12 week old male F344/N rat) (right). *A* Central artery, *F* Follicle, *H* Hilus, *MS* Marginal sinus region, *MZ* Marginal zone, *P* Periarteriolar lymphoid sheath, *RP* Red pulp. [*Republished with permission of SAGE publishing from Cesta, M. F., "Normal structure, function, and histology of the spleen." Toxicologic Pathology, 34:455-465, 2006, Figure 3. Conveyed through STM permission guidelines 2014*]

within the red pulp, surrounding central arteries (central arteriole), consisting of lymphoid tissue and the **periarterial lymphoid sheath (PALS)** a T cell rich area. The border between the red and white pulp is known as the **marginal zone**, with a mantle containing many resting B cells. Plasma cells and macrophages can also be found here. Lymph nodules (lymph follicles) are B cell rich areas located in the white pulp. The direction of blood flow into and out of the spleen is shown below.

Direction of Blood Flow Entering and Exiting the Spleen

Splenic artery enters spleen at hilus → trabecular arteries → central arteries (surrounded by lymphatic tissue) → pencillar arteries → red pulp. In the red pulp, blood flows through sheathed arteries (arterioles) and capillaries to sinusoids (closed circulation) → veins of the pulp → trabecular veins → splenic veins → circulation. In the red pulp, blood flows through sheathed arteries and capillaries and can also enter → splenic cords (open circulation) → reenter blood vessels.

Tertiary lymphoid organs: These are loose collections of lymphocytes, macrophages, granulocytes and mast cells. They may be organized mainly as lymphoid follicles or lymphoid nodules. They contain a large number of antibody producing cells. Tertiary lymphoid tissue serves as the primary defense of tissues in close contact with the environment such as mucosal tissue.

Examples of tertiary tissues and cells include:

Mucosal-associated lymphoid tissue	Diffuse mucosal lymphoid tissue
(MALT):	Intraepithelial lymphocytes (IEL).
Organized mucosal lymphoid tissue	Lamina propria
Tonsils	M cells
Adenoids	Cutaneous-associated lymphoid tissue:
Bronchial associated lymphoid tissue	Skin
Appendix	Intraepidermal lymphocytes
Lymphoid follicles	Keratinocytes
Peyer's patches	Melanocytes
Gut-associated lymphoid tissue (GALT):	Langerhans cells

Peyer's patches are tertiary lymphoid tissue located beneath the mucosal layer of the small intestine, mostly in the ileum of the small intestine. Peyer's patches are part of the mucosal associated lymphoid tissue (MALT) in the gastrointestinal tract (gut associated lymphoid tissue, GALT) (Fig. 5.6). Microfold cells (M cells) capture antigens from the GI lumen for transfer to Peyer's patches. M cells are part of the tertiary lymphoid organ system. They are found in the inductive site and have deeply invaginated pockets containing B, T cells and macrophages. M cells function in MALT and GALT and they express class II MHC antigens. M cells transport antigens to cells in MALT and GALT and activate B cells. The activated B cells differentiate into IgA secreting plasma cells leading to high levels of IgA production at these sites. Lymph nodules and germinal centers form within the Peyer's patches and lymphocytes traffic across HEVs for entry into the Peyer's patches. Follicles develop into germinal centers following antigen contact (Fig. 5.6).

The **appendix** is also tertiary lymphoid tissue, with lymphoid tissue beneath the GI epithelium. Both B and T lymphocytes are located within the appendix. **Tonsils** consist of **palatine** tonsils, **lingual** tonsils and **pharyngeal** tonsils (**adenoids**). The palatine tonsils are surrounded by a hemicapsule which is a thin capsule at the base and sides of the tonsil. Stratified squamous epithelium (SSE) is found in the palatine tonsils. Palatine tonsils possess multiple tonsillar crypts (10–20 crypts) and lymphoid nodules (follicles) that form germinal centers. Diffuse nodular tissue makes up the parenchyma of the tonsils, which are B cell rich. Lingual tonsils are also lined by SSE and possess a single crypt. Pharyngeal tonsils are unencapsulated, have no crypts and are lined by pseudostratified columnar epithelium.

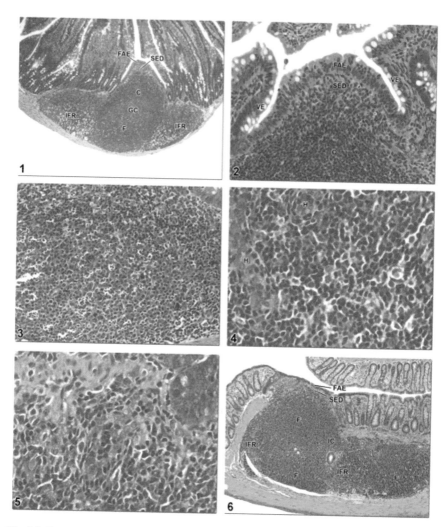

Fig. 5.6 Peyer's Patch from rat (31 day old male Sprague-Dawley rat) small intestine. (**1**) Follicle (F) with germinal center (GC) surrounded by mantle zone or corona (C) is shown. The GC is flanked by interfollicular regions (IFR). The corona is surrounded by the subepithelial dome (SED) and follicle-associated epithelium (FAE). (**5**) High magnification of high endothelial venule (HEV) showing lymphocytes on endothelial cell surface. [*Republished with permission of SAGE publishing from Cesta, M. F., "Normal structure, function, and histology of mucosa-associated lymphoid tissue." Toxicologic Pathology, 34:599-608, 2006, Figures 1 and 5. Conveyed through STM permission guidelines 2014*]

Selected References

Cesta MF (2006) Normal structure, function, and histology of the spleen. Toxicol Pathol 34:455–465

Cesta MF (2006) Normal structure, function, and histology of mucosa-associated lymphoid tissue. Toxicol Pathol 34:599–608

Mescher L (2018) Junqueira's basic histology text and atlas, 15th edn. McGraw Hill Lange

Murphy K, Weaver C (2017) Janeway's Immunobiology, 9th edn. Garland Press, New York

Pearse G (2006) Normal structure, function and histology of the thymus. Toxicol Pathol 34:504–514

Punt J, Stranford SA, Jones PP, Owen JA (2019) Kuby immunology, 8th edn. W.H. Freeman and Company, New York. Chapter 20, Antigen-antibody interactions

Travlos GS (2006) Normal structure and function, and histology of the bone marrow. Toxicol Pathol 34:548–565

Willard-Mack CL (2006) Normal structure, function, and histology of lymph nodes. Toxicol Pathol 34:409–424

Chapter 6
Innate and Adaptive Immunity

Initial exposure of the host to pathogens results in the interaction of host cells with the pathogens through the use of membrane receptors that bind to molecules on the pathogen. Detection of the pathogen by sentinel cells leads to endocytosis or phagocytosis and cytokine secretion by the host cell. Dendritic cells, macrophages or epithelial cells of the mucosa may participate in these response resulting in pro-inflammatory cytokine secretion to initiate innate immune responses. If the pathogen is not cleared, the responses begun in the innate immune responses may activate T and B lymphocytes leading to antibody production and additional cytokine secretion by both cells in the adaptive immune response. Dendritic cells and macrophages classically bridge the responses between innate and adaptive immunity.

Innate immunity: Responses of the innate immune system generally involve cells that participate in phagocytosis of invading pathogens and damaged cells in association with inflammation. In addition, inflammatory cytokines, antimicrobial peptides (AMPs) and acute phase proteins such as C-reactive protein (CRP) produced by the liver are key mediators of innate immunity. Cells of the innate system also express receptors known as pattern recognition receptors (PPRs) that bind to various macromolecular patterns on the cell surfaces of pathogens (pathogen associated molecules or PAMPs), including secreted or excreted products from pathogens and nucleic acids from viruses. The PRRs are distributed on the surfaces of innate cells and within the interior of the cells in the cytoplasm and endosome. Receptor recognition directed at PAMPs is specific and discriminates between the pathogen and host antigens, but receptor binding does not involve binding to specific antigenic determinants or epitopes. Innate responses do not increase in magnitude despite continued exposure to the pathogen. Innate immunity presents a first line of defense against an invading agent that involves the initial "sensing" of the pathogen by sentinel cells present in the skin and mucosal areas of the body. The general features of innate immunity include anatomical barriers of the body, physiological barriers, binding of PAMPs to PRRs, phagocytic cells and inflammatory responses combined with rapid response. We will discuss PRRs in more detail below.

© Springer Nature Switzerland AG 2021
T. Y. Sam-Yellowe, *Immunology: Overview and Laboratory Manual*,
https://doi.org/10.1007/978-3-030-64686-8_6

Anatomic barriers include the skin where Langerhans cells found in the epidermis can take up invading pathogens, ultimately delivering digested pathogen peptides to T lymphocytes in draining lymph nodes. Lactic acid and fatty acids are produced in sweat and sebaceous secretions, urine flow prevents infection in the lower urinary tract, ciliated epithelial cells and mucus in the respiratory tract sweep away debris and bacteria. Within the gastrointestinal tract, mucus produced by goblet cells and overlaying the epithelium along with the presence of microfold (M) and paneth cells present a barrier to invading pathogens. Commensal gut microbiome trapped within the mucus layer present an additional layer of protection as they secrete products that can inhibit the establishment of infection by pathogenic bacteria.

Physiological barriers consist of saliva in the oral cavity, high or low pH in organ compartments, high or low temperature, mucous secretions, lysozyme in tears which degrades mucopeptides on bacterial cell walls, acute phase proteins such as C-reactive protein (CRP), mannose binding protein, serum amyloid P component, histamine, kinins, complement proteins of the alternate pathway, soluble factors such as interferons which prevent viral infections (alpha, beta, gamma), perforins, tumor necrosis factor and granzymes produced by natural killer cells.

Inflammatory responses include cytokine mediated-tissue destruction. Increased blood flow and capillary permeability which leads to increased migration of phagocytic cells to the site of inflammation in response to chemotaxis. The cardinal features of inflammation include redness (*rubor/erythema*), swelling (*tumor*), pain (*dolor*), heat (*calor*) and loss of function (*funcio laesa*). The cells involved in inflammatory responses during innate immunity include neutrophils, monocytes, macrophages, mast cells, basophils and eosinophils.

Phagocytosis is a specialized uptake of particulate antigens such as pathogens. The pathogen is engulfed using pseudopods which are extensions of the plasma membrane. Phagocytosis is performed by specialized cells such as neutrophils, monocytes, macrophages and dendritic cells. The process of phagocytosis involves the migration of cells, adherence of cells through **pseudopods** to the pathogen, engulfment of the foreign particle or pathogen into the cell cytoplasm using pseudopodia to form a phagocytic vesicle known as a phagosome. Fusion of the **phagosome** with a **lysosome** to form a **phagolysosome** results in enzymatic digestion of the foreign particle and elimination through the **endosomal** processing pathway. **Endocytosis** is distinct from phagocytosis and can also involve receptor mediated interaction. Endocytosis includes pathogen-receptor interaction, internalization of the pathogen into an **endocytic** vesicle, fusion of the **endocytic** vesicle to form an **endosome,** fusion of the endosome to a primary lysosome to form a **secondary lysosome,** degradation of the pathogen and recycling of the receptor.

Pattern recognition receptors (PRRs) are expressed on the surface of cells, in the cytoplasm and in endosomes. PRRs serve as receptors for diverse ligands, known as pathogen associated molecular patterns (PAMPs). Toll-like receptors (TLRs), NOD-like receptors (NLRs) and C-lectin like receptors (CLRs) are examples of PRRs important in innate immunity. The PAMPs include cell wall components on bacteria, lipopolysaccharide (LPS) on gram negative bacteria, flagella proteins, mannans on fungi and virus nucleic acids. Binding of PAMPs, to PRRs activate signaling pathways that result in transcription and expression of proinflammatory cytokines and activation of dendritic cells (DCs) which function to bridge innate and adaptive immunity (Fig. 6.1). Cells involved in innate immunity include

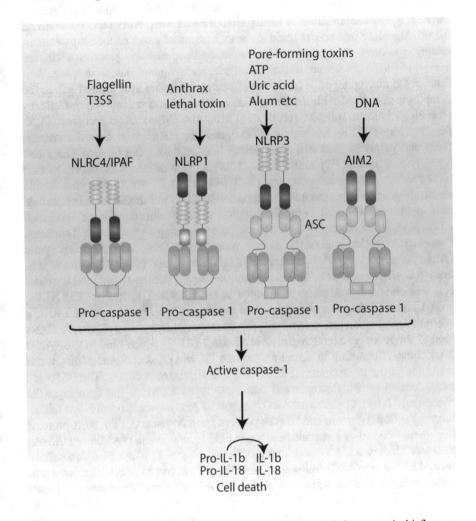

Fig. 6.1 Pattern recognition receptor family members NLR and ALR from canonical inflammasomes. NLR or ALR sensors detect and bind to viral and bacterial PAMPs. NLRC4 is activated by bacterial flagellin and T3SS components, NLRP1b is activated by anthrax lethal toxin and AIM2 is activated by cytosolic dsDNA. NLRP3 is activated by a wide variety of signals including pore-forming cytotoxins, ATP, uric acid and alum. Once activated the receptors form an inflammasome complex with or without the adaptor, ASC and recruits procaspase-1, which is subsequently cleaved into caspase-1. Caspase-1 cleaves precursors of IL-1βand IL_18 into their active forms as well as induces cell death. [*Republished with permission of Elsevier publishing from Vanaja S. et al. Mechanisms of inflammasome activation: recent advances and novel insights. Trends Cell Biol. 25:308-315, Figure 1. Conveyed through STM permission guidelines 2014*]

granulocytes, monocytes, innate lymphoid cells, dendritic cells and macrophages. Epithelial cells lining mucosal surfaces participate in pathogen recognition using PRRs and activation of signaling pathways resulting in the secretion of proinflammatory cytokines and antimicrobial peptides.

Innate immune responses constitute the first line of defense against pathogens. Innate responses are initiated by the ligation of PRRs with PAMPs and DAMPs and the cell signaling that occurs leads to the expression of genes encoding proinflammatory cytokines, chemokines and antimicrobial peptides and proteins. PRRs are expressed on the cell surface of various cells including monocytes, neutrophils, dendritic cells, macrophages, B and T lymphocytes. PRRs are also located within the cytoplasm associated with membranes of endosomes and mitochondria. Cell surface PRRs include Toll like receptors (TLRs) and C-type lectin receptor (CLR) family. Thirteen TLRs are known, with ligands associated with bacteria, viruses, fungi and parasites. Bacterial components like peptidoglycan bind to TLR2 and lipopolysaccharide (LPS) binds TLR4. TLRs also include receptors that are located on the membrane of endosomes such as TLR3 and TLR7 which bind viral double strand RNA and single strand RNA, respectively. TLRs are characterized by leucine rich repeats (LRRs) and homodimerization or heterodimerization of receptors. CLRs bind to carbohydrates on fungi and parasites using dectin 1 on cell surfaces. Cytoplasmic PRRs include NOD-like receptors (NLRs), AIM2-like receptors (ALRs) (Fig. 6.1), RIG-1-like receptor (RLRs) family and cyclic GMP-AMP synthase (cGAS) a member of the nucleotidyltransferase family. NLRs bind bacterial cell wall components such as peptidoglycan and muramyl dipeptides. The NLRs, NOD1 and NOD2 located on endosomal membranes possess C-terminal LRRs, a central NOD-domain and N-terminal caspase recruitment domains (CARDs). NLRs bind to the receptor-interacting protein kinase 2 (RIP2) which bind to the TAK1/TAB complex resulting in signaling through the MAPK and NFκB pathway and activation of the transcription factors AP-1 and NFκB, respectively. The NLRs are multi-domain proteins categorized into three types based on the domain at the N-terminus. NLRCs possess a CARD domain, NLRBs possess a baculovirus inhibitory repeat (BIR) domain and NLRPs possess pyrin domains (PYD). NLR proteins oligomerize once they sense and bind intracellular (endogenous) PAMPs or DAMPs. Receptor binding leads to recruitment of the adaptor protein, apoptosis-associated speck-like protein (ASC) followed by recruitment of pro-caspase-1. The three proteins interact to form an active inflammasome. Autocleavage of pro-caspase-1 leads to activation forming caspase-1 which activates the precursors of the pro-inflammatory cytokines IL-1β and IL-18 resulting in inflammation. The N-terminal domains are used for homotypic protein-protein interactions (NLRPPYD-ASCPYD and ASCCARD-Caspase-1-CARD). Activation of inflammatory responses through the inflammasomes can lead to a type of cell death in the activated cell known as pyroptosis. Swelling of the cell, lysis and release of cellular contents characterizes pyroptosis. NLRP1, NLRP3 and NLRC4 participate in formation of canonical inflammasomes that activate caspase-1 to cleave precursors of IL-1 β and IL-18 (Fig. 6.1).

The RLR family receptors bind to viral dsRNA. RIG-1 binds terminal 5′-triphosphate of the dsRNA and the family member MDA5 binds to the body of dsRNA. RIG-1 recognizes viral RNAs tri-phosphorylated in their 5′ ends. Following binding, the adaptor mitochondrial membrane associated mitochondrial antiviral signaling (MAVS) protein recruits signaling proteins that leads to the activation and translocation of the transcription factors NFκB, IRF3 and IRF7 into the nucleus and secretion of IFNα and IFNβ. MAVS and RIG-1 possess CARD domains with which they interact.

ALRs possess pyrin domains (PYDs) and hematopoietic expression, interferon inducibility, nuclear localization (HIN) domain which binds DNA from viruses. cGAS also binds DNA from viruses. AIM2 and dectin-1 receptors also participate in inflammasome formation. Dectin-1 sensors bind to PAMPs from fungal cell walls and induce non-canonical inflammasome assembly in a caspase-8-dependent manner. Following DNA binding, cGAS changes conformation, becomes activated and synthesizes cGAMP from GTP and ATP. cGAMP, a second messenger binds to the ER membrane associated stimulator of interferon genes (STING). Binding of cGMP to STING leads to IRF3 activation. The signaling molecules recruit and activate transcription factors like NFκB and IRF3 that influence cytokine secretion, including type 1 interferons. The important role of cGAS as a DNA sensor was demonstrated in cGAS knock-out mice. The mice were unable to produce type 1 interferons in the presence of cytosolic DNA from viral infection or from transfected DNA.

TLRs are the most well understood of the PRRs and will be the focus of our discussion on the mechanism of cell signaling following binding to PAMPs. TLRs differ in the signaling pathways that are activated following ligation of receptors with PAMPs. For example TLR1 and TLR2 activate signaling cascades through the adaptor myeloid differentiation factor 88 (MyD88) and recruitment of the IL-1 receptor associated kinase 1 (IRAK1) (Fig. 6.2). TLR3 on the endosomal membrane binds viral ds RNA and activates signaling through the TIR domain-containing adaptor-inducing IFN-β factor (TRIF) which binds to and activates tumor necrosis factor receptor-associated factor 3 (TRAF3) resulting in the exposure of binding sites for the recruitment of the adaptors NEMO and TANK and the protein kinases IKKε and TBK1. Interferon regulatory factor 3 (IRF3) and IRF7 become phosphorylated by TBK1 causing both proteins to dimerize and translocated into the nucleus where they influence the transcription of the type 1 interferons, IFNα and IFNβ. Through the adaptor NEMO, signaling events also lead to NFκB activation and translocation into the nucleus leading to transcription of genes encoding proinflammatory cytokines. In contrast, TLR7, 8 and 9 also on the endosome membrane signal in a MyD88 dependent manner leading to phosphorylation of IR7 which dimerizes and translocates into the nucleus. MAP kinase signaling is also activated by the endosomal TLRs.

Following the binding of PAMPs to TLR1 and TLR2, the receptors dimerize and within the cytoplasm the adaptor protein MyD88 is recruited to the TIR domains of the receptor. IRAK1 and IRAK4 are recruited to MyD88. IRAK1 autophosphorylates itself and TRAF6. Once activated TRAF6 forms a scaffold for binding of the

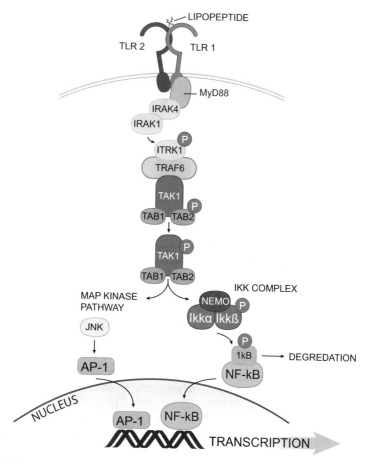

Fig. 6.2 Toll-like receptor (TLR) signaling showing some of the pathways activated following PAMP binding to PRR. Binding of a ligand to the membrane bound TLR1/TLR2 dimerized receptor activates cytoplasmic signaling through the MyD88 adaptor protein. IRAK1 is recruited to the MyD88 and becomes activated by phosphorylation. TRAF 6 is recruited along with TAB1 and TAB2. Activation TAK1 results in the activation of the MAP kinase pathway leading to production of the transcription factor AP-1. Activation of the IKK complex results in the production of the transcription factor NFκB. Transcription factors influence gene expression various molecules including cytokines. Interferon regulatory factors (**IRFs**), IL-1 receptor-associated kinase (**IRAK**), Myeloid differentiation factor 88 (**MyD88**), NFκB essential modifier (**NEMO**), Toll/IL-1 receptor (**TIR**), Transforming growth factor β-activated kinase (**TAK1**), TAK 1-binding protein 1 and 2 (**TAB1** and **TAB2**), Tumor necrosis factor receptor-associated factor 6 (**TRAF6**)

adaptor proteins TAK binding proteins 1 and 2 (TAB1 and TAB2) and the kinase (transforming growth factor β activated kinase 1 (TAK1). IRAK1 phosphorylates and activates TAK1. Additional signaling molecules are recruited and include the IKK complex; NEMO, IKKα and IKKβ. TAK1 phosphorylates and activates IKKβ and also activates the MAP kinase pathway leading to the activation of the transcription factor AP-1 which is translocated into the nucleus. Inactive NFκB is located in the cytoplasm associated with IκB, an inhibitor of NFκB. Phosphorylation of IκB by IKKβ leads to its degradation and dissociation from NFκB, allowing the transcription factor to enter the nucleus where it influences gene expression of cytokines. Transcription factors influence gene expression of various molecules including cytokines.

Adaptive immunity (specific, acquired, induced): These are highly discriminatory responses to foreign substances and pathogens collectively known as antigens, that increase in magnitude, and quality following repeated exposure to the antigen, due to the development of memory to the previous exposure of antigen. Unlike innate immunity, this is an induced immunity that is highly specific for distinct epitopes on the antigen. The acquired or induced immunity amplifies the defense mechanisms of innate immunity. The functional components of the antigen-specific system are not interchangeable. The cell populations involved are subdivided into distinct clones, each responding to a specific antigen in association with accessory molecules. **The clonal selection theory** is the fundamental basis of adaptive immunity that explains T and B lymphocyte antigen receptor expression and clonal expansion following antigen binding. T and B lymphocytes express unique membrane receptors for distinct antigens before antigen exposure. Following antigen contact and cell activation, clones of B and T cells bearing identical receptors to parental cells will bind epitopes on antigen with the same specificity as the parental cells. The general features of adaptive immunity include specificity, diversity, memory, self-nonself recognition and immune regulation. Specificity involves the membrane receptors on the surface of B and T lymphocytes, which bind to specific antigen epitopes leading to cell activation. With diversity the lymphocyte receptors can recognize a large variety of natural and synthetic antigens i.e. the repertoire or capability for antigen recognition is large. In regulation the response to decreased levels of antigens involves feed-back regulation, lymphocyte differentiation and a return to resting state. Self-nonself recognition involves lymphocyte tolerance to self-antigens. Only B and T lymphocytes develop memory. However in recent studies, natural killer cells have been reported to develop memory. Memory cells recognize an antigen upon secondary exposure following a previous initial contact with the same antigen. The development of memory B and T lymphocytes is the basis for vaccine effectiveness in preventing infection. Unlike innate immunity, development of primary adaptive immune responses following exposure to antigen takes 4–5 days.

Macrophages, neutrophils, eosinophils, natural killer cells, cytotoxic T lymphocytes and NKT cells mediate cellular cytotoxicity. Cellular responses are not entirely antibody free since antibody dependent cellular cytotoxicity (ADCC) performed by NK cells and macrophages also occurs through the binding of the Fc region of antibodies to Fc receptors expressed on the surface cells. B lymphocytes recognize antigen using BCR expressed on the cell surface. However, T cells are unable to recognize antigen directly and require the antigen to be processed and presented by antigen presenting cells expressing major histocompatibility complex (MHC) antigens bound to the antigen. This is known as **MHC restriction. T helper cells expressing CD4** interact with **Class II MHC proteins.** This means that TH cells will interact with and respond only to antigen presented in association with class II MHC proteins by the APCs. Cytotoxic T cells expressing **CD8** interact with **Class I MHC proteins.** Tc cells will interact with and respond only to antigens presented in association with class I MHC antigens on the surface of host target cells. **NK cells are not MHC restricted and** can recognize cell surface molecules not associated with MHC proteins. NKT cells recognize lipid antigens bound to CD1 proteins. Although B cells are not MHC restricted in their recognition of antigen, they also process antigen for presentation to T helper cells in association with MHC class II antigens.

An individual may develop immunity in several ways. Immunity can be obtained by **passive immunization**, which is protection resulting from the transfer of pre-formed antibodies from an immune individual to a non-immune individual. This provides short-lived immunity. **Active immunization** provides immunity by protection resulting from an immune response to antigen administration either through infection or through administration of vaccines. Humoral and cell-mediated immune responses are involved and results in memory cells, some of which can be very long-lived. **Adoptive immunization** results in protection from the transfer of cells from an immune individual to a non-immune individual such as bone marrow cells or lymphocyte subpopulations. A form of immunization used in the early days of induced protection involved the inoculation of live small pox virus in a process known as **variolation.** The administration of antigen to induce immunity and stimulate an active immune response is known as **vaccination. Herd immunity** achieved through the administration of vaccines provides protection or immunity of a **whole population** due to the presence of immune individuals in that population, that leads to a decrease or complete prevention of pathogen transmission.

Neuroendocrine Effects on the Immune System

A number of cells in the immune system can produce a variety of neuropeptides and neuroendocrine hormones. Lymphocytes express receptors for many hormones (insulin, thyroxine, somatostatin, growth hormone, neuropeptides, neurotransmitters, steroids and catecholamines (adrenaline and noradrenaline). Lymphocytes produce ACTH in response to corticotophin release factor. The nervous system directly or indirectly controls the release of various hormones during periods of stress which have an immunosuppressive effect on the immune system. There are nerves linked to the Langerhans cells in the skin. Neuropeptide release can depress the APC function of the Langerhans cells. E.g. cases of contact dermatitis and psoriasis worsen with anxiety. Macrophage derived IL-I stimulates synthesis of nerve growth factor in inflammatory sites promoting innervation and nerve healing. An interacting network exists between the nervous system, endocrine system and immune system. Any changes in one system can modulate the activity of the other systems. Factors influencing neuroendocrine effects on the immune system include; Stress (defined physiologically by a significant increase in corticosterone concentration in the serum, with negative effects on the immune system), depression (psychological factors) can induce release of ACTH from the pituitary. This leads to the release of glucocorticoids which are immunosuppressive. Additional effects include, reduced immune responses to mitogens by T lymphocytes (and lymphocytes in general), reduced NK cell activity and reduced IL-2 and IL-2R expression. The reduced immune response reduces the ability of the host to recover from infection. The central nervous system modulates immune function. Most lymphoid tissues (Thymus, spleen, lymph nodes) receives direct sympathetic noradrenergic innervation both to the blood vessels passing through the tissue and to the lymphocytes.

References

Koenderman L, Buurman W, Daha MR (2014) The innate immune response. Immunol Lett 162:95–102
Lanier L (2013) Shades of grey-the blurring view of innate and adaptive immunity. Nat Rev Immunol 13:73–74
Murphy K, Weaver C (2017) Janeway's immunobiology, 9th edn. Garland Press, New York
Netea MG, Schiltzer A, Placek K, Joosten AAB, Schultze JL (2019) Innate and adaptive immune memory: An evolutionary continuum in the host's response to pathogens. Cell Host Microbe 25:13–26
Punt J, Stranford SA, Jones PP, Owen JA (2019) Kuby immunology, 8th edn. W.H. Freeman and Company, New York
Vanaja S, Rathinam VK, Fitzgerald KA (2015) Mechanisms of inflammasome activation: Recent advances and novel insights. Trends Cell Biol 25:308–315

Chapter 7
Leukocyte Homing, Migration and Recirculation

Cell Adhesion Molecules

Lymphocyte homing, trafficking and recirculation ensures maximum contact and interaction of cells with antigen, and correct homing of lymphocytes to appropriate lymphoid microenviromnents. Lymphocytes remain in the blood 2–12 h before homing to organs. Most leukocyte migration occurs across venules (e.g. lymphocytes cross high endothelial venules). The cells migrate for several reasons. These include migration of mononuclear cells into chronic inflammatory sites in response to chemotaxins, migration of activated lymphocytes into inflammatory sites, migration of neutrophils into sites of acute immune response and migration of lymphocytes into secondary lymphoid organs (spleen, lymph nodes). The adherence and movement of cells through the vascular and endothelial spaces, in response to chemotactic factors, chemokines, antigens, or as a result of inflammation is called extravasation (also called diapedisis or transendothelial migration). This process is highly regulated. The cytokines IL-1, IFNγ, and TNFα influence the expression of cell adhesion molecules (CAMs) and vascular addressins (VAs). Lymphocyte homing is influenced by the state of cell activation, for example, the homing properties of naive cells, effector cells and memory cells is different. CAMs expressed by endothelial cells interact with receptors (CAM receptors) on leukocytes to aid the process of cell migration and extravasation. The pattern of cell migration depends on CAMs such as selectins and is also aided by chemokines. A rolling mechanism of migration and diapedesis is used by neutrophils. Neutrophils respond and move up a chemokine gradient as they respond and migrate to sites of inflammation. The chemokine CXCL8 (IL-8) is an important chemoattractant for neutrophils responding to the concentration gradient of the chemokine. Leukocyte adhesion deficiency (LAD) results from a lack of expression of integrins. Leukocytes are not able to diapedese out of the blood vessels into tissue. Neutrophils and monocytes recruited to sites of infection and inflammation remain within the blood vessels. Skin window tests such as the Rebuck skin window test show a failure of leukocyte migration to

© Springer Nature Switzerland AG 2021
T. Y. Sam-Yellowe, *Immunology: Overview and Laboratory Manual*,
https://doi.org/10.1007/978-3-030-64686-8_7

a site of superficial skin abrasion. In the course of LAD, such a skin abrasion would result in the accumulation of leukocytes such as neutrophils and monocytes. Individuals with LAD experience recurrent bacterial infections.

There are four CAM receptor families that include adhesion receptors, homing receptors and CAMs.

1. **Immunoglobulin superfamily:** These are cell adhesion molecules that interact with $\beta2$ integrins. Examples include intracellular adhesion molecule (ICAM-1, ICAM-2), mucosal addressin cell adhesion molecule-1 (MAdCAM-1) and vascular cell adhesion molecules (VCAM). Expression of family member CAMs can be induced by IL-1β, TNFα and IFNγ. ICAM-1 binds to LFA-1. Binding to integrins mediates adhesion and cell migration. MAdCAM-1 possesses both mucin-like and Ig family domains and is a mucosal addressin that binds both L-selectin and integrins on lymphocytes. MAdCAM-1 is expressed on endothelial cells in blood vessels and facilitates diapedesis of lymphocytes migrating and homing into mucosal tissues. MAdCAM-1 is expressed on high endothelial venules (HEVs) of Peyers patches and mesenteric lymph nodes. Lymphocytes migrating into the gut mucosa binding to MAdCAM-1 on the HEVs using $\alpha4\beta7$ expressed on the cell surface. The c-type lectin receptor, dendritic cell-specific intracellular adhesion molecule-3-grabbing non-integrin (DC-SIGN) expressed on dendritic cells and macrophages binds to ICAM-3 on naïve resting T cells. The adhesion between the two cells mediates proliferation in the resting T cells.

2. **Integrin family:** Integrins bind ICAMs and VCAMS, the former using R (Arg) G (Gly) D (Asp) sequences. Integrins are heterodimeric molecules, being composed of α and β chains bound in a noncovalent association. They interact using their extracellular domains to molecules in the extracellular matrix. VLAs (Very Late Antigens) are $\beta1$ integrins that bind VCAMS. Leukocyte functional antigens (LFAs) are example of integrin molecules of the $\beta2$ integrins. They consist of a CD11a and a CD18 chains. LFA-1 (CD11a/CD18) is important for migration of lymphocytes across the endothelium and for cell adhesion during T cell interaction with B and dendritic cells. Vascular cell adhesion protein-1 (CD 106) is expressed on endothelial cells and binds to $\alpha4\beta1$ (VLA-4) on leukocytes including lymphocytes and monocytes. Other examples include complement receptor 3 CR3 (CD11b/CD18) expressed on all mononuclear phagocytes and CR4 (CD11c/CD18 expressed on tissue macrophages. CD11 is the $\beta2$ integrin chain shared by the three molecules. Integrins exist in active and inactive states. They bind strongly to their ligands in the active state, and weakly in the inactive state. Ligand binding is associated with talin which connects the integrin molecule to the actin cytoskeleton.

3. **Selectin family:** Selectin molecules bind to mucin-like molecules. They are membrane glycoproteins that possess lectin-like domains used to bind carbohydrates on mucin-like cell adhesion molecules. Selectins generally enhance the "stickiness" or adhesion of leukocytes to the endothelia. TNFα secreted by macrophages activates endothelial cells and results in degranulation of granules knonw as Weibel-Palade bodies which release P-selectin and E-selectin. Both

selectin molecules bind a blood group antigen protein also expressed on neutrophils known as sulfated sialyl-Lewis^x (s-L^x), facilitating extravasation (diapedesis). L-selectin (CD62-L) is expressed on lymphocytes and neutrophils (on most leukocytes) and functions in diapedesis of naïve T lymphocytes across the high endothelial venules (HEVs) of secondary lymphoid organs. CD62-L binds mucins on endothelial cells. Memory T cells use cutaneous leucocyte antigen (CLA) to bind E-selectin and direct migration into the skin. Pselectin and E-selectin are also expressed on the vascular endothelium and have lectin-like domains which bind carbohydrates on leukocytes.

4. **Mucins:** The mucins bind to sialylated moieties on selectins expressed on the endothelia. They are richly glycosylated molecules comprising serine and threonine rich proteins. Examples include the sialomucins CD34 and CD43, MAdCAM1 and glycosylation-dependent cell adhesion molecule 1 (GlyCAM1) expressed on hematopoietic cells, mast cells and HEVs in peripheral lymph nodes. GlyCAM1 binds L-selectin expressed on the surface of naïve T cells, facilitating their homing and migration out of the blood vessels into lymph nodes where they bind HEVs as they enter the lymph nodes. CD43 expressed on TH17 cells was shown to be important for recruiting cells to sites of inflammation. CD43 binds E-selectin on endothelial cells.

Cell Migration

The key features of cell migration include; contact, rolling, activation, arrest and adhesion and extravasation (diapedesis or transendothelial migration) in response to chemokines. Neutrophil and lymphocyte extravasation are most widely investigated.

Neutrophil extravasation: Neutrophils responds to chemoattractants due to inflammation, bind to the endothelial layer, penetrate the layer and migrate into the underlying tissue using an end-over-end rolling mechanism. The process is activated by platelet derived growth factor, including signaling through G proteins. No HEVs are required for neutrophil migration. In the absence of inflammation, neutrophils do not adhere to endothelia or migrate into tissues.

Lymphocyte extravasation: Lymphocyte migration is chemokine-directed and HEVs are required for lymphocyte entry into lymphoid organs. Antigen simulation is required to maintain HEVs. Homing receptors are required to bind vascular addressins, integrin receptors bind CAMs on HEVs and the lymphocyte extravasates. Chemokines produced by lymphocytes, APCs and cells within lymph nodes bind to chemokine receptors on lymphocytes. Chemokine receptors are G-protein receptors and following binding to chemokines, signals are transduced within the cell which facilitate binding of integrins to intracellular adhesion molecules on endothelial cells. Entry of lymphocytes into lymph nodes is aided by autotaxin, an enzyme secreted by HEVs and other signals that enhance reorganization of the cell cytoskeleton and endothelial cell adhesion, allowing lymphocytes to "squeeze" through the endothelia. Lymphocytes migrate in response to inflammation and also enter specific areas within lymphoid tissue and organs, such as the spleen and lymph nodes for antigen contact.

Monocyte extravasation: Monocytes differentiate into macrophages in tissue. They migrate in response to chemokines (chemoattractants) to sites of infection and inflammation. In the absence of inflammation, monocytes also migrate to tissues to repopulate the tissues with macrophages and dendritic cells. The various cells and their migratory patterns in response to chemokines, function in both the innate and adaptive immune responses.

Selected References

Gibson NJ (2011) Cell adhesion molecules in context. Cell Adhesion and Migration 5:48–51

Lawrence T (2009) The nuclear factor NF-κB pathway in inflammation. Cold Spring Harb Perspect Biol 1:a001651

Murphy K, Weaver C (2017) Janeway's immunobiology, 9th edn. Garland Press, New York

Punt J, Stranford SA, Jones PP, Owen JA (2019) Kuby immunology, 8th edn. W.H. Freeman and Company, New York. Chapter 20, Antigen-antibody interactions

Takeuchi O, Akira S (2010) Pattern recognition receptors and inflammation. Cell 140:805–820

Chapter 8
Apoptosis

Cell death by **apoptosis** serves as an important regulatory mechanism to eliminate cells following differentiation in the bone marrow and also during embryogenesis and organ development. Cytotoxic T cells and NK cells induce apoptosis in target altered host cells. Apoptosis also known as programmed cell death or cellular suicide is a process of cell death that involves a defined death pathway as a result of extrinsic and intrinsic signals effective in the cell, resulting in cell death. This process is distinct from other causes of cell death such as **necrosis, autophagy** and **pyroptosis**. Programmed cell death is accompanied by distinct structural, morphological and biochemical changes in the dying cell. The activation of the suicide program within the cell is a gene directed mechanism. The process of apoptosis is conserved among multicellular organisms. It is a highly regulated process that requires maintenance of a critical balance between cell survival and cell death. Apoptosis is of critical importance during morphogenesis, tissue homeostasis, elimination of self-reactive clones from the immune system, elimination of damaged and altered host cell. Altered host cells include neoplastic cells and cells infected by intracellular pathogens. During normal embryonic tissue development, cell proliferation and differentiation is accompanied by programmed cell death as tissue is formed and shaped for various effector functions of the tissue. Apoptosis is important during synapse formation in the nervous system. Apoptosis is as important for regulation of cell number as mitosis. Similarly, during hematopoiesis, apoptosis is a critical factor in regulating blood cell populations. Apoptosis is one of the regulatory processes used to eliminate blood cells as different cell lineages terminally differentiate in response to growth factors, colony stimulating factors and cytokines. In the thymus during T cell development and maturation thymocytes that fail positive and negative selection die by apoptosis. Among the general features of apoptosis is the observation that apoptosis varies with the type of tissue and type of cell undergoing apoptosis. The mechanisms of intrinsic and extrinsic pathways for apoptosis are shown in Fig. 8.1.

© Springer Nature Switzerland AG 2021
T. Y. Sam-Yellowe, *Immunology: Overview and Laboratory Manual*,
https://doi.org/10.1007/978-3-030-64686-8_8

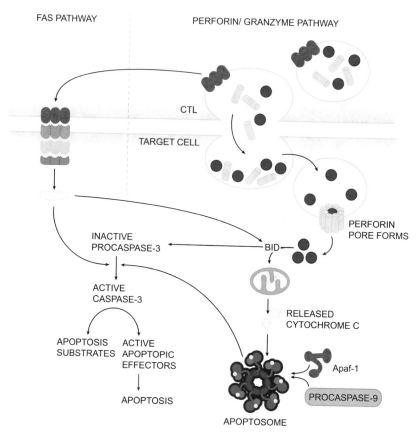

Fig. 8.1 Apoptosis induced by cytotoxic T lymphocytes (CTL) can occur through the Fas or per-forin granzyme pathways. In the Fas pathway, Fas on the target host cell binds to Fas ligand (FasL) on the CTL. The adapter protein FADD binds to Fas, inactive caspase 8 is recruited to the adapter resulting in activation of caspase 8 and events leading to apoptosis within the target cell. Perforin and granzyme are released from granules in the CTL and taken up by the target cell. Perforin forms pores in the endocytic vesicle releases granzyme which activates Bid, a proapoptotic protein and procaspase 3. Bid induces cytochrome c release from the mitochondria. Cytochrome c, Apaf-1 and procaspase 9 assemble to form the apoptosome, where caspase 9 is activated and also cleaves procaspase 3. Active caspase 3 along with cytochrome c initiate apoptosis in the target cell

Characteristics of Apoptotic Cells

Apoptotic cells show distinct morphological and biochemical features such as plasma membrane blebbing, cytoplasmic and nuclear condensation, chromatin deg-radation and fragmentation, decreased cell volume and changes in the orientation of phospholipids in the plasma membrane. Membrane blebbing results in the forma-tion of apoptotic bodies which are phagocytized by macrophages. Chromatin frag-mentation results in characteristic DNA cleavage resulting in 50–300 kilobase (kb) bands and 180–200 base pairs (bp) (monomers, multimers) in formed oligonu-cleosomal fragments resolved following electrophoresis on agarose gels. Increased

levels of clusterin form, activation of type II transglutaminase occurs, which cross-links proteins to apoptotic bodies. Phosphatidylserine (PS) becomes accessible on the outer layer of the plasma membrane, changed in orientation from the normal distribution in the inner layer of the plasma membrane. Diverse signals can activate or suppress apoptosis. These signals include lineage specific signals, ionizing radiation, viral infection, extracellular survival factors, hormones and cell interactions. IL-1β-converting enzyme (ICE/caspase 1), a cysteine protease causes apoptosis when overexpressed in the cell. During apoptosis, cysteine aspartyl-specific proteases known as caspases become activated by extrinsic factors such as the interaction of Fas on altered host target cells with Fas ligand (FasL) on cytotoxic T lymphocytes (CTLs) or TNF interaction with the TNF receptor. Intrinsic signals such as cytochrome c released from the mitochondria following DNA damage, oxidative stress or hypoxia can activate the death pathway leading to caspase activation and eventual cell death. The caspases are categorized as initiator caspases and executioner caspases. Caspases 2, 8, 9, and 10 make up the initiator caspases, while caspases 3, 6, and 7 constitute the effector or executioner caspases.

Intrinsic Pathway (Mitochondrial Pathway)

The intrinsic pathway of apoptosis is regulated by the B cell lymphoma-2 family of proteins which possess both pro-apoptotic and anti-apoptotic activity. The pro-apoptotic proteins of the Bcl-2 family include Bad, Bak, Bax, Bcl-X, Bid, Bik, Bim and Hrk. Other pro-apoptotic molecules include Puma and Noxa. The anti-apoptotic proteins include Bcl-2, Bcl-W, Bcl-X_L, Bfl-1 and Mcl-1. Inhibition of the anti-apoptotic protein Bcl-2, results in apoptosis. Inhibitors include Bcl-X_L (bcl long). Bcl-2 is produced in large amounts by some cancer cells leading to the inhibition and blocking of apoptosis. In healthy cells Bcl-2 binds Apaf-1 which binds to caspase 9 forming a trimer known as the apoptosome. Following cell damage, the heterodimer Apaf-1-caspase is released leading to sequential activation of other caspases. Structural proteins are digested, chromosomal DNA is degraded and the cell enters the death pathway. Bcl-2 homology domain 3 (BH3) containing proteins Bad, Bik, Bid and Bim also inhibit anti-apoptotic proteins. Bac and Bax oligomerize, resulting in the release of cytochrome c and second mitochondria-derived activator of caspase (SMAC).

Lack of cell survival signals such as growth hormones and cytokines, initiate activation of pro-apoptotic signals within the cell. Pro-apoptotic molecules like Bax, Puma and Noxa become activated and initiate the intrinsic pathway. These intracellular signals are also known as negative signals. Stimuli originating from within the cell due to DNA damage, oxidative stress or hypoxia lead to mitochondrial permeability with the opening of the mitochondrial permeability transition (MPT) pore and the release of cytochrome c, apoptosis inducing factor (AIF), SMAC and DIABLO (direct inhibitor of apoptosis (IAP) binding protein with low pI) into the cytoplasm. Activation of CTLs leads to the release of granzymes and perforins from intracellular granules. A similar release of granzymes occurs from NK, NKT and some TREG cells. Entry of granzymes into target cells through pores

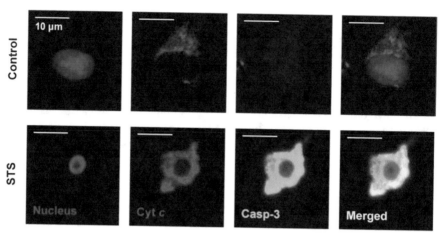

Fig. 8.2 Detection of mitochondrial outer membrane (OM) permeabilization in H1975 cancer cells treated with 1µM staurosporine (STS) for 12 h followed by immunofluorescence staining. Antibodies specific for Cyt *c* and active caspase-3 (Casp-3), as well counterstaining with Hoechst (which marks chromatin) were used to stain cells. In control cells (upper panels), Cyt c is detected in the intermembrane space (IMS). A "tubular" pattern of fluorescence was observed and caspase-3 was detected. STS-induced mitochondrial membrane permeabilization (lower panels), shows Cyt *c* released into the cytosol and observed as diffuse staining) where it leads to the activation of caspase-3. The pyknotic nucleus detected is characteristic of cells undergoing apoptosis. White scale bars represent 10 µm. [*Republished with permission of SpringerNature publishing from Galluzi, L., Zamzami, N., de La Motte Rouge, T., Lemaire, C., Brenner, C. and Kroemer, G. (2007), "Methods for the assessment of mitochondrial membrane permeabilization in apoptosis." Apoptosis, 12:803-813. Figure 1. Conveyed through STM permission guidelines 2014*]

formed by perforin or through endocytosis of surface bound granzymes results in cleavage of procaspase 3 and Bid. Caspase 3 induces the release of cytochrome c from mitochondria. Once in the cytoplasm, cytochrome c activates caspase 3 leading to the formation of the apoptosome. H1975 cancer cells treated with staurosporine (STS) to induce apoptosis and then processed for immunofluorescence using caspase-3 and cytochrome c specific antibodies show the distribution of both proteins within the cytoplasm and demonstrate permeabilization of the mitochondrial outer membrane (Fig. 8.2). Cytochrome c binds to the adapter protein apoptotic protease activating factor-1 (Apaf-1), deoxy ATP (dATP) and procaspase 9 to form the apoptosome. Procaspase 9 binds to the caspase recruitment domain (CARD domain) of Apaf-1 following a change in conformation of the CARD domain following reception of apoptotic signals. Cytochrome c binds to the WD domain of Apaf-1 monomers resulting in conformational changes that expose a nucleotide binding and oligmerization domain that binds to dATP. Deoxy ATP binding leads to the recruitment of several Apaf-1 molecules which together form the apoptosome complex. Conversion of procaspase 9 to active caspase 9 occurs within the apoptosome as the exposed CARD domains in the center of the apoptosome bind to procaspase 9. The activated caspase 9 cleaves procaspase 3 converting it to caspase 3. SMAC inhibits the activity of inhibitors of apoptosis proteins (IAPs) to prevent inhibition of caspase 9 activation. The executioner (effector) caspases become activated by caspase 9, resulting in cell death (Fig. 8.1).

Extrinsic Pathway

Binding of proteins in the tumor necrosis receptor (TNFR) family to their ligands, initiates cell signaling leading to cell death using the death receptor pathway. Fas ligand (FASL/CD95L) binding to the death receptor Fas (FAS/CD95) results in the recruitment of the Fas-associated protein with death domain (FADD), an adaptor protein. The death receptors (DR) belong to the tumor necrosis factor (TNF) super-family and include TNF receptor (TNFR). Binding of TNF to TNFR leads to the recruitment of the TNFR-associated death domain (TRADD). Procaspase 8 binds to FADD or TRADD and forms the death-inducing signaling complex (DISC). Procaspase 8 is activated by DISC to caspase 8, leading to activation of the execu-tioner caspases and resultant cell death. Several monomers of procaspase 8 are recruited to DISC where they become dimerized and activated. Both perforin and Fas-FasL systems are necessary for induction of apoptosis by CTLs. CTLs are pro-tected from damage and death by the apoptotic pathway through the expression of serpins. Proper regulation of apoptosis is essential for ensuring cell death in cells with pro-apoptotic signals and promoting cell survival in cells with anti-apoptotic signals (Fig. 8.3).

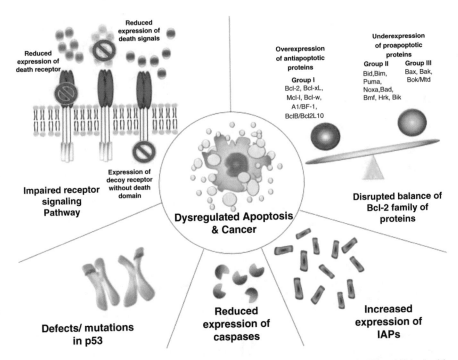

Fig. 8.3 Mechanisms contributing to evasion of apoptosis and carcinogenesis. [Republished with permission of SpringerNature publishing from Wong, R. S. Y. (2011) "Apoptosis in cancer: from pathogenesis to treatment." Journal of Experimental & Clinical Cancer Research, 30:87, Figure 2. Conveyed through STM permission guidelines 2014]

Selected References

1. D'Arcy MS (2019) Cell death: A review of the major forms of apoptosis, necrosis and autophagy. Cell Bio Int 43:582–592
2. Galluzi L, Zamzani N, de La Motte Rouge T, Lemaire C, Brenner C, Kroemer G (2007) Methods for the assessment of mitochondrial membrane permeabilization in apoptosis. Apoptosis 12:803–813
3. Murphy K, Weaver C (2017) Janeway's immunobiology, 9th edn. Garland Press, New York
4. Punt J, Stranford SA, Jones PP, Owen JA (2019) Kuby immunology, 8th edn. W.H. Freeman and Company, New York. Chapter 20, Antigen-antibody interactions
5. Wong RSY (2011) Apoptosis in cancer: from pathogenesis to treatment. J Exp Clin Cancer Res 30:87

Chapter 9
Antigens

An immune response is generated within the host as a result of exposure to or encounter with a pathogen (various microbes, viruses, parasites), or any *agent* that is recognized by host immune cells to be "different" or foreign to host tissue. The agent may be natural or synthetic or it may be altered host molecules unrecognizable to host immune cells as self. Collectively, the term used for pathogens, foreign macromolecules or altered host molecules is **antigen**. Exogenous (**extracellular**) **antigens** are found on and in invading pathogens found in blood or other tissue and also found on transplanted tissue (**alloantigens**). **Endogenous (intracellular) antigens** are found in pathogens invading host cells or antigens expressed by cancerous cells and **autoantigens** (self-antigens) are antigens on host cells that can be recognized by the immune system leading to autoimmunity. An antigen is also any substance, free in solution or membrane bound that is capable of inducing an immune response and interacting with the antigen binding site of an antibody molecule (B cell receptor) or T cell receptor. This type of antigen is called an **immunogen**. Antigens have properties that determine if they can stimulate a response and bind to products of the response. The antigenic properties also determine the type of response that will be generated. For example, an **allergen** will stimulate a hypersensitive reaction or allergic reaction while a **tolerogen** will induce a specific non response. **A hapten** is a small antigenic molecule that by itself cannot induce an immune response due to its small size but can combine with the antigen binding site of an antibody molecule or T cell receptor. Haptens are typically conjugated to large protein molecules known as carriers, for use in immunizations. The clinical importance of haptens is demonstrated by drug-induced hypersensitivities. For example, penicillin and naproxen acting as haptens, can bind to proteins on red blood cells and induce antibody formation. Antibody binding to the hapten forms circulating immune complexes or leads to hemolysis of red blood cells. Haptens can mediate antibody dependent and cellular hypersensitivities by binding to proteins in the body. The binding sites or binding pockets of the receptor molecules on B and T cells cannot accommodate the entire antigen but can bind to discrete amino acid sequences on the antigen. Those discrete sites are known as **antigenic**

© Springer Nature Switzerland AG 2021
T. Y. Sam-Yellowe, *Immunology: Overview and Laboratory Manual*,
https://doi.org/10.1007/978-3-030-64686-8_9

determinants or **epitopes**. Epitopes are the immunologically active regions of antigens. B and T lymphocytes recognize epitopes on antigens differently. However, both cell types must recognize the same antigen, in the context of their particular epitopes in order to stimulate a coordinated immune response. B lymphocytes can recognize conformational epitopes on surface antigens, discontinuous epitopes and hydrophilic molecules. T lymphocytes recognize internal peptides, linear epitopes and hydrophobic molecules.

There are molecules such as haptens that possess antigenic properties i.e. have the potential to induce an immune response, but by themselves cannot induce a response. When antibodies or T cell receptors interact with an antigen the binding typically takes place on the epitopes. B cells can recognize antigen directly using immunoglobulin receptors in association with accessory molecules on the cell membrane (B receptor complex). Following receptor binding the bound antigen is internalized leading to B cell activation and differentiation. T cells cannot recognize antigen directly.

Recognition and binding of antigen by the T cell receptor/CD3 complex is possible only when the antigen is presented by antigen presenting cells (APCs). The antigen is presented on the surface of APCs associated with major histocompatibility complex proteins. In order to fully understand antigens and antigenic properties we need to examine **immunological properties** of antigens. The properties listed below demonstrate how we will discuss antigens in the rest of the chapters.

Immunogenic: An immunogenic antigen is an immunogen that can induce a humoral (HI) or cell-mediated immune (CMI) response and combine with products of the response such as antibodies or T cell receptor (for CMI). Immunogenicity is not an intrinsic property of antigens.

Antigenic: An antigen that cannot by itself induce an immune response but can combine specifically with products of the immune response. An example of such a molecule is a hapten. Haptens are very small antigens possessing antigenic properties but by themselves cannot induce an immune response. They must be covalently attached to large protein carrier molecules in order to achieve immunogenicity.

Allerogenic: An antigen that induces an allergic response such as a type I or IgE-mediated hypersensitivity. Allergens activate TH2 cells.

Tolerogenic: An antigen that induces specific tolerance leading to a non-response of the immune system for humoral as well as cell-mediated immunity.

An immunogen is an antigen but an antigen is not an immunogen. In order to study antigens it has been necessary to make antibodies against different antigens and then to use the antibodies to define antigen properties. Haptens have been the most widely used antigens for this purpose. Karl Landsteiner pioneered several studies in this area. Haptens chemically coupled to carriers stimulate antibodies to epitopes on the carrier as well as antibodies to the hapten. Conclusions from Landsteiner's studies demonstrated the specificity of the immune system and the ability of the immune system to recognize diverse antigenic determinants. Various factors influence immunogenicity. These factors include, foreignness, molecular size, chemical heterogeneity, and degradability, genetic control of the immune response (MHC genes), route of antigen exposure and antigen inoculum or dosage. For example, the route of entry of a pathogen determines which lymphoid organs and which cell populations will contact antigen. The type of antigen will also determine which T helper subsets will be polarized to become effector cells for the antigen response. **Adjuvants** are also important in stimulating the immune response to achieve a strong immune response following administration of an antigen for **immunization.** Adjuvants prolong the retention of antigen at injection sites within **granulomas,** they increase the effective size of the antigen and adjuvants promote an influx of macrophages and lymphocytes to the site of injection. Examples of adjuvants include aluminum hydroxide and Freund's adjuvant.

Examples of Haptens and Carrier Proteins Used in Studies
Haptens:

Trinitrophenyl (TNP)
Benzene arsonate
Glucose (monomeric)
Lactose (oligomeric)
Pentalysine (oligomeric)
Dinitrophenyl (DNP)
Aminobenzene (aniline) derivatives

Carrier proteins:

Bovine gamma globulin (BGG) 150 kDa
Bovine serum albumin (BSA) 68 kDa
Hen egg lysozyme (HEL) 15 kDa
Ovalbumin (OVA) 44 kDa
Keyhole limpet (KHL)
hemocyanin (~8000 kDa)

The studies by Landsteiner involved a number of approaches. These included the use of equilibrium dialysis using pure hapten without carrier proteins, immunoprecipitation using hapten coupled to different non-cross reactive carriers and performing inhibition of precipitation with free hapten. Experiments using aminobenzene derivatives with a carboxyl group in the ortho, meta and para positions demonstrated the exquisite specificity of antibodies. The antigen binding sites on the antibodies could discriminate among the different haptens. The bulk and shape of the hapten and the overall configuration of the hapten was different and so antibodies did not cross react but were specific only to individual haptens. In experiments using aminobenzene with different substitutions in the para position (p-toluidine, p-chloroaminobenzene, p-nitroaminobenzene), the overall configuration of the hapten was kept the same and so antibodies raised against each hapten, cross reacted with other haptens. The slight structural difference achieved by substituting a chlorine for a methyl group still permitted the antibodies to recognize and bind the hapten.

Antigen Characteristics

Proteins typically make better immunogens. However carbohydrates, lipids and nucleic acids can also be immunogenic. We typically think of protein antigens as more immunogenic with nucleic acids being the least immunogenic as shown below.

Proteins > polysaccharides > lipids > nucleic acids

However, proteins complexed to polysaccharides (glycoproteins), lipids (lipoproteins) and nucleic acids (nucleoproteins) can be potent immunogens. Glycolipids can also induce strong immune responses. T cells can interact with antigens generated from any of the four macromolecules presented with MHC or CD1 molecules for lipid antigens. The immune system recognizes the macromolecular components of pathogens and infectious agents and responds through lymphocyte activation.

As we discuss antigens and epitopes, you may wonder what the size of an epitope is. Is there an upper or lower limit to the size of an epitope in antigens and the ability of the antigen to stimulate an immune response? Earlier experiments using saccharide units demonstrated that units of hexasaccharides and heptasaccharides saturated antigen binding sites suggesting that an epitope was about the size of 6–7 monomer sugar residues also equivalent to approximately 7 amino acid residues. Additional studies showed that an epitope could be the size of a small peptide containing as many as 5–15 amino acids. The structure of the antigenic determinants on carbohydrates depend on the sequence and linkage of monomer units and not on the conformation. What are the differences between B and T cell epitopes? Remember that the TCR and BCR bind to the epitopes on antigens. B cell epitopes can be conformational, with discontinuous amino acids, hydrophilic amino acids and easily accessible residues on the surface of cells. B cells are not MHC restricted and the BCR can bind to antigen directly. However, T cell epitopes are linear internal peptides, hydrophobic, having been processed within endosomes by antigen presenting cells for MHC class II presentation to TH cells or processed in proteasomes for MHC I presentation to Tc cells. T cells are MHC restricted. In response to an antigen, 10^9 different antibodies can be produced. Up to 10^7 clones of B and T cells each expressing unique BCRs and TCRs can be produced following cell activation as a result of antigen binding.

Mitogens are used in experimental studies to investigate lymphocyte activation and signaling. They are known as polyclonal activators and can induce cell division in B and T cells. Mitogens activate many clones of B and T cells independent of antigen specificity. Most of the common mitogens are lectins, proteins derived from plants. Lectins bind to membrane glycoproteins on cell surfaces leading to agglutination or clustering of cell surface receptors. This leads to cell activation. Concanavalin A (Con A) is mitogenic for T cells and lipopolysaccharide (LPS) is mitogenic for mouse B cells. Mitogens along with phorbol esters are used in studies of cell division, activation and signaling. Phorbol esters are not mitogens in the strict sense. However, they activate cells by activating protein kinase C (PKC) and are used in T cell activation studies alone or with the calcium ionophore, ionomycin to understand the cell signaling mediated by antigen binding to the TCR Superantigens are potent T cell mitogens. They bind to the V beta domain of the T cell receptor and to other molecules outside the antigen binding pocket. Cross-linking of the receptor in an antigen independent manner leads to activation of the T cell, resulting in excess cytokine gene expression and secretion. Staphylococcal enterotoxins (SES) and Toxic shock syndrome toxin 1 are examples of superantigens.

The B cell receptor (BCR), T cell receptor (TCR) and major histocompatibility (MHC) antigens are all products of a family of ancestrally related genes whose products bind antigens. This family is the immunoglobulin superfamily. The proteins are organized into domains of approximately 100 amino acids typically encoded by a single exon with one intradomain disulfide bond. Each domain assumes a secondary conformation of anti-parallel strands forming beta pleated sheets. Antigen sources vary and can include cell surface, membrane, excreted and secreted antigens of pathogens. Secreted antigens can comprise exotoxins, superantigens and allergens, particularly from helminth parasites. Other antigens are histocompatibility proteins, cluster of differentiation antigens, autoantigens, alloantigens and blood group antigens which are naturally occurring antigens from commensal bacterial in the human GI tract. Immune response to pathogens and mechanisms of immune response include cellular recognition of pathogen, antigen processing and presentation. There are generally six groups of pathogens that cause infectious diseases. These include viruses, bacteria, protozoa, helminths, fungi and prions. In order for a pathogen to establish an infection within a host, the barriers providing innate protection have to be breached. The pathogen may escape immune recognition by host cells due to its intracellular location, such that infection within host cells lead to sequestration of the pathogen from immune cells. Membrane antigens may be shed or the pathogen may be covered by host or parasite derived molecules that mimic those of the host. Pathogens can also suppress the host immune response selectively or have surface antigens that continually vary resulting in antigenic variation. Accumulated point mutations as a result of **single nucleotide polymorphisms (SNPs)**, nucleotide sequence deletions, insertion or transpositions, genetic diversity or large changes in genes leading to changes in expressed surface antigens can result in the generation of antigenic variants leading to changes in the virulence of pathogens. Both innate and adaptive immune responses are made in response to antigens from pathogens. Depending on the pathogen, life cycle stages of the pathogen and the site of infection, innate or adaptive responses may predominate.

Antigenic variation: This is a process used by infectious disease organisms (parasites, viruses, bacteria) to evade products of the immune system. It is caused by either minor or major changes in amino acid sequences of the antigen. Antigenic variation in influenza virus results in changes in the hemagglutinin (H) and neuraminidase (N) glycoproteins found in the viral envelope. Two major types of variation occur, known as **antigenic drift** and **antigenic shift**. In antigenic drift minor amino acid changes due to point mutations in the genes and in antigenic shift major amino acid changes that may be due to gene recombination can lead to antigenic variation because new antigenic epitopes are created. A few of the predominant antigens found in different pathogen groups are discussed below. Immune responses to different pathogen groups will also be examined. Important bacterial antigens are found in the cell wall (O antigens), flagella (H antigens) and capsule (K antigens). Lipopolysaccharide (LPS) from gram negative bacteria induces strong immune responses and also possesses mitogenic properties for mouse B lymphocytes. The O and K antigens are useful in serotyping bacteria. Viral antigens include capsid antigens, spike proteins, newly synthesized viral proteins and nucleoproteins. Viral proteins from influenza virus stimulate protective cell mediated immunity. Parasite antigens elicit immune responses following extracellular and intracellular infections from protozoan and helminth parasites. Different life cycle stages of parasites including trophozoites, cysts, eggs (ova) and adult parasite stages, induce stage specific immune responses. Parasite antigen sources include surface coat proteins, tegument proteins, flagella and newly synthesized proteins. Fungal antigens include both yeast and hyphal antigens. Spore antigens may also induce immune responses. Innate immunity is made to fungal antigens. New or altered antigens appear on the surface of tumor cells resulting in an antigenically different cell. Developmental antigens may be expressed on mature cells such as carcinoembryonic antigen (CEA). These are known as tumor associated antigens (TAAs). Unique antigens expressed by tumor cells, that are used as marker antigens for the tumor are known as tumor specific antigens (TSAs) virus-related antigens or antigens found normally on other cells.

Immunity to Bacteria

The immune response to bacteria depends on whether the infection is extracellular or intracellular. The immune response is also determined by whether the bacteria are gram positive, gram negative or gram variable as observed with Mycobacteria which are acid-fast. Antibody responses are most effective for extracellular infections because organisms can be neutralized by the antibodies. Cell-mediated immunity, specifically delayed-type hypersensitivity is most effective for intracellular organisms. TH1 cells possessing DTH effector functions secrete IFNγ which can activate macrophages to carry out more effective killing of bacterial pathogens. TH1 cells can also assist cytotoxic T lymphocytes in targeting and killing intracellular infected host cells. Antibody-mediated activation of the complement system can also induce localized production of immune effector molecules that can generate an enhanced inflammatory response. Complement split products such as C3a and C5a, acting as anaphylatoxins can induce local mast cell degranulation which leads to vasodilation and extravasation of lymphocytes or the products may be chemotactic and lead to infiltration of neutrophils causing an accumulation of phagocytic cells at the site. Bacteria may secrete toxins that can stimulate antibody production (immunogenic toxins). **Endotoxin** or LPS is a component of the cell wall of gram negative bacteria. Exotoxins are proteinaceous molecules secreted by bacteria that can also induce strong humoral immunity. If the pathogen secretes a toxin, this may be neutralized by antibody and the immune complex formed cleared by phagocytic cells.

Immunity to Viruses

Innate immune response to virus infection occurs following interaction of virus nucleic acids with PRRs in the cytoplasm and within endosomes. Dendritic cells secrete IL-12 which mediates natural killer cell cytotoxicity targeting virus infected cells. Type I interferons (IFNα and IFNβ) are produced following signal transduction through PRR signaling pathways leading the blocking of virus replication. Interaction of type I interferons with specific receptors leads to expression of nucleic acid degrading enzymes such as RNases, the formation of inflammasomes, IL-12 activation of natural killer cell cytotoxicity. Humoral immunity is generally effective against viral infection. On mucosal surfaces secretory IgA is produced and blocks viral attachment to mucosal epithelial cells. Immunoglobulin M and IgG antibody isotypes are produced against virus proteins. The antibodies can neutralize virus particles and also enhance opsonization and agglutination of viruses. Antibodies specific for virus receptor molecules can block fusion to host cell membranes and check the spread of virus during acute infection. Influenza virus binds sialic acids on glycoproteins expressed on host cell membranes, Epstein-Barr virus binds to complement receptor 2 (CR2) on B cells, SARS-Cov-2 virus spike protein binds to human angiotensin-converting enzyme 2 (ACE2) and rhinovirus bind to intracellular adhesion molecules (ICAMs). Antibodies against surface receptor molecules can effectively neutralize or agglutinate virions and prevent or block binding of virus particles to the host cell. The antibody may also function as an opsonin thus mediating Fc or C3b mediated virus phagocytosis. The antibody may activate the complement pathway leading to lysis of the virus infected cell. Once infection by the virus is established, cell-mediated immune responses become a more effective way of eliminating the infection. CD8⁺ Tc cells and CD4⁺TH1 cells mediate antiviral defense. IL-2 and IFNγ produced by TH1 cells enhance NK cell and CTL activation.

Immunity to Fungi

Fungi are eukaryotic organisms that can cause infections ranging from superficial cutaneous infection to systemic deep mycoses that can be fatal. The site of infection determines the type of immune responses generated. Three sites of fungal infection are cutaneous, subcutaneous and deep mycosis. In deep mycoses, fungi are transmitted by inhalation, ingestion and entry of fungi into the blood stream. Infection in the lungs, central nervous system and bones can lead to deep mycosis and systemic infection. Ringworm infections of the skin, hair and nails make up cutaneous infections caused by fungi. Exposure to molds of *Aspergillus, Fusarium* and *Mucor* species can lead to opportunistic infections. Infections by *Cryptococcus neoformans* and *Histoplasma capsulatum* can lead to serious infection. Encapsulated *C. neoformans* can evade immune attack due to the capsule. Innate immune responses control most fungal infections. PRRs on host cells recognize PAMPs on fungi leading to their elimination. Breaches of barriers in the skin and mucosal areas of the body can lead to infections by fungi. Dysbiosis in the host microbiota can lead to reduction in commensal bacteria populations that control pathogens, including fungi, leading to overgrowth of *Candida albicans*. Immunosupressed hosts due to HIV infection, drug therapy or neutropenia are predisposed to fungal infections. COVID-19 patients have also been reported to have fungal infections such as mucormycosis and aspergillosis. Cell wall components of fungi are recognized by dectin-1 a C-type lectin receptor leading to cell signaling that results in proinflammatory cytokine secretion. Beta-glucan binding to Dectin-1activates the spleen tyrosine kinase pathway (Syk) resulting in NFκB activation. Syk activation also produces NFAT in a calcium dependent pathway. Proinflammatory cytokines and chemokines are secreted as a result of Dectin-fungal PAMP binding. Important PAMPs on fungi include β-glucans, mannans and chitin composed of N-acetylglucosamine. Toll-like receptors 2, 4 and 6 bind fungal PAMPs. Fungal cell wall components also fix complement. TH cells binding to fungal antigens presented on MHC class II proteins and B cells become activated and secrete antibodies. TH1 cells are associated with mild infections compared to TH2 which involve humoral immunity and severe disease. TH17 cells play a regulatory role. However, deficiencies in RORγt affect IL-17 secretion and protection against fungal infections.

Selected References

Landsteiner K (1962) The specificity of serological reactions. Dover Publications, New York

Murphy K, Weaver C (2017) Janeway's immunobiology, 9th edn. Garland Press, New York

Punt J, Stranford SA, Jones PP, Owen JA (2019) Kuby immunology, 8th edn. W.H. Freeman and Company, New York. Chapter 20, Antigen-antibody interactions

Roberts LS, Janovy J Jr, Nadler S (2013) Gerals D. Schmidt & Larry S. Robert's foundations of parasitology, 9th edn. McGraw Hill, New York

Song G, Liang G, Liu W (2020) Fungal co-infections associated with Global COVID-19 Pandemic: A clinical and diagnostic perspective from China. https://doi.org/10.1007/s11046-020-00462-9

Underhill DM, Perlman E (2015) Immune interactions with pathogenic and commensal fungi: A two-way street. Immunity 43:845–858

Chapter 10
B Cell Development, Activation and Immunoglobulin Structure

B Cell Development

Antibody production is the hallmark of humoral immunity in the adaptive immune responses. B lymphocytes produce antibodies (immunoglobulins) specific to antigens. B cell development occurs in the bone marrow. Unlike T cells which develop and mature mostly in the thymus, B cells begin development in the bone marrow and begin expression of immunoglobulin (Ig) and expression of B cell surface markers in the bone marrow. In this chapter, we will highlight the features that distinguish B cells from T cells and discuss the markers that define developmental stages of B lymphocytes and allow for the cells to be isolated and studied. A major event that occurs during B cell development is the generation of the variable region of the antibody molecule in the genes that encode the heavy and light chain polypeptides. The antigen binding regions of the antibody molecule are found in the variable regions in the heavy and light chains. Three germ-line genes recombine and rearrange to form the variable region. The heavy (H) chain gene is composed of V (variable), D (diversity) and J (joining) genes. The light (L) chain gene is composed of V and J genes. B lymphocytes differentiate from the common lymphoid progenitor (CLP), with the transcription factors Ikaros, purine box factor 1 (PU.1), early B cell factor-1 (EBF-1) and E2A driving B cell commitment into the B cell lineage. Maturation of the B cell continues following migration and homing of the B cells into secondary lymphoid organs. B cells exhibiting autoreactivity are deleted and negatively selected like the T cells in the thymic medulla, resulting in central tolerance within the bone marrow. Following rearrangement of Ig, autoreactivity is further prevented by receptor-editing of Ig and B cell anergy. B lymphocytes transition through pre-pro, pro and pre B cell stages. Each stage is marked by expression of specific molecules that define the developmental stage.

B cell development progresses through the pre-pro B stage with the expression of B220+, EBF1 without Ig VDJ rearrangement. Next is the early pro B stage where rearrangement of DJH occurs and progresses to the late pro B stage and VDJ

© Springer Nature Switzerland AG 2021
T. Y. Sam-Yellowe, *Immunology: Overview and Laboratory Manual*,
https://doi.org/10.1007/978-3-030-64686-8_10

rearrangement to form the pre B cell receptor (preBCR). Under the influence of the Pax5 transcription factor, VDJ recombination takes place along with CD19 and Ig alpha/Ig beta expression. Large preB cells differentiating from late proB cells express CD25 and IL-2R and decrease expression of preBCR as they differentiate to small preB cells. The preB cell receptor is formed during the preB cell stage. The heavy (H) chain combines with VpreB and lambda 5 (surrogate light chain, SLC). Light chain gene rearrangement occurs in the small preB cell stage and as immature B cells develop, IgM expression takes place. The immature B cells express IgM, B220$^+$, CD25$^+$, IL-7R$^+$, Ig alpha/Ig beta and CD19. As the B cell migrates to secondary lymphoid organs, transitional stages of B cells expressing different gene products and responding to different signaling molecules can be identified. The cells enter the secondary lymphoid organs as transitional (T) stages T1 and T2 and complete maturation within the secondary organs. Transitional stage 3 (T3) cells have been described and express CD93$^+$, mIgD^{high}, mIgM^{low} and CD23$^+$. B cells are categorized as B-1, B-2 and MZ (marginal zone) cells.

B-1 cells further categorized as B-1a and B-1b cells, bind self-antigens and are thought to be derived from a different developmental lineage. They are self-renewing cells with limited diversity for antigen binding and bind to carbohydrate antigens. In mouse studies, B-1 progenitor cells were detected in fetal liver of mice that were unable to produce hematopoietic stem cells (HSC). The mice lacked B-2 cells.

B-2 cells enter lymphoid follicles and organs and respond to antigen with T cell help. They depend on IL-7, BAFF, are highly diverse in antigen recognition, express high levels of IgM/IgD, and undergo class switching and somatic hypermutation (SHM). B-2 cells recirculate between blood and secondary lymphoid organs, produce antibodies and have a half-life of 4–5 months in the periphery. MZ B cells are located in the white pulp of the spleen and are important for recognizing blood borne antigens. MZ B cells can recognize both protein and carbohydrate antigens.

Antibodies

Immunoglobulins (Ig) also known as antibodies, are serum glycoproteins that are secreted from plasma cells and found in serum or membrane bound on B cells. In serum, immunoglobulins are associated with the gamma globulin fraction of serum. Following immunization, antiserum subjected to electrophoresis shows a highly elevated gamma globulin peak. Incubation of the antiserum with specific antigen and evaluation of the serum by electrophoresis following removal of the immune complex results in a diminished gamma globulin peak. Initial studies looking at antibody structure involved the use of myeloma proteins (**Bence Jones Proteins**), homologous immunoglobulin light chains secreted in urine.

Most studies employing antibodies for antigen detection use polyclonal or monoclonal antibodies. An antibody is a globular serum glycoprotein with a defined specificity for an epitope at the antigen binding site of the molecule made up of constant and variable domains of the heavy and light chains. Antibodies are secreted only by differentiated B cells i.e. plasma cells. Five antibody classes or isotypes are secreted by plasma cells (IgM, IgG, IgE, IgA, IgD). B lymphocytes interact with antigen by using the B cell receptor complex (BCR). The mIg is generated as a result of gene rearrangements. The B cell receptor complex consists of mIg associated with a heterodimeric alpha/beta chain (Ig alpha, a product of the mb-1 gene and Ig beta, a product of the B29 gene). The cytoplasmic tails of both molecules are sufficiently long to facilitate signal transduction through the phosphorylation of ITAM domains within the tails. The BCR is found only on B lymphocytes, it is not class specific and all mIgs are associated with the same heterodimeric signaling complex.

B Cell Activation

Antigen binding to the membrane Ig (mIg) receptor on the surface of B cells leads to cell signaling and gene transcription within the cell that results in a variety of effects that include, actin-cytoskeletal reorganization, inhibition of apoptosis, cell survival, cytokine and cytokine receptor expression, antigen presentation to T helper cells and differentiation to **antibody secreting plasma cells (antibody forming cells, AFCs)**. In addition to mIg, coreceptor molecules that make up the B cell receptor complex include the Igα/Igβ (CD79a/CD79b) heterodimer, CD19, CD21 (CR2) and CD81 (TAPA-1) (Fig. 10.1). Following antigen binding to mIg, coreceptor proteins and membrane associated enzymes cluster within lipid rafts. The src family kinases, Lyn and Fyn become activated by phosphatases in the lipid rafts. Lyn becomes activated by autophosphorylation and then phosphorylates the ITAMs on the Igα/Igβ coreceptors and CD19 in the BCR complex. Antigen bound to the Ig molecule may also be bound to the complement protein C3d on CD21. Recruitment of Syk, Tec family kinases and the adaptor molecule BLNK follows as attachment sites for the SH2 motifs on BLNK become exposed. B-cell linker protein (BLNK) and B-cell adapter protein (BCAP) are phosphorylated by Syk following its autophosphorylation and activation. Phosphorylation of BLNK and BCAP leads to recruitment of Bruton's tyrosine kinase (Btk) and phospholipase Cγ2 (PLCγ2), which become activated by phosphorylation. Vav is recruited to the adaptor BLNK followed by binding to the small GTPases Rho, Rac and Cdc42. Phosphatidylinositol 3-kinase (PI3 kinase) is recruited to the membrane. The production of phosphatidylinositol triphosphate (PIP3) and the recruitment and activation of PDK1 and AKt to the membrane follows, resulting in the inactivation of Bax and Bad and inhibition of apoptosis. PLCγ2 cleaves phosphatidlylinositol bisphosphate (PIP2) to generate inositol triphosphate (IP3) and diacylglycerol (DAG). Calcium release from intracellular stores is mediated by IP3 followed by calcium binding to calmodulin, leading to the dephosphorylation of the transcription factor NFAT by calcineurin and NFAT translocation into the nucleus. The MAP kinase pathway is activated following DAG interaction with PKC and Ras-GRP resulting in the activation of the transcription factors Elk-1, Erg-1, CREB (cAMP response element binding protein) and Jun. The transcription factors influence transcription and gene expression of

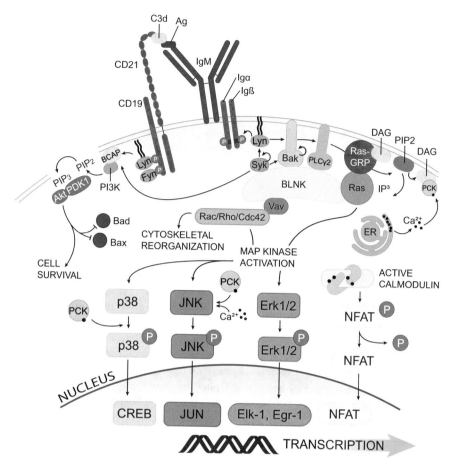

Fig. 10.1 B lymphocyte activation. Antigen binding to membrane immunoglobulin (Ig) leads to phosphorylation of Igα/Igβ and CD19 by Lyn, followed by recruitment and activation of Syk and Btk (signalosome) through phosphorylation. Following phosphorylation of the adaptor proteins BLNK and BCAP, phosphatidylinositol 3-kinase is recruited to BCAP and Vav to BLNK resulting in PIP3 formation and MAP kinase activation, respectively. The guanine nucleotide exchange factor Vav mediates cytoskeletal reorganization. PLCγ2 recruited to BLNK is activated by Syk-mediated phosphorylation leading to the cleavage of phosphatidylinositol bisphosphate (PIP2) and generation of diacylglycerol (DAG) and inositol triphosphate (IP3). The MAP kinase pathway becomes activated once DAG binds to the GTP exchange factor RasGRP and PKC enhanced by IP3-mediated release of calcium from calcium stores. The transition factors cyclic-AMP responsive element binding protein (CREB), Jun, Ets-like-1 (Elk1), early growth response 1 (Egr1) and nuclear factor of activated T cells (NFAT) become activated and translocate into the nucleus. Elk1 and Egr1 are activated down-stream of extracellular signal-regulated kinase1/2. PDK1 and Akt localize to the membrane, activated Akt phosphorylates and inactivates Bax and Bad resulting in inhibition of apoptosis and enhancement of cell survival

cytokines, cytokine receptors, chemokines, chemokine receptors, antibodies and other growth factors required for B cell survival and memory B cell production. In the next section we will discuss the antibody structure and examine the features used for antigen interaction.

Antibody Structure

The antibody structure consists of 2 heavy and 2 light chain polypeptides. The light (L) chain in combination with the N-terminus of the heavy (H) chain form the antigen binding site. The constant light chain domains can be either kappa (κ) or lambda (λ) on a single antibody molecule. A naturally synthesized single antibody molecule cannot have both types of light chains on one molecule. The constant region of the H chain defines the **isotype** or **class** of the antibody. The domain that is responsible for biological activity, known as the **Fc**, is contained in the C-terminus of the H chain. The antigen binding site is formed by a combination of the variable regions in both H and L chains known as the **Fab** region (fragment of antigen binding) (Fig. 10.2).The isotypes denoted by Greek letters indicate individual antibody

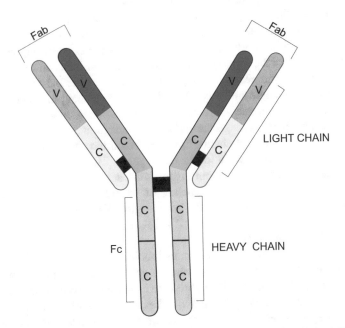

Fig. 10.2 Antibody structure consisting of 2 heavy (H) chains (blue/green) and 2 light chains (orange/yellow). Both H and L chains contain variable (V) regions in the amino terminus and constant (C) regions in the carboxyl terminus of the antibody molecule. Carbohydrate molecules are associated with the H chain constant region (not shown) at the second C domain (CH2) of the H chain. The antigen binding domain of the antibody molecule is composed of the VL and VH regions known as the Fab fragment. The constant region of the H chain is known as the Fc region and is important for binding to Fc receptors on cells expressing the Fc receptor

isotypes. The designations are alpha (α) for IgA, delta (δ) for IgD, epsilon (ε) for IgE, gamma (γ) for IgG and mu (μ) for IgM. The formula for a typical IgG molecule is designated $\gamma 2\lambda 2$ or $\gamma 2\kappa 2$. Each H chain has a variable (V) region and a constant (C) region separated into 3–4 domains. Each light chain has a variable region and a constant region. The variable region is in the N terminus of the polypeptide chain in both H and L chains. Variable regions contain amino acid residues that differ or vary among antibody molecules within the same individual and between different individuals. **Hypervariable regions** within V regions make up the antigen combining regions. Amino acid variation is highest in this region. The **VH** region makes an important contribution to epitope contact with the antibody molecule. **Framework regions** contain less variable amino acid sequences on either side (flanking) of the hypervariable regions. Constant regions contain amino acids that do not vary but remain the same among antibodies within the same individual or between two different individuals.

Within the variable region are domains that are referred to as **"hot spots"** or **hypervariable regions**. These regions are also known as **complementarity determining regions (CDRs)**. The epitope combines with the CDR. There are six CDRs per antibody molecule (3 on the H chain and 3 on the L chain). A minimum of 4 CDRs mostly from the variable H chain make contact with the epitope on the antigen. The less variable regions of the framework regions act as scaffolding and generate beta pleated sheets important in maintaining the overall conformation of the region. Genes encoding the variable region and constant region are expressed and combined to form the mature antibody molecule. The genes encoding the variable and constant regions of the antibody molecule are present in embryonic DNA. During B cell development, the genes rearrange to produce the variable region. Proteins combining to form a single antibody molecule comprise 2 heavy chain polypeptides and 2 light chain polypeptides. Structurally, the variable region genes are different from the constant region genes, ensuring that antigen binding will occur in the variable region of heavy and light chains. Epitope recognition appears to be the driving force behind the structural evolution of the V genes. The primary, secondary, tertiary and quaternary levels of protein organization determines the final form of an antibody molecule. The compact structure of an antibody is formed by folded immunoglobulin domains known as the immunoglobulin fold. The secondary structure consists of anti-parallel beta plated sheets stabilized by disulfide bonds, H bonds and hydrophobic interactions.

Initial studies to determine the immunoglobulin structure was performed using Bence Jones Proteins. These proteins were the sole source of homogeneous immunoglobulins at the time. In 1975 the hybridoma technology was described by Kohler and Milstein. Since then monoclonal antibodies have been used to investigate antibody structure. Non-covalent interactions between domains occur between identical domains e.g. CH2/CH2, CH3/CH3 and CH4/CH4. Non-identical interactions occur between VH/VL and CH1/CL. The variable regions consist of the VH/Vλ and VH/ Vκ. Hypervariable regions occur in the variable domains with three regions in the VH/VL chain. CH1/CL also contributes to diversity of the variable region. In experiments where the variable regions of one antibody (Ab A) were mixed with variable regions from a second antibody (Ab B), homogeneous complexes were obtained with variable regions VH and VL from Ab A, combined. Similarly, VH and VL from Ab B combined. When the experiment was repeated with the inclusion of the constant chains, both homogeneous and heterogeneous complexes were obtained. Variability plots established the presence of hypervariable regions in the H and L chains of the Ab. The heavy chain (VH) provides important contributions to epitope contact. Framework regions (FR) are found in the variable domains but contain less variable sequences flanking hypervariable regions. The CH1/CL domains stabilize VH/VL interactions. A hinge region is present in γ, δ, α between CHI and CH2. For ε and μ there is no hinge, just the CH2 domain and an extra CH4 domain after the CH3 domain. The Fc region on the H chain is responsible for binding to self-molecules. The self-molecules represent the receptors on host cells. The Fc region possesses the biologic and physiologic properties of the Ab molecule.

As we discussed earlier, many early studies to investigate antibody function and antigen properties utilized haptens as the antigen. The small size of the haptens enables them to fit into grooves and pockets created by the VH and VL domains. However, large proteins cannot fit into pockets and grooves and so extend onto the surface of the antibody such that an epitope on a large antigen (one larger than the antibody) or an antigen with similar size to the antibody molecule can still bind to the Fab regions. In this type of binding, amino acid sequences comprising the framework regions may also become involved in the binding. Each antibody molecule has a different shape in the Fab fragment to accommodate the variety of antigen epitopes that the immune system will come in contact with.

Subisotypes exist for the H chain and are the result of gene duplications denoting more recent events in evolution. When subisotype sequences are compared, the H chain subisotyes showed a greater sequence similarity. Affinity labeling experiments were performed to show the differences in how large and small (haptens) proteins bind within the CDR. The experiments showed that a minimum of 4 CDRs (most from VH chain) make contact with the epitope. The presence of specific antibodies against immunoglobulins and the availability of amino acid sequences led to the identification of serological characteristics in the antibodies. The antibody molecules possess antigenic determinants that can be identified serologically. These became identified as **allotypic, isotypic** and **idiotypic** differences. **Isotypic determinants** are found in all individuals at the CH 1–4 and CL domains, found across species. Species-specific antisera can be prepared against a specific isotype. The antisera are useful in identifying the specific isotype. Antibody conjugates prepared using this type of antisera, have a central role in numerous immunoassays performed in the laboratory. **Allotypic determinants** are found in some individuals, differences are due to polymorphisms leading to variations in the alleles (allotypic variation is also known as allelic variation) for the isotype genes. Allelic variations refer to polymorphisms. There are minor variations of 3–6 amino acids among antibody molecules of the same isotype within a species. Variants are found among racial groups. Allotypic determinants used to be employed in forensics but the variations are not as clear as using DNA. **Idiotypic determinants** are found in all individuals.

These determinants are found in the antigen binding domains. These are the determinants of the variable region. This correlates with antigen binding specificity. The idiotope is antigenic and anti-idiotype antibodies are made against the antibodies within an individual. The idiotope is the antigenic determinant of the variable region. These differences are found in all individuals but correlate with the antibody binding specificity.

Antibodies can recognize a vast diversity of antigens, either natural or synthetic. Diversity of the antibody molecule contributed by the antigen binding domain is a result of several features which function in combination to produce a unique antibody molecule. Some examples of features contributing to diversity include, antibody gene recombination, different variable and constant regions of the H and L chains, multiple gene families for the H and L chains, random joining of the H and L chains and the use of identical V regions for different isotypes. Studies performed using enzymes and reducing agents led to the determination of the antibody structure. Incubation of IgG with papain generated 2 Fab fragments of 45 kDa each and 1 Fc fragment of 50 kDa. These studies were performed by Rodney Porter. In the studies by Alfred Nisonoff, IgG was incubated with pepsin resulting in the cleavage and generation of 1 F(ab')2 fragment of 100 kDa plus small fragments of the Fc region. The presence of interdisufide bonding between the H and L chains of the antibody molecule was demonstrated by Gerald Edelman in studies using 2-mercaptoethanol treatment of IgG. 2-mercaptoethanol disrupted the disulfide bonds generating 2 H chain molecules migrating electrophoretically at 50 kDa and 2 L chain molecules at 25 kDa.

Selected References

Cyster JG, Allen CDC (2019) B cell responses: Cell interaction dynamics and decisions. Cell 177:524–540

Edelman GM, Cunningham BA, Gall WE, Gottlieb PD, Rutishauser U, Waxdal MJ (1969) The covalent structure of an entire gammaG immunoglobulin molecule. Proc Natl Acad Sci U S A 63:78–85

Gearhart P (2002) The roots of antibody diversity. Nature 419:29–31

Heesters BA, van der Poel CE, Das A, Carroll MC (2016) Antigen presentation to B cells. Trends Immunol 37:844–854

Kohler G, Milstein C (1975) Continuous cultures of fused cells secreting antibody of predefined specificity. Nature 7:495–497

Murphy K, Weaver C (2017) Janeway's immunobiology, 9th edn. Garland Press, New York

Nisonoff A, Wissler FC, Lipman LN (1960) Properties of the major component of a part of a peptic digest of rabbit antibody. Science 132:1770–1771

Porter RR (1973) Structural studies of immunoglobuins. Science 180:713–716

Punt J, Stranford SA, Jones PP, Owen JA (2019) Kuby immunology, 8th edn. W.H. Freeman and Company, New York. Chapter 20, Antigen-antibody interactions

Treanor B (2012) B-cell receptor: From resting state to activate. Immunology 136:21–27

Yang J, Reth M (2016) Receptor dissociation and B cell activation. Curr Top Microbiol. Immunol 393:27–43

Yoshikawa K et al (2002) AID enzyme-induced hypermutation in an activelytranscribed gene in fibroblasts. Science 296:2033–2036

Chapter 11
Immunoglobulin and T Cell Receptor Gene Rearrangements

The antigen binding receptor molecules on B and T lymphocytes are synthesized and expressed on the surface of the cells during development in the bone marrow for B cells and in the thymus for T cells. The genes encoding the B cell receptor and T cell receptor undergo rearrangements and recombination with the aid of lineage specific recombinases which together with DNA repair enzymes facilitate the recombination of the variable genes of heavy and light chain genes of BCR and TCR. RAG (recombination activating genes)-1 and -2 encode recombinases that initiate recombination and rearrangements of the immunoglobulin (Ig) in B cells and T cell receptor (TCR) in T cells. A deficiency of RAG-1 and RAG-2 genes leads to severe combined immunodeficiency (SCID), with no mature B and T cells in the periphery. Missence mutations in the RAG genes can lead to Omenn syndrome with no B lymphocytes and severe reduction in T lymphocyte populations. The heavy (H) and light (L) chain genes for immunoglobulins are located on different chromosomes. The H chain genes are located on chromosome 14 in humans and chromosome 12 in mice. The kappa gene in humans is on chromosome 2 and in mice on chromosome 6. The lambda gene in humans is on chromosome 22 and in mice on chromosome 16. Rearrangements of the variable genes in H and L chains occurs in B and T lymphocytes to generate receptors that can bind to diverse antigens leading to adaptive immune responses. Receptor specificity is important for antigen recognition and reactivity. In addition to multiple variable genes available for recombination and nucleotide additions that generate new binding sites for epitopes on antigens, only one H chain and one L chain bind to form an Ig. The process of allelic exclusion ensures antibody specificity by having only one H and L chain synthesized. In B cells following H chain recombination, a surrogate light chain is synthesized and combines with the H chain, followed by L chain recombination and the expression of a mature Ig molecule. Human Ig molecules contain more V lambda genes in the L chain than mouse Ig. Up to 40% of the L chain variable genes are lambda compared to 5% in mice. How is variable gene diversity obtained in the antigen binding receptors of B and T cells? We will discuss the mechanisms involved below. It will be important to note that the mechanisms are very similar in both cell

© Springer Nature Switzerland AG 2021
T. Y. Sam-Yellowe, *Immunology: Overview and Laboratory Manual*,
https://doi.org/10.1007/978-3-030-64686-8_11

types with the use of the same recombinases and recombination rules. Differences unique to T and B cells will be highlighted. The mechanisms for Ig recombination will be examined first.

General Mechanisms of Rearrangements in B and T Cell Antigen Receptor Genes

Variable (V), diversity (D) and joining (J) genes are required to generate the H chain variable region (Fig. 11.1). The process of recombination involves B and T cell specific proteins as well as non B and T lymphocyte specific proteins involved in nonhomologous end-joining (NHEJ) DNA repair mechanisms. For the light chain, V and J genes are required (Fig. 11.2). Recombination signal sequences (RSSs) flank each Ig gene fragment. Each RSS has conserved nonamer (nine) and heptamer (seven) sequences. In between nonamer-heptamer sequences are 12 or 23 bp spacer sequences. 12 bp RSSs pair with 23 bp RSS for recombination. This is known as the 12/23 joining rule. Heavy chain genes are recombined and expressed first. Products of RAG1/RAG2 genes initiate the recombination of Ig by binding to the RSSs and cleaving DNA. Epigenetic modifications on histones affects DNA access by RAG1/

ANTIBODY HEAVY CHAIN VARIABLE REGION REARRANGEMENT

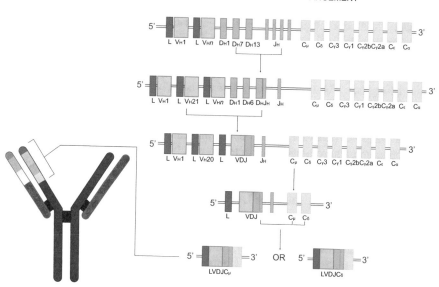

Fig. 11.1 Germline organization and rearrangement of the antibody H chain gene. From multiple V (D) J genes, recombination and rearrangements take place in H chain gene to generate the variable region for antigen binding. The V regions are combined with constant region genes to encode the full H chain

ANTIBODY LIGHT CHAIN VARIABLE REGION REARRANGEMENT

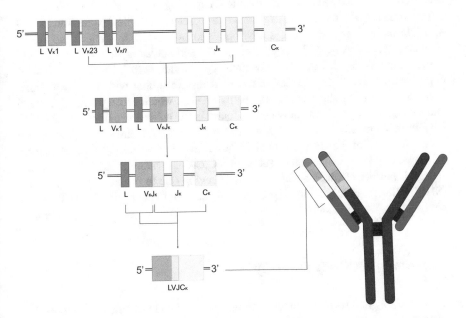

Fig. 11.2 Germline organization and rearrangement of the antibody L chain gene. From multiple VJ genes, recombination and rearrangements take place in L chain gene to generate the variable region for antigen binding. The V regions are combined with constant region genes to encode the full L chain. Antibody molecules can have either a κ or λ L chain combined with the H chain

RAG2 combined with HMGB1/2 which provides stability of the DNA for cleavage. RAG1/RAG2 cleaves DNA at the 5′ border of heptamers flanking V and J gene segments. A hairpin loop forms between non-coding strands of V and J segments forming coding and signal joints. Cleavage of the hairpin loop results in a recombined coding joint and a signal joint. The signal joint will either be excised or degraded. The signal end joins ends of heptamer RSS sequences remaining from the original V, J coding sequences. The hairpin loop is cleaved by Artemis, generating 3′or 5′ overhangs or a blunt end. The DNA binding proteins Ku70/80 at the DNA double strand breaks enable DNA-PKcs to bind to the DNA hairpin ends. DNA-PKc is an NHEJ kinase required for the activation of Artemis. Cleavage of the hairpin generates sites for complementary nucleotide addition during repair by DNA repair enzymes. Nucleotide additions added to palindromic sequences are known as P-additions. Nucleotide additions are added to complementary bases using template and non-template DNA. These are known as N-additions. In addition to TdT, DNA polymerase λ and DNA polymerase μ participate in the non-template insertion of nucleotide bases. DNA segments at the coding joint are ligated (joined) using XRCC4 activated DNA ligase IV. Exonuclease and endonuclease trimming occurs at the V-region joints and can lead to productive as well as unproductive rearrangements. Autoreactive Ig is edited to generate rearrangements that bind foreign antigen. The Ig is either membrane bound (anchored) or secreted. Membrane anchored or secreted Ig is obtained by mRNA splicing. Removal of the exon encoding the transmembrane region of Ig leads to a secreted molecule. Expression of IgM and IgD or IgM or IgD alone is also obtained by mRNA splicing at the spacer sequence between VDJ and C region sequences and polyadenylation. If RNA polymerase transcribes IgM and IgD constant region, then both IgM and IgD will be expressed. In T cells recombination mechanisms are similar with VDJ recombination occurring in the beta and delta chains of TCR which are equivalent to the H chain of Ig. The Ig L chain equivalent is found in the alpha and gamma chain which have both VJ recombination. Within the V region of delta genes, D-D joining can occur. Activity of Tdt is prominent in N-nucleotide additions following hairpin cleavage. Unlike Ig which can be secreted, TCR is only membrane bound and is not secreted. Further changes occur in the Ig V region due to somatic hypermutations (SHM) following antigen binding to Ig. This does not occur with the TCR. In the next section, we will examine the generation of antibody diversity in more detail.

Generating Antibody Diversity

There are roughly 100,000 standing clones of B cells at any one time. On each B cell, there are again roughly 100,000–200,000 antibody molecules on the surface of the cell, each with identical antigen binding sites. This creates a "dynamic inventory" of receptors on the surface of B cells. The progeny of each B cell will possess the identical antibody receptors found on their respective parental cells. In silico experiments identified 1688 genes for immune responses. In 1965, Dryer and Bennett proposed that multiple V genes and one constant gene were present in embryonic DNA, and one V gene was joined to the constant region gene to generate an antibody molecule (two genes, one protein hypothesis) in B cells. Additional investigations by Hozumi and Tonegawa using restriction enzyme analysis and DNA sequencing confirmed the presence of multiple V genes and identified J genes, both of which are required to generate the variable region of a light chain molecule. V and J genes recombined to form the variable region of a light chain. Further experiments identified a similar process of recombination for the variable region of the heavy chain. Instead of two genes for generating the heavy chain variable region, three genes were identified; V, D and J genes. Somatic hypermutation in mature B cells was also described, demonstrating that after BCR interaction with antigen resulting in antibody production, mutations occur in the V region of antibody genes to further diversify the receptor repertoire, with increase in the affinity of binding to antigen. Somatic gene recombination in the DNA of V, D, J genes is followed by transcription, RNA splicing and protein synthesis. The recombination that occurs here involves non-homologous gene segments. The rearranged Ig genes and the products encoded possess enormous diversity specifically at the V region of the Ig. Lymphocyte specific recombinases which are products of recombination activation genes 1 and 2 (RAG 1/2), recognize conserved recognition sequences in the introns flanking the 3′ end of V genes, 5′ end of J genes and the 3′ and 5′ ends of D genes. These recognition sequences have a specific pattern of nucleotide organization. The recognition sequences consist of nonamer (nine nucleotides) or heptamer (seven) sequences. The nonamer-heptamer sequences are separated or interspersed by nucleotide sequences consisting of 12 or 23 non-conserved bases known as spacers (12/23 bp joining rule).

Components involved:
- V (D) J genes

Recombination signal sequences

B and T lymphocyte specific molecules:
- Recombination activating genes encode lymphocyte specific recombinases (RAG1/2)

Terminal deoxyribonucleotidyl transferase (TdT)

Non-B and T lymphocyte specific molecules involved in NHEJ mechanisms:
- High mobility group B proteins 1 and 2 (HMGB 1/2)

Artemis

Ku70/80

DNA-PKcs

DNA polymerases μ and λ

DNA Ligase IV

XRCC4

XLF

Features Contributing to Antibody Diversity

1. **Multiple V(D)J genes in germ-line DNA:** Random somatic DNA recombination of the V, D and J genes leads to increased diversity of antibodies and allows interaction with a range of diverse antigens. Imprecise joining of the VDJ genes can occur as the genes are brought close together.
2. **Combinatorial joining of the V(D)J genes:** All the V genes (approx. 50) can potentially combine with all the D genes (27) as well as with all the joining genes (6) to give a large number of diverse antibodies.
3. **Junctional flexibility:** Joining can be productive resulting in the production of a functional molecule or non-productive as a result of the production of a non-functional molecule. When recombination signal sequences (RSSs) join there is precision to the joining. These are the sequences that flank the exons (coding sequences). When the exons join there is some "sloppiness" at the ends of the exons. This provides flexibility in the joining of the exons and generates differences in the DNA sequence at the joints which leads to differences in the amino acids encoded from these regions. Junctional flexibility contributes to the high variability found in the CDR region of the H chain.

Junctional diversity refers to the diversity found in the collection of the antibody molecules. Diversity is maximum in the CDR region.

Recombination signal sequences (RSS) are located in the intervening sequences (introns) flanking gene segments. AT rich palindromic sequences are involved in rearrangements of the DNA.

V(D)J recombination:

12/23 bp joining rule e.g. prevents two V genes or two J genes from combining

12 bp = 1 turn of the DNA helix.

23 bp = 2 turns of the DNA helix

Conserved heptamer and nonamer sequences.

Joining involves 1–2 turns of the DNA helix:

V-J joining

V-D joining

D-J joining

Mechanisms of joining:

Synapsis

Cleavage

Ligation/joining

Recombinase activating genes 1 and 2 (RAG- I and RAG-2), found in pre-B cells and in thymocytes (immature T cells) are absolutely essential for rearrangements. The recombinases cut 3′ of the gene and 5′ of the joining region. They engineer breaks in the DNA then allow joining DNA sequences to be reordered. Intervening sequences are circularized and removed then exon ends are joined and ligated. DNA is transcribed and polyadenylated, RNA is spliced and the transcript taken into the cytoplasm on the ER.

Sequence of events leading to antibody synthesis:

Germline DNA → rearranged DNA in nucleus → Transcription → splicing → mature mRNA → Translation on the ribosomes in the ER in the cytoplasm.

B cell commitment

(a) D-J joining commits cell to B lineage

(b) V-DJ joining occurs

(c) VDJ - C joining completes the rearrangement

4. **N-nucleotide additions:** Additional nucleotides are added to the ends of exons by the enzyme terminal deoxynucleotidyl transferase (TdT), when V (D) J rearrangements are taking place. These bases are not found originally in the germline. Cells without functional TdT cannot carry out N-nucleotide additions.

5. **P-nucleotide additions:** Additional nucleotides (palindromic sequences) are added by DNA repair enzymes following single stranded DNA cleavage at the junctions of V gene and RSS sequences. Hairpin loops form after the junctions between the V genes and RSSs are cleaved. The nucleotide bases on the single stranded DNA formed by the cleavage loop back on the strand to form a hairpin loop. The hairpin loop can form at different positions on the DNA sequence. Endonucleases such as Artemis cleave the hairpin and short strands of DNA

formed by this second cleavage are soon filled with complimentary nucleotides. Note, that the endonuclease can cleave at different positions of the hairpin. So that the nucleotides added during repair will contribute different nucleotide bases and lead to different amino acids that will be encoded by the DNA sequence at the coding joint. All of these changes add variability to the final Ig product.

6. **Association of H and L chains (kappa or lambda):** Each generated L chain is capable of combining with each generated H chain. Roughly 2 million H and L chain combinations are possible. Note, that for the light chains this means both kappa and lambda L chains.

7. **Somatic hypermutation and Receptor editing**: Following antigen exposure and B cell activation, additional mutations occur in the variable region of the antibody leading to generation of additional variability and increased affinity of the antibody for its cognate epitope. The mutations occur predominantly in the complementarity determining regions (CDRs) in the variable regions of the H and L chains. As discussed above, there are three CDRs each per chain. Hypermutation at these sites leads to **affinity maturation and better "fit" between antibody and antigen.** The enzyme activation-induced cytidine deaminase (AID) is essential for the mechanisms leading to mutations in the variable region genes of antibodies. AID deaminates deoxycytidine residues found in single stranded DNA forming deoxyuridine and creating U-G mismatches. DNA repair mechanisms such as mismatch or base excision is initiated, leading to mutated DNA. Depending on the extent of mutations it is possible to also develop loose affinity for antigen. The overall benefit of somatic mutation is that B cells possessing high affinity antibodies will be selected because of their increased binding affinity for a specific antigen. The antibody affinity increases in a secondary response, so that the affinity can be 10–10,000× higher than that of the primary response. Somatic hypermutation occurs in a T cell assisted response i.e. with T-dependent (TD) antigens in the **germinal centers** of spleen, lymph nodes, lymph nodules and lymph patches. In such a response, class switching occurs, memory cells develop and somatic mutations will occur in the variable region of the Ig H and L chains.

Four points to remember regarding B cell development and somatic hypermutation in the germinal center:

(a) Generation of additional variation on the antibody molecule
(b) B cell selection
(c) B cell proliferation
(d) Plasma cell generation

8. **Allelic exclusion:** This process does not contribute to antibody diversity. However, it ensures antibody specificity. During B cell development, rearrangement takes place on one chromosome at a time for H and L chain rearrangements. So that rearrangements do not occur simultaneously on both the paternal and maternal derived chromosomes. This is important in ensuring specificity of the antibody molecule. It is thought that if rearrangements on one chromosome are non-productive then rearrangements will take place on the homologous chromosome. If both are non-productive, then that cell undergoes apoptosis. However,

if productive rearrangements occur leading to antibody synthesis, the antibody product acts as an "inhibitory signal" to prevent additional rearrangement.

9. **Class (isotype) switching:** The constant region of the heavy chain is changed during a class switch so that the new isotype is associated with the same variable region that was on the previous isotype. For example, when IgM is changed to IgG, Cμ is changed to Cγ. This is known as class switch recombination (CSR). The variable region that was associated with Cμ becomes associated with Cγ with the resultant loss of the Cμ segment. Switch sites/switch regions flank the constant heavy genes except for Cδ. There are class specific recombinases that participate in the recognition of the switch sites. Class switching results in a change in biological function of the antibody. The same H chain V region is combined with a different C region. There is no class switching in L chains. The action of the recombinases is very precise. There are specific switch sites in switch region genes that bring into contiguity the switch gene with the constant gene. Heavy chain DNA is cut from one isotype, and rejoined to the 5' of the constant region of another isotype except for Cδ. Recombination occurs between donor and acceptor switch regions upstream of the constant heavy region of each isotype except for Cδ. AID plays a role in isotype switching. The enzyme targets specific sites in the switch region, deaminates deoxycytidine residues leading to cytidine to uridine conversion which are repaired by mismatch or base excision repair mechanisms. In AID knock-out mice, somatic hypermutation and class switch recombination do not occur demonstrating the essential role of AID in the mechanism of class switching and somatic hypermutation. Fibroblasts transfected with the AID gene underwent somatic hypermutation and class switching underscoring the major role of the enzyme in the mechanism for SHM and CSR. Switching can only occur to classes downstream for the eventual switch. Classes upstream cannot be used because the DNA that is looped out during the switch is lost. Cytokines influence specific isotype switching. For example IL-2 is involved in switching to IgG subclasses. Interleukin-4 is involved in IgG, IgA and IgE switching and TGF beta influences switching to IgA. A single B cell can switch isotypes more than once. The same primary transcript can give rise to μ or δ chain. The same transcript can also give rise to membrane bound or secreted antibody. Antigen triggers secretory events such as plasma cell formation. This occurs at the level of RNA processing. Cμ and Cδ genes are on the same transcript and are co-expressed by differential transcription. They become separated before expression. Combinatorial joining occurs due to sloppiness at the ends of genes during joining.

Nucleases cleave at the ends of the genes resulting in differences at the junctions. This increases diversity. Antibodies exist as either membrane bound or secreted molecules. Membrane bound Ig is expressed on mature, naive antigen committed B cells. Immunoglobulin is secreted from differentiated B cells which become plasma cells following antigen contact. Two exons, M1 and M2 encode the membrane and cytoplasmic segments of Ig, respectively. Membrane bound Ig has a membrane domain, it contains more hydrophobic amino acids and no carbohydrates. Exon M1 encodes the transmembrane segment of Ig. Secreted Ig has no membrane domain. Carbohydrates are added posttranslatioally, making it more soluble. Exon M2 encodes the cytoplasmic segment of Ig.

Germinal Center Formation

Antigen stimulated B cells enter follicles in peripheral lymphoid organs and differentiate into antibody secreting plasma cells (antibody forming cells, AFCs). Following antigen stimulation, B cells differentiate into plasmablasts; cells still expressing BCR, proliferating and beginning to secrete antibody. Further differentiation occurs to form plasma cells which secrete large amounts of antibody with no BCR expression. Plasma cell survival is supported by dendritic cells and monocytes which secrete IL-6 and APRIL, cytokines which promote plasma cell survival in the lymph nodes. IgM is first secreted by plasma cells and is followed by IgG secretion 5–6 day after immunization with antigen. Within follicles, antigen stimulated B cells divide rapidly, continue differentiation and form evanescent structures known as germinal centers (GCs). Within GCs follicular dendritic cells (FDC), T follicular helper cells (TFH) and macrophages interact to sustain antigen delivery to B cells and specifically allow TFH-B cell interaction and cooperation to take place. A mantle zone forms around the follicles and contains IgM/IgD expressing B cells. The B cells begin to lose IgD expression as they migrate toward the GC. The size of the GC is dependent on the type of antigen expressed by a pathogen or used for immunization. Formation of the GC peaks within 7–12 days after antigen exposure and persists for up to 4 weeks. High levels of somatic hypermutation in the V regions of Ig occur in the GC resulting in selection of high affinity antibodies. Isotype switching also occurs within the GC resulting in a switch from IgM to other antibody isotypes except for IgD.

Histologically, GC are described as having a dark zone (DZ) and light zone (LZ) due to the presence of large numbers of cells in the DZ which stain more intensely with dyes, compared to the LZ. Large numbers of proliferating B cells known as centroblasts are located in the DZ, an area that is close to T cell rich areas of the lymphoid organ. B cells in the LZ, known as centrocytes have decreased levels of proliferation and are associated with FDCs and TFH. Centrocytes express high levels of activation markers such as CD86. In contrast to centrocytes, centroblasts express high levels of CXCR4 and bind to CXCL12 secreted by DZ stromal reticular cells leading to centroblast retention within the DZ. Centroblasts also express high levels of AID and DNA polymerase η (eta) essential for SHM and CSR. Follicular dendritic cells secrete CXCL13 which binds to CXCR5 expressed on centrocytes and othe GC B cells. Upon formation of the GC, B cells move from DZ to LZ every 4–6 h where the mutated BCR is tested for high affinity binding to antigen. B cell interaction with TFH cells using CD40 on B cells with CD40L on TFH results in cell signaling that enhances helper cell signaling such as cytokines from TFH cells and B cell re-entry into the DZ for further rounds of SHM. B cells expressing low affinity BCR and autoreactive BCR die by apoptosis. Germinal center B cells express an inhibitory sphingosine 1-phosphate (SIP) receptor, SIP_2-type receptor for SIP binding leading to the formation of GCs containing tight clusters of cells.

Memory B Cells

Following clonal expansion of B cells after antigen stimulation, effector and memory B cell populations are formed. Memory B cells are a heterogeneous population of cells that have responded to T dependent antigens. Phenotypic and morphological differences have been observed between memory B cells and long-lived plasma cells (LLPCs). The LLPCs are larger than memory B cells. The cells also differ in their distribution in tissues. Before GC formation, IgM^+ memory B cells with low affinity for antigen are produced. These are followed by a second population of memory B cells that develop in GCs with isotype switched antibodies and SHM in the V region. This second population of memory B cells can home to different tissues in the body. Long-lived plasma cells return to the bone marrow and persist in secretion of antigen specific antibodies, supported by APRIL-secreting eosinophils and megakaryocytes. The cytokine binds to the B cell maturation antigen (BCMA) receptor on plasma cells. Stromal cells in the bone marrow secrete the chemokine CXCL12 which binds the CXCR4 receptor on the LLPCs. Follicular dendritic cells and TFH cells also help to maintain memory B cell populations within the lymphoid organs.

Selected References

Abbas AR, Baldwin D, Ma Y, Duyang W, Zgurney A, Martin F, Fong S, Campagne MV, Godowski P, Williams PM, Chan AC, Clark HF (2005) Immune response in silico (IRIS): Immune-specific genes identified from a compendium of microarray expression data. Genes Immunity 6:319–331

Hozumi N, Tonegawa S (1976) Evidence for somatic rearrangement of immunoglobulin genes coding for variable and constant regions. Proc Natl Acad Sci U S A 73:3628–3632

Murphy K, Weaver C (2017) Janeway's immunobiology, 9th edn. Garland Press, New York

Punt J, Stranford SA, Jones PP, Owen JA (2019) Kuby immunology, 8th edn. W.H. Freeman and Company, New York. Chapter 20, Antigen-antibody interactions

Rodgers KK (2017) Riches in RAGs: Revealing the V(D)J recombinase through high resolution structures. Trends Biochem Sci 42:72–84

Roth DB (2014) V(D)J recombination: Mechanism, errors, and fidelity. Micobiol Spectrum 2(6):MDNA3-0041-2014

Ru H, Chambers MG, Fu T, Tong AB, Liao M, Wu H (2015) Molecular mechanisms of V(D)J recombination from synaptic RAG1-RAG2 complex structure. Cell 163:1138–1152

Yang J, Reth M (2016) Receptor dissociation and B cell activation. Curr Top Microbiol Immunol 393:27–43

Chapter 12
Major Histocompatibility Complex Genes

Antigen binding by B cells occurs directly with the BCR recognizing epitopes on antigens. T cell recognition of antigens cannot occur unless the antigens are bound to **major histocompatibility complex (MHC)** proteins. A deficiency in MHC class I or II proteins results in failure of T cells to express CD4 or CD8 molecules in the thymus. The MHC genes encode proteins responsible for diversity of the immune response in individuals. The MHC genes are the most polymorphic in the human genome and include genes encoding glycoproteins responsible for recognition of alloantigens on foreign tissue such as transplantation antigens. MHC is a cluster of genes encoding class I, II and III proteins. Both class I and II MHC proteins are responsible for T cell restriction in its recognition of antigen. The gene clusters of class I and II are closely linked in all species. The genes are highly **polymorphic**, closely linked and therefore inherited together. The MHC genes contain many alternate forms referred to as alleles. The alleles are codominantly expressed and inherited as a set of alleles from each parent. Each set is known as a haplotype. There is no self/non-self-discrimination in the interaction with antigens. The selection pressures responsible for maintaining the close link are not well understood. The class III locus contains a cluster of unrelated genes encoding proteins that have importance in immunity but do not directly bind antigens. The MHC gene order on chromosomes varies from mouse to humans. All vertebrate species possess MHC or MHC-like collection of genes. MHC proteins are essential for both CD4+ and CD8+ T cell effector functions. Unlike B lymphocytes, which can recognize antigens directly, and can recognize epitopes that are conformationally constrained, T lymphocytes cannot recognize antigens directly and require that the antigens be processed to reveal internal hydrophobic peptides. These peptides bind to MHC molecules and the MHC-peptide complex becomes expressed on the surface of antigen presenting cells (APCs). In humans, MHC proteins are also known as human leukocyte antigens (HLA).

Class I MHC proteins are located on almost all somatic cells (nucleated cells and platelets), and are responsible for binding altered self-antigens and antigens expressed by intracellular pathogens. Class II MHC genes encode proteins that are

© Springer Nature Switzerland AG 2021
T. Y. Sam-Yellowe, *Immunology: Overview and Laboratory Manual*,
https://doi.org/10.1007/978-3-030-64686-8_12

responsible for foreign antigen recognition and are located on specific immune cells known as antigen presenting cells (APCs). The MHC genes are codominantly expressed. There is no allelic exclusion. An APC may express six class I molecules and six class II molecules. The MHC functions in humoral and cell mediated immunity and plays a central role in immune response development and in autoimmunity. Class III MHC genes encode a number of different proteins also involved in the immune response. Examples of these proteins are complement components C4 and Factor B, cytochrome P450, tumor necrosis factor (TNF), heat shock proteins, enzymes involved in corticosteroid metabolism and molecules involved in inflammation. The MHC locus is the most polymorphic locus in the germline DNA. As many as six different class I MHC proteins can be displayed at one time. On the average 4–6 different types can be displayed. All different alleles have the potential for expression. The function of the class I and II MHC molecules is to present antigen to T lymphocytes, in the form of oligopeptides approximately 8–22 amino acids in length, that reside within the antigen binding groove of MHC molecules. Unlike the antigen binding site of mIg and TCR, the MHC antigen binding site is not the result of gene rearrangement. Recognition of antigen by T lymphocytes in association with MHC antigens is known as MHC restriction.

A few of the genes are expressed and a large number form a loose cluster that is maintained as part of the MHC. Pseudogenes, unexpressed genes and genes encoding proteins with unclear function have been identified in the MHC loci. Both expressed and unexpressed genes form a cooperative group. The MHC protein possesses a **histotope** for binding the TCR/CD3 complex and the **desetope** for combining with the peptide. The antigen possesses an **epitope** for binding to the TCR/CD3 or Ig and an **agretope** for combining with the MHC protein. MHC diversity appears to protect a species from a wide range of infectious disease. The class I MHC proteins play an important role in foreign tissue rejection. This is due to immune responses generated to cell surface antigens on the foreign tissue. Why is polymorphism needed for effective immune response? One explanation is that gene conversion (GC) occurs allowing for the exchange of short DNA segments between homologous regions of chromosome pairs in class I. This allows class I genes to maintain large pools of potential restricting residues. GC could also explain why polymorphism is maintained and why there are close links between the closely related class I and II genes. Another suggestion is that polymorphism of class I and II molecules is needed to maintain diversity and dispersion of the germ line V region genes of the T cell receptor (TCR). There are differences between the two classes. Both structural and molecular differences are present in both proteins. Mutations can also occur to generate polymorphisms e.g. single point mutations and multiple point mutations along the DNA can occur and lead to changes in encoded protein. Small blocks of genetic material can be exchanged between different class II genes. Class I MHC proteins are found on all nucleated cells and are responsible for cell surface recognition, identified by **cytotoxic T cells**. Class I MHC presents antigen from altered self-cells to cytotoxic T cells.

Initial isolation of class I molecules was difficult because of low level expression (compared to other surface molecules), and the fact that they were membrane bound.

The use of membrane solubilizing detergents such as nonidet P40 (NP-40) and the use of protease digestion (papain) and lectin affinity column chromatography made isolation possible. In humans the major class I MHC proteins are designated as HLA-A, B and C. Other class I molecules include HLA-E and G which encode class I-like molecules, HLA-F found differentially expressed on resting cells in the skin and HLA-H and HLA-X. In mice the major class I MHC proteins are designated H-2K, H-2D and H-2L. Other class I MHC proteins include Q, T and M found 3' to the K and D loci. The three are non-polymorphic. Q is secreted and T is found expressed on thymocytes, activated T cells, thymic leukemia cells, on regulatory and immature lymphocytes and on hematopoietic cells. Many of the genes in Q and T region are pseudogenes. Class I MHC proteins are expressed on all nucleated cells, responsible for Ag presentation to CD8$^+$ cells, endogenous antigens processed through the proteasome. The structure of class I and II MHC proteins is shown in Fig. 12.1.

Structure of Class I MHC Proteins

The MHC class I molecule consists of a single α chain with three domains (α1, α2 and α3 domains) associated with β$_2$ microglobulin. The α chain is a transmembrane protein glycosylated in the extracellular domain. The peptide binding pocket consists of closed ends, with the peptide binding domain located between α1 and α2 (Fig. 12.1), in a "hamburger in a bun" motif. The pocket fits peptides of 8-10 amino acids, preferentially nonamers. Each allele encoding MHC class I protein binds distinct peptides. The α3 domain is highly homologous to beta2 microglobulin and is highly conserved in class I proteins. The α3 domain also has homology to the constant region of Ig. This domain also contains the binding site for CD8.

Experiments using Daudi cells (tumor cell line) show the essential requirement for β2 microglobulin. This cell line cannot synthesize β2 microglobulin. However, the transcript for the α chain is present in the cells. MHC class I is translated but the protein is not expressed on the cell surface. Transfection of beta 2 microglobulin gene led to surface expression of MHC class I proteins.

Two types of experiments were performed to determine the type of peptides bound by MHC proteins. Antigens were digested and incubated with cells expressing class I proteins. The question asked was, what type of peptide and what length of the peptide binds to the binding pocket? In a second type of experiment for class II, MHC-Ag complexes were isolated from cell surfaces, purified and denatured to release bound peptides. The rationale for the second experiment was similar to that for class I MHC proteins. The experiment sought to determine the type and the length of peptides that bind to the class II MHC binding pocket. X-ray crystallography experiments were also performed to determine the structure of the binding pockets for both MHC proteins. The experiments identified specific peptide motifs that fit the binding pockets of class I and class II MHC. The peptide-MHC interaction was found to be very stable with very low dissociation. The peptides bound to

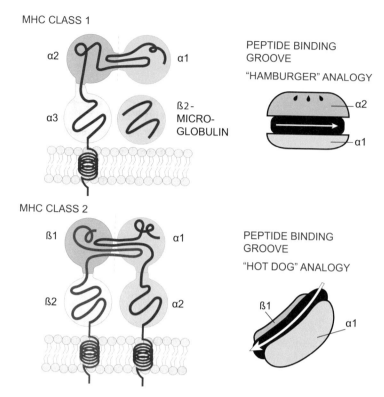

Fig. 12.1 Structure of the class I and class II MHC proteins. Class I MHC consists of a membrane protein α chain organized in three domains and associated with β2-microglobulin. The α1 and α2 domains make up the closed antigen binding pocket that fits peptides of 8–10 amino acid residues, with nine residues being the optimum length. A longer peptide would buckle to fit the binding pocket. The "hamburger in the bun" analogy used here shows the peptide confined within the binding groove or pocket. Class II MHC consists of α β membrane proteins associated as a heterodimer. The antigen binding pocket is made up of α1 and β1 domains. Longer antigen peptides can fit into the pocket with the ends of the peptides protruding out of the pocket in a "hot dog in a bun" analogy

MHC class I had conserved hydrophobic and basic residues at the C termini and were mostly nonamers. The peptides binding MHC class II were more variable and longer. The length of peptides binding to the class II MHC pocket ranged from 13 to 18 amino acids in length. Unlike the closed-ended binding pocket of class I MHC proteins, the binding pocket of class II MHC proteins was found to be open-ended, allowing the peptides to protrude out of the pocket on either end similar to a "hot dog in a bun" (Fig. 12.1). Class II MHC proteins are responsible for cooperation and interaction between cells of the immune system. Class II MHC proteins present antigen to helper T cells and are found on B cells, monocytes, macrophages, dendritic cells and some epithelial cells.

Structure of Class II MHC Proteins

The class II MHC protein consists of $\alpha\beta$ polypeptide chains in a heterodimer of $\alpha1$ and $\alpha2$ domains and $\beta1$ and $\beta2$ domains. Each polypeptide possesses a transmembrane domain that anchors the proteins to the cell membrane. The peptide binding pocket is open-ended, located between $\alpha1$ and $\beta1$ domains and fits peptides of 13–18 amino acids in length. In humans class II MHC proteins are designated HLA-D. The three major HLA-D proteins are HLA-DP, DQ and DR. Each contains one α and one β gene. Additional HLA-D proteins include DO, DX, DV, DM, DN and DZ, non-classical class II molecules. The α and β genes of DM are invariant. They function in the loading of peptide onto MHC II. DM behaves like an enzyme and facilitates the ligand dissociation from the binding pocket of MHC class II. DM induced dissociation is related to the affinity of the ligand within the binding pocket. An additional protein Ii (invariant chain) is found associated with the MHC II heterodimer in the endoplasmic reticulum (ER). CLIP (class II associated invariant chain generated from Ii cleavage) can be easily removed in the presence of DM because of its weak affinity. Functionally both class I and class II molecules are similar i.e. both display antigens and allow antigen recognition by T cells at the variable region of TCR (VTCR). The VTCR gene pool does not dictate differences in antigen recognition. Antigenic determinants found on class I proteins may also be found in class II proteins. The non-MHC molecule CD1 also binds antigen, specifically lipid antigens.

Genes encoding molecules responsible for transporting peptides from the cytoplasm into the lumen of ER for association with class I proteins map in the class II MHC region between HLA-DP and HLA-DQ e.g. TAP genes, genes encoding low molecular weight proteins (LMP) 2 and 7, genes important for regulation of interferon gamma. The class II transactivator (CIITA) functions in the transcription of genes involved in MHC function.

In mice H2-A (structurally similar to DQ) and H2-E are structurally similar to HLA-DR, they possess two loci, each encoded by alpha and beta genes. There are also non-classical genes Oα, Oβ, Mα and Mβ. The combinatorial pairing of alpha and beta chains generates a large number of class II restriction specificities. This may be an important mechanism for generating antigenic diversity/polymorphism when compared to gene conversion in class I proteins. The diversity generated in class II molecules is in excess of what is needed for the immune response. The H2-E beta chain is not polymorphic in some strains of mice. In some strains it is not expressed. In Syrian and golden hamsters, the class I locus appears to be monomorphic while the class II locus is polymorphic. Antigens can still be presented and histocompatibility antigens are still recognized. In studies to determine the structure and function of the MHC proteins, inbred strains of mice were used. Repeated crossings of successive generations of mice generated mice with identical pairs of chromosomes. The studies confirm the increased polymorphism (many alternate forms of the genes, alleles) of MHC genes. The studies also showed that genes in the MHC loci are closely linked with very low frequency of recombination (0.5%).

The alleles encoded by the closely linked genes are inherited as 2 sets from either parent. Each set of alleles is known as a haplotype. The type of mice used include, syngeneic, congenic and recombinant congenic mice. Class I and II MHC proteins possess different types of specificities. The use of serology to map the MHC revealed the presence of public and private specificities. Public specificities are determinants common to several different class I molecules or haplotypes. Private specificities are determinants unique to a particular molecule or haplotype. Antigens of insufficiently defined specificity are known as workshop antigens.

Functional Assays for Class I MHC Proteins

Cell-Mediated Lympholysis (CML) (^{51}Chromium Release Assay)

This is an assay used for measuring the activity of CTLs generated to allogeneic cells.

Splenic lymphocytes from an immunized animal are incubated with allogeneic cells (that were used for immunization) labeled with ^{51}chromium. If CTLs within the splenic population recognize surface antigens on the allogeneic cells, they attack the cells resulting in the release of ^{51}chromium. The amount of ^{51}chromium released is proportional to the cytotoxic activity of the CTLs. In mice the activity of the CTLs maps to H-2K or H-2 D region indicating class I MHC involvement.

Functional Assays for Class I and II MHC Proteins

Mixed Lymphocyte Response (MLR)

This is an assay that measures the functional activity of helper T cells. Class II MHC antigens also function in the T cell response to antigens on allogeneic cells. The MLR will also measure the intensity of the cell response by measuring the proliferation of helper T cells.

Two-Way MLR (e.g. Typing Tissue for Transplantation)

Donor lymphocytes (Responder) are mixed with recipient lymphocytes (Stimulator) and cultured for four days. Both sets of cells are allogeneic cells. Tritiated thymidine (^{3}H-thymidine) is added to the culture and incubated an additional 18–24 h. The cells are harvested and the incorporation of thymidine measured. The extent of cell proliferation is proportional to the amount of ^{3}H-thymidine taken up by the cells. The greater the proliferation, the greater the sensitization i.e. recognition of "foreign antigen". In the two-way assay both responder and stimulator cells are allowed to proliferate.

One-Way MLR

In the one-way assay the stimulator cells from the recipient lymphocytes are treated with irradiation (X-ray) or with mitomycin C to prevent cell proliferation. Antigens on the cell are still present. The stimulator cell population is mixed with responder cells and incubated as in the two-way assay. In this assay only the activity of the responder and stimulator cell will be measured individually. The advantage of the one-way to the two-way test is that interpretation of results is "cleaner" since the activity of one cell population will be measured at a time.

MHC and Disease

Most individuals are heterozygous at the MHC loci e.g. six class I genes expressed, twice for HLA-A, B and C. The significant point here is whether recognition of self-antigens will be maximized or minimized. Six MHC class I molecules (alleles of the three HLA antigens) seems a reasonable compromise between maximizing and minimizing recognition of self-antigens. Homozygosity at any one of the three class I loci will reduce the number of alleles from six to five leading to a 16% drop. This will result in a loss of immune capability. With increased MHC expression (variations), there is an increase in negative T cell selection. The limiting factor in resistance to infectious disease is related to the efficacy of the antigen binding by each of the alleles. MHC polymorphism within species will generate different patterns of responsiveness and unresponsiveness to different antigens. The structure of the MHC determines the strength of binding with the antigen. This is known as the **determinant-selection model.** Elimination of self-reactive T cells for MHC/peptide or foreign antigens closely resembling self-antigens leads to elimination of those cells. This is the **holes-in-the-repertoire model.** MHC gene polymorphism resulting in diversity of antigen binding provides protection of populations from disease.

No single MHC allele is found present at very high frequencies and combinations of some alleles are advantageous to the host. Mutations in the MHC genes may increase or decrease resistance to disease. Extensive polymorphism has several advantages to the host. Each member of the population is different at MHC class I or II loci. This is needed to control the spread of pathogens. A given population should contain as many different MHC molecules as possible. This increases the ability of the MHC proteins to combine with different peptides. The observed frequency for a particular combination of haplotypes does not match the expected frequency of the individual haplotypes. This is known as **Linkage disequilibrium.** This is important in disease associations. There may not be enough crossover events to permit each to reach equilibrium. There may also exist "hot spots" of recombination in the DNA. Positive selection may favor some alleles. The frequency of a particular allele in a patient is higher than the allele frequency in the general population. The frequency of the allele may be associated with a particular autoimmune disease. This is known as **relative risk.**

Relative Risk Calculations

Relative risk (RR also sometimes referred to as risk ratio) will be evaluated to understand the association of MHC alleles with autoimmune disease. Relative risk is also referred to as the Odds Ratio. However both terms have different uses. We will calculate RR using 2 x 2 contingency tables to evaluate the risk of having the MHC antigen (i. e. particular MHC haplotype) and also having the disease.

For example:

Individuals that have the particular MHC allele and have the disease versus the risk for not having the particular MHC allele but having the disease

$$\frac{a}{a+b} \times 100 \tag{12.1}$$

Individuals that do not have the MHC allele but have the disease

$$\frac{c}{c+d} \times 100 \tag{12.2}$$

The **relative risk** (disease risk associated with having the MHC allele) is as follows:

$$\frac{\frac{a}{a+b}}{\frac{c}{c+d}} \text{ same as } \frac{\text{Probability}(p)(\text{disease / MHC allele} +)}{\text{Probability}(p)(\text{disease / MHC allele} -)} \tag{12.3}$$

2 × 2 contingency table for relative risk/odds ratio calculation

	MHC+	MHC−
Disease +	a	b
Disease −	c	d

The **odds ratio (OR)/relative risk (RR)** calculation multiplies across the table.

$$\frac{ad}{bc} \tag{12.4}$$

The odds ratio calculation is used to estimate a population's relative risk for disease (in retrospective studies), due to disease exposure etc. and is important and used in case-controlled studies. Examples are cases of food poisoning and exposure to infectious disease agents or pathogens. The ratio of MHC antigen frequency in a disease population can be compared to the frequency of MHC antigen in a control population. The relative risk calculation requires incidence data. In our examples we can use the OR = RR calculation shown below to determine the RR for an individual having a particular MHC allele and the association for developing a particular autoimmune disease.

RR = 1	the disease risk in the same in individuals having or not having the MHC allele (disease is same in exposed or non-exposed group i.e. for exposure to pathogen)
RR > 1	Individuals with the MHC allele have a higher risk for developing disease (individual with exposure has a higher risk of disease)
RR < 1	Individuals has a lower risk of developing disease (exposed group has lower risk of developing disease)

Example: A clinical study is being performed to evaluate the risk associated with the presence of HLA-B27 and an Unknown syndrome (UnkS). The study population consists of 112 individuals with UnkS and HLA-B27, 80 individuals with UnkS without HLA-B27, 350 individuals without UnkS and HLA-B27 and 67 individuals without UnkS that have HLA-B27. What is the relative risk (odds ratio) associated with having HLA-B27 and developing UnkS?

	MHC+	MHC−	Total
Disease +	a	b	
Disease −	c	d	

Total				

Antigen Presenting Cells

Antigen presenting cells (APCs) function in phagocytosis, antigen processing and presentation. These are a morphologically and functionally diverse group of cells derived from the bone marrow that are specialized in processing and presenting antigen in association with class II MHC antigens to helper T lymphocytes. Their mechanisms of antigen uptake and effector function are different. All APCs express MHC Class I and II antigens. The class II MHC antigens are either constitutively expressed or induced by specific cytokines. Constitutive expression of MHC class II proteins is found on macrophages, dendritic cells, B cells, Langerhans cells, vascular endothelial cells, dendritic and epithelial cells in the thymus. Induced expression of MHC class II proteins is found on glial cells, skin fibroblasts and beta cells in the pancreas. Some APCs secrete cytokines that induce specific functions in the T cells. APCs also express essential surface accessory molecules required by the T cell e.g. CD80. In addition to APCs directly presenting antigens to T cells, nanovesicles (exosomes) derived from endosomes in APCs are also implicated in antigen presentation.

Monocytes are found in peripheral blood, they are phagocytic for opsonized antigen on C3b or Fc receptors, and express Class II MHC antigens, CD14, CD35 (FcγRI) and CD64. Macrophages are located in various solid tissues. They are differentiated monocytes and are phagocytic. Examples include Kupffer cells in the liver and splenic macrophages. They express Class II MHC antigens, CD35 and CD64. Both macrophages and monocytes are important in chronic inflammatory lesions. Following activation by T cell cytokines, they can kill phagocytized pathogens using products of respiratory (oxidative) burst. Both cells also mediate cytotoxic killing. Langerhans cells are found in the skin and express class II MHC antigen, CD35 and CD64. Dendritic cells are resident in solid organs of the immune system. They are potent APCs that activate T cells. In B cell rich areas and lymph nodes follicular dendritic cells are present. Dendritic cells express CD35, CD64 and CD80/CD86 in addition to class II MHC proteins. In T cell rich areas and lymph nodes interdigitating dendritic cells are present and also express the class II MHC antigen. B lymphocytes also present antigen to CD4⁺ T cells following capture of antigen by the BCR complex. T-B cell cooperation leads to more efficient antigen clearance.

Antigen Processing

Antigen binding receptors on B and T lymphocytes bind to epitopes on antigens. For T lymphocytes, internal peptides generated from protein antigens in APCs are recognized by the TCR. B lymphocytes can recognize peptides as well as epitopes on tertiary conformations of proteins. Major histocompatibility complex (MHC) proteins determine how and when T lymphocytes interact with antigenic peptides during an immune response. Two types of MHC proteins interact with peptides for antigen presentation to T cells. Class I MHC proteins combine with endogenous or intracellular antigenic peptides processed in proteasomes located within the cytoplasm of altered or infected host cells. The peptides associated with class I MHC are presented to cytotoxic T lymphocytes (CTLs) which recognize and bind the peptide using the T cell receptor. Class II MHC proteins combine with exogenous or extracellular antigenic peptides processed in the endosome of antigen presenting cells (APCs) such as dendritic cells or macrophages (Fig. 12.2). The APCs present the antigenic peptides to helper T cells which recognize and bind to the peptide using the TCR. We will examine below how intracellular and extracellular antigens are processed and discuss how the peptides generated from processing combine with MHC proteins for presentation to T cells.

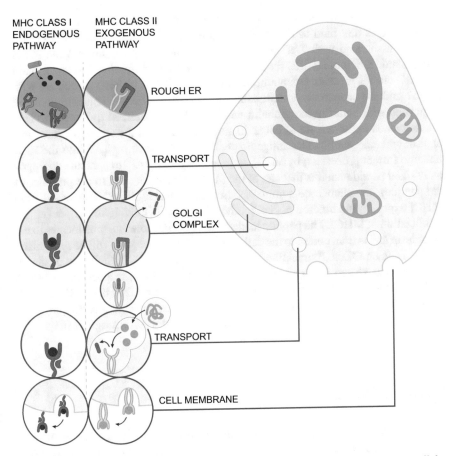

MHC CLASS I
ENDOGENOUS
PATHWAY

MHC CLASS II
EXOGENOUS
PATHWAY

ROUGH ER

TRANSPORT

GOLGI
COMPLEX

TRANSPORT

CELL MEMBRANE

Fig. 12.2 Antigen processing and presentation. Endogenous antigens produced by intracellular pathogens or through changes in protein expression due to neoplastic growth are processed in immunoproteasomes. Peptides generated are transported to the ER where they interact with MHC class I proteins. MHC class I bound proteins are transported to the host cell surface where they are recognized by CD8+ cytotoxic T cells. Exogenous antigens are phagocytosed or endocytosed by dendritic cells or macrophages. Phagocytic vesicles fuse with lysosomes to form phagolysosomes. MHC class II proteins synthesized in the ER associate with the invariant chain protein, the invariant proteins becomes cleaved leaving CLIP in the antigen binding site and becomes transported into the endosome where antigenic peptides are located. CLIP is exchanged for antigenic peptide and MHC class II bound to antigen peptide is transported to the surface of the antigen presenting cell for recognition by CD4+ T helper cells

Endogenous Antigen

Antigens destined for CTL recognition associate with ubiquitin before entry into proteasomes. Due to increased protein expression and secretion from intracellular pathogens or cells undergoing neoplastic growth, cytokine induced formation of immunoproteasomes occurs. Enzymatic cleavage of ubiquitinated antigens takes place within the cytosolic proteasomes and immunoproteasomes resulting in peptide fragments that bind to transporter associated with antigen processing (TAP). Peptides associated with TAP are transported from the cytoplasm into the rough endoplasmic reticulum (RER) for association with MHC I proteins. The alpha chain of MHC class I proteins are synthesized in the RER and become associated with ERp57 and the chaperone protein calnexin. The MHCI-ERp57-calnexin complex associates with beta 2-microglobulin which is also synthesized in the RER. This binding leads to the release of calnexin and the binding of the chaperone proteins, tapasin and calreticulin. The antigenic peptides transported by TAP into the RER undergo further processing by an ER aminopeptidase, ERAP1to generate appropriately sized peptide lengths that can fit the MHCI binding pocket. In the presence of the peptides, the chaperone complex, calreticulin-tapasin-ERp57 is released from MHCI exposing the binding pocket to allow for peptide binding to the pocket and stabilization of MHCI. The peptide loaded class I MHC molecule translocates to the cytoplasm and is transported to the cell surface where the peptide will be recognized by the TCR on CTLs. Extracellular antigens recognized by TH cells are phagocytized or endocytosed into phagocytic or endocytic vesicles, respectively. Class II MHC proteins and the invariant chain (Ii, CD74) are synthesized in the RER. The Ii binds to the binding pocket of class II MHC molecules, preventing premature binding of peptide to the binding pocket. The Ii also provides sorting signals in its cytoplasmic tail to guide the MHCII protein to the endosome.

Exogenous Antigen

Following the uptake of extracellular antigens, endosomal vesicles fuse with lysosomes to become early endolysosomal vesicles possessing a pH of 6.0–6.5. Endolysosomal vesicles become increasingly acidic as antigen is enzymatically degraded, reaching a pH of 4.5–5.0 in late endosomes. The MHCII-Ii complex in the RER is packaged into vesicles and transported from the RER to the Golgi. The Ii becomes cleaved within the endosome, leaving a fragment still associated with the binding pocket. This fragment is known as the class II-associated invariant chain (CLIP). To facilitate peptide binding to the MHCII binding pocket, HLA-DM exchanges CLIP for the peptide. Once peptide is bound to the MHCII binding pocket, MHCII-peptide is transported to the cell surface of the APC. The antigen processing discussed above deals with protein antigens. Lipid antigens are also processed for presentation to NKT cells.

Lipid Antigens

Glycolipid antigens associate with CD1 and MRI (MHC class I-related protein) proteins. The MRI are non-classical class I molecules. There are five human CD1 proteins and one MRI. The CD1 proteins are structurally similar to MHCI molecules but function in a manner similar to class II MHC molecules. CD1 molecules have a reduced polymorphism for antigen binding and possess a deeper binding pocket formed by the alpha chain. The alpha chain is associated with beta 2-microglobulin, which like the class I MHC proteins does not interact with peptide. MRI has been shown to present non-peptide antigens to mucosal-associated invariant T (MAIT) cells and may be important in responses generated in mucosal surfaces of the host and for maintaining homeostasis in mucosal barriers. In a process influenced by cytokines, cross-presentation of antigen can occur with dendritic cells involved with presenting exogenous antigen to TH cells also presenting exogenous antigen through the endocytic pathway to CTLs. Dendritic cells are "licensed" by cytokines to perform cross-presentation of antigen to CTLs.

Selected References

Bahr A, Wilson AB (2012) The evolution of MHC diversity: Evidence of intralocus gene conversion and recombination in a single-locus system. Gene 497:52–57

Komov L, Kadosh DM, Barnea E, Milner E, Hendler A, Admon A (2018) Cell surface MHC class I expression is limited by the availability of peptide-receptive "empty" molecules rather than by the supply of peptide ligands. Proteomics 18:1700248

Santbrogio L, Sato AK, Fischer FR, Dorf ME, Stern LJ (1999) Abundant empty class II molecules on the surface of immature dendritic cells. Proc Natl Acad Sci U S A 96:15,050–15,055

Taxman DJ, Cressman DE, Ting JP (2000) Identification of class II transcriptional activator-induced genes by representational difference analysis: Discoordinate regulation of the DNα/Doβ heterodimer. J Immunol 165:1410–1416

Chapter 13
T Cell Development and T Cell Receptor Structure

T Cell Development

B and T lymphocytes differentiate from the common lymphoid progenitor in the bone marrow. While B cells develop in the bone marrow, thymocytes differentiated from the common lymphoid progenitor migrate from the bone marrow into the thymus, and enter the cortex of the thymus from blood vessels located in the cortico-medullary junction. The thymocytes lack T cell markers and are therefore $CD4^-CD8^-$ or double negative (DN) for both coreceptor molecules. Recombination activating genes (RAG) 1 and 2 expression begins in the early lymphoid progenitor stage. Products of the RAG1/2 genes are essential for T cell receptor gene rearrangement. Four stages of DN development occur. DN1 cells express $CD44^+CD25^-$, DN2 cells express $CD44^+CD25^+$, DN3 express $CD44^-CD25^+PreTCR$ and DN4 express $CD44^-CD25^-preTCR^+$. Within the subcapsular cortex of the thymus, the TCR gene rearrangement is initiated at DN2 and is followed by expression of the coreceptor molecules, resulting in the development of double positive (DP) cells expressing both $CD4^+$ and $CD8^+$ molecules. $\gamma\delta$ and β genes rearrange and at the DN3 stage, β chain selection occurs along with preTCR expression. Rearrangement is completed at the DN4 stage with the rearrangement of the α gene resulting in DP cell development. $\gamma\delta$ TCR expressing T cells migrate out of the thymus very early as DN T cells. With T cell commitment the double positive T cells expressing $CD4^+CD8^+TCR^+$ further develop into single positive T cells with the expression of either CD4 or CD8 with the TCR. Double positive thymocytes can develop into NKT cells, intraepithelial lymphocytes (IELs) or regulatory T cells (TREGs).

© Springer Nature Switzerland AG 2021
T. Y. Sam-Yellowe, *Immunology: Overview and Laboratory Manual*,
https://doi.org/10.1007/978-3-030-64686-8_13

Positive and Negative Selection of T Cells

T cells undergo positive and negative selection in the thymus to produce mature T cells capable of interacting with antigen under major histocompatibility complex (MHC) restriction and to have T cells that have developed tolerance to self-antigens, respectively. Cells positively selected express the chemokine receptor CCR7, allowing them to migrate into the thymic medulla. Positive selection establishes MHC restriction for thymocytes capable of binding self-MHC proteins with low affinity. A large number (95%) of thymocytes die by apoptosis ("death by neglect") due to failure of becoming positively selected. Thymocytes binding with high affinity to self-MHC-peptide complexes are not selected. Negative selection of thymocytes also occurs leading to central tolerance. In this case, potentially autoreactive thymocytes are not selected. Central tolerance is established by the non-selection of thymocytes binding with high affinity to self-MHC-peptides. Negatively selected cells undergo clonal deletion and die by apoptosis. Thymocytes that successfully undergone positive and negative selection receive an additional layer of scrutiny to prevent autoreactivity, before emigrating from the thymus. Medullary thymic epithelial cells express tissue specific proteins induced by autoimmune regulator (AIRE) protein. Upregulation of the transcription factor FOXO1 leads to the expression of klf2 which upregulates sphingosine-1-phosphate (SIP) receptor, which is an important molecule required for emigration of T cells from the thymus. FOXO1 also upregulates IL-7R a survival signal for thymocytes. In classic experiments demonstrating MHC restriction of T cells and the requirement of the thymus for establishing positive selection, F1 progeny of A×B mice possessing $H2^{a/b}$ haplotype were irradiated to destroy hematopoietic cells which also resulted in the destruction of the mouse's immune system. The mice were also thymectomized and a thymus from parental B strain was used to replace the thymus in the F1 mice. Hematopoietic cells obtained from sibling F1 mice were used to re-establish the immune system. The reconstituted A×B F1 were challenged with virus-infected cells from parental strains A and B mice. Cells from A×B F1 were unable to destroy virus-infected cells from strain A, but destroyed virus-infected cells from strain B. This demonstrated that positively selected T cells were MHC restricted in the thymus from parental strain B and therefore recognized the MHC on strain B infected cells.

T Cell Receptor

The T cell receptor (TCR) is a heterodimeric membrane protein with defined specificity for an epitope on an antigen molecule. Like the antibody molecule, the antigen binding site is made up of variable domains in the alpha and beta chains of the TCR. The TCR is produced as a result of gene rearrangements with considerable diversity for antigen binding in the variable region. The TCR is found either as an αβ or γδ heterodimer in association with CD3. The CD3 molecule is a transmembrane protein that consists of five subunits, γδεζη. The γ, δ and ε subunits exist as monomers while ζ exists as a homodimer in 90% of TCR. The η subunit exists as a heterodimer with ζ in 10% of TCR only on T lymphocytes. The CD3 molecule is essential for TCR activity. Transmembrane domains of the CD3 molecule contain an aspartic acid residue for interaction with lysine on αβ or γδ polypeptide chains. Phosphorylation of CD3 is required for T cell activator leading to cell differentiation and cytokine production.

The genes for antibodies are found on separate chromosomes in three loci, κ and λ L and H chains. Each of the genes contains multiple gene segments encoding polypeptides separated by noncoding regions. The noncoding regions or introns contain regulatory sequences that control gene recombination. During B cell development and maturation the DNA encoding antibody expression undergoes a number of recombination events which generate specificity in the variable region at the N terminus resulting in diversity in antibody recognition of antigen. The TCR genes undergo similar gene rearrangements. Both antibody and TCR genes have multiple variable (V), diversity (D) and joining (J) gene segments. Following recombination, the rearranged variable region joins the constant region genes of the antibody or TCR molecule. Four multigene families encode the αβ and γδ TCR polypeptide chains. Each chain consists of V and C regions.

The α and γ gene families contain V and J genes used to form the variable region of the TCR. Both β and δ gene families contain V, D and J genes in the variable region of the TCR (Fig. 13.1). Each TCR polypeptide contains two constant region

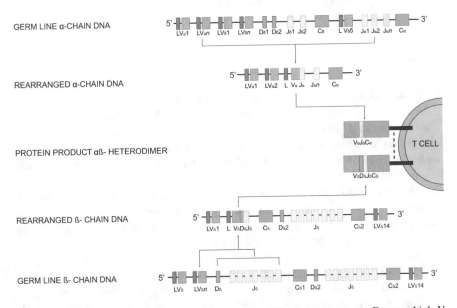

Fig. 13.1 Germline organization and rearrangement of αβ T cell receptor genes. From multiple V (D) J genes, recombination and rearrangements take place in the α and β genes to generate the variable region for antigen binding. The V regions are combined with constant region genes to encode the full α and β chains

genes with the TCR expressed in association with CD3. In order to generate the level of antibody and TCR diversity required for antigen binding, multiple germline V, D and J genes are used to form the variable region on TCR polypeptides. Recombination between V, D, and J gene segments forms the H chain in the antibody molecule and in the beta and delta polypeptide chains in TCR. Recombination between V and J gene segments forms the L chain in the antibody molecule and in the alpha and gamma polypeptides of TCR. The delta chain D, J and C genes lie in between V alpha and J alpha genes. In TCR recombination, multiple D joining occurs (VDDJ). Insertion of N nucleotide additions (non-germ line) and varied combinations of heavy and light chain polypeptides occur. Somatic hypermutations (SHM) of V chain occurs in B cells but does not occur in T cells.

Alpha/Beta TCR

TCR alpha/beta heterodimer associates with gamma/delta/epsilon CD3 core complex in the ER and then moves to the Golgi for modification of N-linked oligosaccharides and then to the plasma membrane. The core CD3 complex is synthesized in excess while the zeta (ζ) chain is synthesized in limited amounts. The cytoplasmic protein ω (omega = TRAP; T cell receptor associated protein) associates with incompletely assembled TCR/CD3 complex. TRAP is thought to control the assembly and transport of the TCR/CD3 complex.

Gamma/Delta TCR

The second TCR, also highly diverse, also CD3 associated, has extracellular lg-like V domains and C domains, hinge region, transmembrane and cytoplasmic domains. Transmembrane regions of $\gamma\delta$ contain (+) charged lysine δ chain like α chain contains (+) arginine residue. Amino acid sequence of γ is most like β chain and amino acids of δ most like α. The $\gamma\delta$ heterodimer exist in disulfide and non-covalently linked forms in humans. In mice only the disulfide linked forms are reported. Experiments to study $\gamma\delta$ TCR centered on determining the location and function of cells expressing the receptor. In addition, investigators were interested in finding out what the $\gamma\delta$ TCR recognized. $\gamma\delta$ TCR gene rearrangements occur earlier than $\alpha\beta$ TCR. $\gamma\delta$ TCR expressing cells appear to be a distinct lineage. Mature $\alpha\beta$ T cells may contain unrearranged or aberrantly rearranged gamma/delta genes. Most $\gamma\delta$ T cells are not MHC restricted or are restricted by non-polymorphic MHC I molecules. In mice and chickens $\gamma\delta$ T cells are found within epithelia and dermis e.g. in the small bowel mucosa in intraepithelial lymphocytes and dendritic epidermal cells respectively. The location of the cells suggests that the $\gamma\delta$ TCR is involved in recognition of antigens coming in contact with epithelial boundaries exposed to the environment. It appears they initiate immune responses to commonly encountered microbial antigens. A non-specific cytotoxic role has been proposed for the $\gamma\delta$ T cells.

Naive or unprimed T cells have high homing tendencies, they extravasate through HEVs into lymph nodes where they make antigen contact. Following activation and blast cell formation. Cells proliferate and then differentiate into effector and memory cells. The effector cells secrete cytokines (TH), e.g. IL-2 known as T cell growth factor or become cytotoxic (Tc). Effector cells die by apoptosis as IL-2 levels decrease. T cell immunity also known as cell mediated immunity generally involves the clearance of intracellular pathogens e.g. viruses, parasites, foreign grafts, tumor cells, and fungi. Cytotoxicity is induced by antigen specific mechanisms. Non-antigen specific cells such as NK cells also participate. This is in contrast to B cell immunity (humoral immunity) that is involved in the clearance of extracellular antigens such as bacterial pathogens. TCR diversity is obtained in the same manner as described for antibody molecules except that somatic hypermutation does not occur in T cells and N-nucleotide terminal additions play a more significant role in generating diversity. RAG- I and RAG-2 genes also play a significant role in TCR rearrangements as in BCR rearrangements. As with B cells, the level of gene rearrangements define the stage of development for the T cell.

T Cell Activation

Naive T lymphocytes become activated following an antigen signal, which is the first signal. The TCR binds to antigen on MHC proteins. For B cells antigens with conformationally defined epitopes or contiguous amino acid sequences bind to the mIg-BCR complex. For T cells the antigen is an internal peptide in association with self MHC. The second signals required for activation are generated from accessory molecules expressed on the surface of the APC such as CD80/CD86 and cytokines such as IL-I secreted from the APC. Expression of CD40 on B cells for interaction with CD40 ligand (CD40L) on T cells also generates cytoplasmic signals required for T cell activation. Adhesion molecules such as LFA-1 on T cells binds to ICAM-1 on APCs. CD2 on T cells binds to LFA-3 on APCs and CD28 on the T cell binds to CD80/CD86. In T cells the TCR has short cytoplasmic tails so that cell signaling is mediated through CD3 subunits whose cytoplasmic tails contain the sequence motif called immunoreceptor tyrosine based activation motif, **ITAM** (Fig. 13.2). Signaling is also mediated through the accessory molecules CD2 and CD45 or through the coreceptors CD4 on T helper cells and CD8 on cytotoxic T cells. Signal transduction occurs through a series of protein phosphorylation–dephosphorylation events which lead to an increase in intracellular calcium levels and activation of transcription factors. Naïve T helper cells undergo differentiation due to polarizing cytokines received from antigen presenting cells like DCs. With the activation of specific transcription factors, polarized T helper subsets secrete effector cytokines that characterizes the helper subset and determines the function of the cell. For example, THI cells are polarized by IL-18, IFNγ and IL-12, and are activated by the master

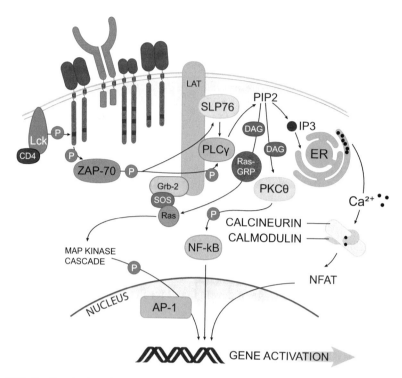

Fig. 13.2 T cell activation. Antigen binding to the T cell receptor (TCR) leads to the phosphorylation of the tyrosine kinases Lck and ZAP-70, leading to the phosphorylation of tyrosines on the ITAMS of the TCR coreceptor molecule CD3 and the adaptor proteins LAT and SLP-76. Docking sites exposed following phosphorylation leads to recruitment of signaling molecules possessing SH2 domains, such as Grb2 and phospholipase Cγ (PLCγ). Phosphorylation and activation of PLCγ leads to the cleavage of PIP2 and the release of IP3 and DAG. The second messenger IP3 stimulates the release of calcium from calcium stores, which binds calmodulin. The phosphatase calcineurin becomes activated by dephosphorylation allowing calcineurin to activate the transcription factor NFAT. DAG binds to protein kinase C theta (PKCθ). The transcription factor NFκB becomes activated by phosphorylation. The adaptor molecule Grb2binds to LAT and recruits members of the Ras pathway activating the MAP kinase (MAPK) pathway. MAP kinases such Erk activates the transcription factor AP-1. The transcription factors translocate into the nucleus and influence the expression of cytokine and cytokine receptor genes

transcription factor T-bet. Effector cytokines secreted by TH1 cells are IFNγ and TNFα. THI cells activate macrophages and promote cell killing of intracellularly infected cells by CD8⁺ cytotoxic T cells. TH2 cells are polarized by IL-4 and the master transcription factor GATA-3 is activated such that TH2 cells secrete the effector cytokines IL-4, IL-5 and IL-13 and activate eosinophils. TH2 responses are made against allergens from helminths with IgE secretion. Other TH subsets include: TH9 with the polarizing cytokines of IL-4 and TGFβ. TH9 cells have the master transcription factor PU.1 and secrete IL-9 as an effector cytokine. TFH cells are polarized by IL-6 and IL-21, express the master transcription factor Bcl-6 and secrete the effector cytokines IL-4 and IL-21. TH17 cells are polarized by TGFβ,

IL-6 and IL-23, express the master transcription factor RORγt and secrete the effector cytokines IL-17A, IL-17F and IL-22. TH22 cells are polarized by IL-6 and TNFα. The master transcription factor is AHR and the effector cytokine secreted is IL-22. TREG cells are polarized in peripheral lymphoid tissue by IL-2, TGFβ and the vitamin A metabolite retinoic acid (RA). Peripheral TREGs (pTREG) express the master transcriptional regulator FoxP3 and secrete the effector cytokines IL-10 and TGFβ. Both cytokines are anti-inflammatory, antitumor and inhibit antigen presenting cells. They can also suppress T cell activity. The absence of pTREGs has been shown to result in autoimmunity.

Following antigen binding to TCR, activated tyrosine kinase Lck phosphorylates tyrosine residues on ITAMs located in the cytoplasmic tails of the TCR coreceptor CD3, leading to the exposure of docking sites for proteins with Src homology 2 domain (SH2 domain) such as the tyrosine kinase ZAP-70. Lck is first dephosphorylated by CD45, a membrane-associated tyrosine phosphatase. This positions Lck to become activated by phosphorylation by other Lck molecules. Lck phosphorylates and activates CD3 and ZAP-70 which phosphorylates the adaptor protein linker protein of activated T cells (LAT) and SH2 domain containing leukocyte protein of 76 kDa (SLP-76). Docking sites exposed on LAT and SLP-76 provide SH2 domain containing proteins like phospholipase Cγ interaction sites as they get recruited to the LAT providing access to phosphatidylinositol 4,5-biphosphate (PIP2) in the membrane. Growth factor receptor bound protein 2 (Grb2), also an adaptor molecule, uses an SH2 domain to bind LAT leading to recruitment of members of the Ras pathway and activation of the MAP kinases RAF, MEK, and ERK. The Ras guanine-nucleotide exchange factor, son of sevenless (SOS) becomes associated with Grb2. The MAP kinases phosphorylate serine residues resulting in activation of the transcription factor AP-1. Phospholipase Cγ hydrolyzes inositol phospholipids such as PIP2 leading to generation of diacylglycerol (DAG) which activates protein kinase C theta (PKCθ) which phosphorylates various cellular substrates to mediate the release of the nuclear factor NFκB, and soluble inositol I,4,5-triphosphate (IP3) which triggers an increase in intracellular calcium followed by the activation of the calmodulin-dependent phosphatase calcineurin.

Calcineurin dephosphorylates the inactive cytosolic form of NFAT which is in the phosphorylated form (T cell specific nuclear factor). Cyclosporin A and FK506 (tacrolimus) inhibit dephosphorylation of NFAT and thereby inhibits T cell activation. This leads to a depressed immune response. Signal transduction and second messenger generation lead to activation of tyrosine and serine/threonine protein kinases and protein phosphatases. These kinases and phosphatases catalyze the phosphorylation and dephosphorylation, respectively, of several signal transducing proteins which result in the activation of cytoplasmic transcription factors such as NFAT and NFκB which become translocated into the nucleus resulting in their binding to 5′ regulatory regions of genes e.g. IL-2 gene, IL-2R gene, essential to cell activation. NFAT associates with AP-1 in the nucleus and then binds the IL-2 enhancer. Transcription of the genes leads to protein synthesis. A similar pathway of signaling occurs in B cells. In B cells ITAM sites are present on the cytoplasmic tails of Igα/Igβ. These ITAMs associate with members of the Src and Syk family of tyrosine kinases. Antigen contact with the mIg on B cells leads the BCR to associate with tyrosine kinases resulting in the activation of the B cell.

T Cell Activation Signals

Signal 1: Interaction of Ag/MHC with TCR/CD3
Signal 2: Antigen non-specific co-stimulatory signal from CD28 on the T cell and CD80 on B cell or APC and/or CTLA-4 on the T cell and CD86 (high affinity interaction)
Signal 3: Cytokine secretion from APCs and T cells

B Cell Activation Signals

Signal 1: for T-independent (TI) antigens, TI-1 and TI-2 antigens is the cross-linking of Ag to mIg, for TD antigens interaction with mIg provides a weak first signal, i.e. competence signal
Signal 2: for TI-1 and TI-2 cytokine mediated progression signal which leads to extensive cell proliferation. For TD antigens an additional signal is provided through interaction of CD40 with CD 154 (CD40L, gp39) on TH cell. Membrane receptors are expressed for cytokines, and the interaction of the cytokines with membrane receptors leads to proliferation and differentiation of the B cell.

B-T Cell Cooperation

B cell presentation of antigen to T cells becomes important when Ag concentration is low. At high antigen concentrations Macrophages and dendritic cell are the major APCs.

Antigen-MHC binding to TH cell leads to formation of the T-B conjugate. The Golgi apparatus and microtubule organizing center reorganizes leading to a directional release of TH cytokines to the B cell and the expression of CD154 on the T helper cell. The CD40-CD154 interaction provides contact dependent help-signal 2 for the B cell. In the germinal center, follicular T helper (TFH) cells provide costimulation through CD40 to B cells which also process and present antigen through MHC class II proteins to the TFH. LFA-1 interaction with ICAM-1 provides adhesion between T and B cells. In addition, receptors of the signaling lymphocyte activation molecule (SLAM) family such as SLAMF1, CD84 (SLAMF5), Ly108, Ly109 and SLAM associated protein (SAP) in T cells induce cell signaling and cell activation in the B-T association. Activation and translocation of the transcription factor NFκB into the nucleus, is essential for somatic hypermutation and class switch recombination (isotype switching). In order for cell differentiation to occur, cytokines also need to be present. The cytokines IL-6, and IL-21 induce cell proliferation of B and TFH cells. In B cells, IL-21 promotes isotype switching. Genetic defects or deficiencies in CD40 or CD154 lead to a lack of germinal center formation, isotype switching and decreased somatic hypermutation.

Memory T Cells

Antigen stimulated T helper cells under activation, proliferate and clonally expand to produce effector and memory cells. Memory cells produced vary in tissue location and effector function. Memory T helper and cytotoxic T lymphocytes are produced following antigen activation. Four categories of memory T cells are formed. Central memory T cells (T_{CM}), effector memory T cells (T_{EM}), resident memory T cells (T_{RM}) and stem cell memory T cells (T_{SCM}). T_{EM} and T_{RM} respond rapidly to reinfection, becoming activated, secreting cytokines and able to engage with B cells for antibody production. Each population of memory cells is characterized by the expression of cell surface molecules that allow migration or retention within tissues. T_{CM} cells express CD62L and CCR7 and are localized within secondary lymphoid organs. T_{RM} express CD69 for retention within tissues and CCR7 for retention in lymphoid tissue. T_{EM} express CD62L but not CCR7. T_{SCM} are self-renewing and can develop into other memory T cell populations. They express Fas (CD95) along with other T cells and IL-2Rβ (CD122).

Accessory Molecules for T Cell Activation

Proper T cell activation is dependent on other surface molecules in addition to the TCR/CD3 complex. These are known as accessory molecules and they are non-polymorphic and invariant. Functions of accessory molecules include specifically binding to other ligands on APCs or target host cells. Some accessory molecules increase the strength of adhesion between the T cell and APC and between T cell and host target cell, they may transduce biochemical signals to the interior of the cell, they may function in the regulation of the immune responses enhanced by cytokines and they may also bind to extracellular matrix vascular endothelium. Accessory molecules are members of the integrin or immunoglobulin gene superfamily and they are useful cell surface markers for T cells in pathologic lesions.

Examples of Accessory Molecules

CD2

Single glycosylated 50 kD protein, high degree of homology among species, 60% of homology in cytoplasmic tail.

Has N-linked extracellular domain, transmembrane region, proline-rich cytoplasmic domain. Binds LFA-3, recognizes homologous glycoprotein on sheep red blood cells (SRBCs). This is the basis for the SRBC rosetting assay for the identification of T cells. Functions in signal transduction in association with TCR/CD3.

CD4

55 kD transmembrane glycoprotein, monomer on peripheral T cells and in thymocytes, invariant, binds non-polymorphic part of MHC class II in beta 2 domain. Also on macrophages in humans. Possesses four extracellular lg domains, transmembrane, long cytoplasmic tail that can be phosphorylated. A cell-cell adhesion molecule, may function in signal transduction. CD4 associates with p55lck, bringing it closer to ITAMS. Required for functional T cell response to class II MHC. An important molecule when there is a low TCR affinity when its adhesive property becomes critical. Point of attachment and receptor for HIV virus.

CD8

Exists as disulfide linked alpha/beta heterodimer, alpha/alpha homodimer or as multimers in association with CD1. The structure varies among species, varies at different stages of T cell maturation. The CD8 binds to alpha 2/alpha 3 domain of MHC class I. Each chain consists of a single extracellular lg, transmembrane region, cytoplasmic tail with phosphorylation sites. Same function as CD4. Increased avidity of cell-cell interactions. Possesses regulatory function, i.e. associates with T cell specific tyrosine kinase, bringing it in close proximity with the TCR/CD3 zeta chain. Both CD4 and CD8 can be phosphorylated by protein kinase C following antigen activation of T cells.

CD45 [CD45R]

Binds to CD22 on APC. Known as leukocyte common antigen with a variable molecular weight of 180–240 kD.

Possesses three isoforms (alternatively spliced forms); CD45RO, CD45RA. Differential splicing events generate eight transcripts. Complex regulation of splicing events with O-glycosylation contributing to different functional epitopes seen on different cell types. CD45 is a membrane associated tyrosine phosphatase found in different leukocytes, but important for T cell activation due to its activity in dephosphorylating the tyrosine kinase Lck and initiation of the activation of signaling molecules following antigen binding to the TCR. CD45 possesses a large cytoplasmic domain, functions in transmembrane signaling, associated with cytoskeleton. Anti-CD45 antibody inhibits T cell activation and regulates signal transduction.

Other accessory molecules with co-stimulatory function during cell activation include **B7-1 (CD80)**, **B7-2 (CD86)** which binds to **CD28** on naïve T cells, inducible costimulatory **(ICOS)** which binds **ICOSL** on memory and effector T cells but not on naïve T cells. **CD154 (CD40L)** on T cells binds to **CD40** on APCs. CD19, CD21 and CD22 are costimulatory molecules on B cells.

CTLA-4 is a coinhibitory receptor molecule that binds to CD80/CD86. Programmed cell death 1 **(PD-1, CD 279)** is another inhibitory molecule that binds **PD-L1** (B7-H1) and **PD-L2** (B7-DC). B and T lymphocytes attenuator (BTLA or CD272) is expressed on diverse cells mostly on B cells. BTLA binds to herpes virus entry mediator (HVEM).

Adaptors

Linker protein of activated T cells (LAT)
  SH2 domain containing leukocyte protein of 76 kDa (SLP-76)
  Growth factor receptor-bound protein 2 (Grb2)

Second Messengers

IP3 (see above) enters the endoplasmic reticulum and causes calcium release from internal stores.
  DAG (see above) causes kinase release and activates kinases
  Calcium

Tyrosine Kinases

Lck
  Zeta-chain-associated protein kinase 70 (ZAP-70)
  Guanine nucleotide exchange factor
  Son of sevenless (SOS)
  G proteins are in active (ON) conformation when binding GTP and inactive (OFF) when binding GDP. In the off position components are separate. When in the on position components are induced to assemble.

Selected References

Bhattacharyya ND, Feng CG (2020) Regulation of T helper cell fate by TCR signal strength. Front Immunol 11:624. https://doi.org/10.3389/fimmu.2020.00624

Den Haan JMM, Arens R, van Zelm MC (2014) The activation of the adaptive immune system: Cross-talk between antigen-presenting cells, T cells and B cells. Immunol Lett 162:103–112

Detre C et al (2010) SLAM family receptors and the SLAM-associated protein (SAP) modulate T cell function. Semin Immunopathol. 32:157–171

Murphy K, Weaver C (2017) Janeway's immunobiology, 9th edn. Garland Press, New York

Ngoenkam J, Schamel WW, Pongcharoen S (2017) Selected signalling proteins recruited to the T-cell receptor-CD3 complex. Immunology 153:42–50

Punt J, Stranford SA, Jones PP, Owen JA (2019) Kuby immunology, 8th edn. W.H. Freeman and Company, New York. Chapter 20, Antigen-antibody interactions

Seo W, Taniuchi I (2016) Transcriptional regulation of early T-cell development in the thymus. Eur. J. Immunol. 46:531–538

Zhu J, Paul WE (2008) CD4 T cells: Fates, functions, and faults. Blood 112:1557–1569

Chapter 14
Cytokines

Innate and adaptive immune responses are coordinated by cytokines and their interactions with cytokine receptors on a variety of cells including dendritic cells, B and T lymphocytes. Cell signaling due to ligation of cytokines with their receptors results in cell growth, differentiation and cell migration. Cytokines are small proteins secreted by cells in the body. Most are secreted by leukocytes and have a variety of functions in the immune system. Interleukins (IL) and interferons (IFN) are examples of cytokines produced by cells following infection by pathogens such as bacteria, viruses and parasites. Cytokines are antigenically nonspecific, low molecular weight proteins possessing regulatory functions. Picomolar concentrations of cytokines can mediate biological activity. The intensity and duration of the immune response is regulated by cytokines. Cytokines participate in signal transduction and intercellular communications. Cytokines mediate effects on target cells in ways similar to hormone action on cells and are therefore considered molecular messengers that facilitate communication between and among cells at varying distances from the source of secretion. The same cell secreting a cytokine can express receptors to bind to the cytokine in an **autocrine** manner. Secreted cytokines may exert their effects on neighboring cells or cells in the vicinity, in a **paracrine** manner or cytokines may be secreted directly into the blood stream and transported to target cells distant from the source of secretion in an **endocrine** manner. Cytokines mediate effector functions on target cells by binding to receptors expressed on the surface of target cells. Following the binding of cytokines to their receptors, signals are transduced to the interior of the cell (signal transduction) leading to the activation and translocation into the nucleus of transcription factors that influence the expression of genes in the cell. Genes expressed can cause cells to grow, proliferate, migrate or adhere to cells and tissue. Gene expression mediated by cytokine binding can lead to the secretion of additional cytokines and expression of cytokine receptors in the target cells, leading to cascades of cell activation that are involved in functions such as hematopoiesis, inflammation and apoptosis. Several cytokines can act on a target cell to effect the same function such as causing the cell to divide or proliferate. This is known as **redundancy** of cytokine function. Cytokines can also

© Springer Nature Switzerland AG 2021
T. Y. Sam-Yellowe, *Immunology: Overview and Laboratory Manual*,
https://doi.org/10.1007/978-3-030-64686-8_14

mediate inhibitory or **antagonistic** effects on cell activity. A single cytokine can mediate the same effect or **pleiotropic** effects on different cells. Additionally, two or more cytokines can act **synergistically** on the same target cell to exert the same effect.

Cytokine Receptor Families

All known cytokines are categorized into six families based on the type of receptors used by the cytokines. The interleukin-1cytokine family contains proinflammatory cytokines that are secreted by monocytes, macrophages and dendritic cells. The IL-1 receptor consists of membrane bound dimers possessing a cytoplasmic domain (TIR domain) used for signal transduction. Soluble receptors also exist in the family. Members of the IL-1 family include IL-1α, IL-1β, IL-18 and IL-33. The largest family of cytokines is the hematopoietin or class 1 family. Family members share receptors that consist of multiple subunits. Many are secreted by T lymphocytes and have effects during hematopoiesis and cell development, proliferation and differentiation of T and B lymphocytes following antigen binding and antibody secretion by B cells. Examples of class 1 cytokines include; IL-2, 3, 4, 5, 6, 7, 9, 12, 13, 15, granulocyte-monocyte colony stimulating factor (GM-CSF). Some members of the family share common receptor subunits γc, βc and gp130 (forming subfamilies within this large family) that associate with an α subunit. A characteristic structural feature of class 1 family members is the presence of four helix bundles in the protein structure and the WSXWS (Trp-Ser-Xaa-Trp-Ser) motif found in the extracellular domain of the receptor (Xaa can be any other amino acid). The interferon or class 2 family consists of cytokines important in innate immunity of viral infections and mediation of cell-mediated immunity. The receptor for class 2 cytokines is a heterodimer, with similar signaling cascades found in class1 receptors. Class 2 receptors share conserved cysteine residues. Some of the cells secreting class 2 cytokines are also antigen presenting cells (APCs), involved in presenting antigen to naïve T lymphocytes. In the APCs, expression of major histocompatibility complex (MHC) proteins expression is enhanced by the interferons. Three types of interferons are represented within the family. The type 1 interferons include IFNα and IFNβ secreted by macrophages and dendritic cells, type 2 interferon is IFNγ secreted by T lymphocytes and natural killer cells and type 3 interferon is IFNλ secreted by plasmacytoid dendritic cells. Members of the TNF family include TNFα, TNFβ (Lymphotoxin, LTα), CD40L, CD95L, BAFF and APRIL. Macrophages, lymphocytes, fibroblasts are examples of cells secreting TNF family cytokines. The family includes both soluble (decoy receptors) and membrane bound cytokines mediating proliferation and survival signals as well as death signals for apoptosis (programmed cell death). Trimers of cytokines bind to trimerized receptors on the target cells. Signal transduction mediates cell adhesion, differentiation, inflammation and apoptosis. Chemokine receptors possess a 7 transmembrane domains; 7-pass membrane proteins coupled to a G protein (G-protein coupled receptors, GPCRs) through which signaling occurs. Conserved cysteines in the receptor, define the class of receptor within the chemokine family. Chemokines have chemoattractant properties which influence cell movement (chemotaxis) and adhesion to the endothelia and to tissues. CCR chemokine receptors bind to corresponding CC chemokines. For example, CCL2 (monocyte chemoattractant protein 1, MCP-1), binds CCR2B and recruits monocytes, dendritic cells, T cells, NK cells and basophils. CCL3 (macrophage inflammatory protein 1α, MIP-1α) secreted by monocytes and T cells binds to CCR1, CCR3 and CCR5 and results in the recruitment of monocytes, dendritic cells and T cells. CCL5 (regulated upon activation, normal T cell expressed and secreted, RANTES) binds CCR1, CCR3 and CCR5. CXCR chemokine receptors bind to corresponding CXC chemokines. CXCL1 secreted by monocytes attracts neutrophils expressing CXCR2. CXCL8 (IL-8) is secreted by endothelial and epithelial cells, monocytes and macrophages and recruits T cells and neutrophils expressing CXCR1 and CXCR2. The receptor CXXXCR (CX_3CR1) expressed on monocytes and T cells binds to CX3CL1 (fractalkine) secreted by monocytes endothelial cells and microglial cells. Several types of leukocytes including B and T lymphocytes and granulocytes secrete chemokines. The newest cytokine family is the IL-17 receptor family. IL-17 interaction with the IL-17 mediates inflammatory reactions. Cytokine function is mediated through binding of the cytokine to cytokine receptors and the induction of cytoplasmic signaling resulting in nuclear translocation of transcription factors. Cytokine signaling pathway is discussed in Chap. 15.

Selected References

Huang L, Avery A (2015) The signaling symphony: T cell receptor tunes cytokine-mediated T cell differentiation. J Leukoc Biol 97:477–485

Liongue C, Sertori R, Ward AC (2016) Evolution of cytokine receptor signaling. J Immunol 197:11–18

Murphy K, Weaver C (2017) Janeway's immunobiology, 9th edn. Garland Press, New York

Olsen JG, Kragelund BB (2014) Who Climbs the tryptophan ladder? On the structure and function of the WSXWS motif in cytokine reeptors and thrombospondin repeats. Cytokine Growth Factor Rev 25:337–341

Punt J, Stranford SA, Jones PP, Owen JA (2019) Kuby immunology, 8th edn. W.H. Freeman and Company, New York

Chapter 15
Lymphocyte Signals

Signal Transduction in Lymphocytes

Cell communication is not just in the immune system. Signal transduction is universal. We have discussed cell signaling in the innate (TLR signaling) and adaptive immune response (T and B cell signaling) and by now we notice that the signaling pathways are very similar. The final event in the signaling pathway is effecting a change that affects gene expression through the activity of transcription factors. **The receptor–ligand interaction is the first step. The receptor amplifies and transfers the message to the cell interior**. What is important to know about each signaling pathway? Knowing the type of cell and the receptor expressed, coreceptors, the location of the cell, initiator signaling molecules, adaptor platform, recruited molecules and the transcription factors generated. It all begins with the ligand binding to its receptor. For example, antigen to BCR, antigen to TCR, cytokine to cytokine receptor, IgE to FcεRI, lipopeptide to TLR1/TLR2 and Fas to FasL. In this chapter, we review the key aspects of the major signaling pathways in lymphocytes. Figure 15.1 shows the key aspects of cytoplasmic signaling following ligand binding to membrane receptors. We review those features again to highlight features that are similar and those features that are unique to each cell type. We discuss cytokine signaling and Fc receptor mediated signaling in mast cells to emphasize the universality of the general aspects of the pathways. When there are no signals the pathways are OFF, meaning only basal activity is present in the cells for the pathways. The pathway of signal transduction follows this general scheme: Ligand binds receptor → signal is transduced though receptor → adaptor proteins (contain SH2, SH3 domains) are recruited → recruit other signaling proteins and bring them to receptor → activate kinases → activate transcription factors → transcription factors translocate into nucleus → gene transcription.

© Springer Nature Switzerland AG 2021
T. Y. Sam-Yellowe, *Immunology: Overview and Laboratory Manual*,
https://doi.org/10.1007/978-3-030-64686-8_15

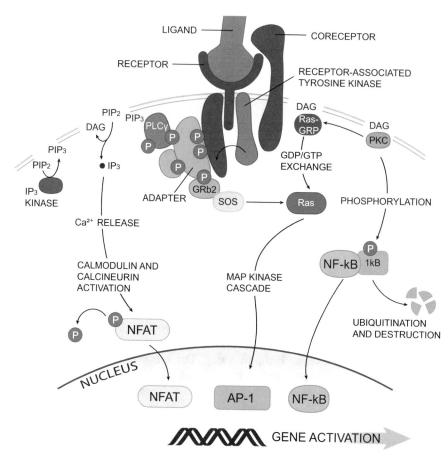

Fig. 15.1 Lymphocyte signaling is initiated by ligand binding to membrane receptors, many of which are associated with coreceptor molecules that may possess long cytoplasmic tail containing ITAMs suitable for phosphorylation and activation to induce cytoplasmic signal transduction. Receptor binding leads to clustering of signaling molecules in the membrane to form lipid rafts. Easy access and exposure of activated domains following phosphorylation by serine-tyrosine kinases leads to recruitment of adaptor molecules, which are also activated and serve as platforms for the binding of other signaling molecules. Some common themes include the cleavage of PIP2 by PLCγ and the generation of the second messengers, DAG and IP3. Calcium release by IP3 leads to binding to calmodulin, which binds to the phosphatase calcineurin. Calcineurin dephosphorylates NFAT, a transcription factor that translocates into the nucleus. Diacylglycerol (DAG) activates PKC leading to events that activate the cytosolic molecule NFκB allowing its translocation into the nucleus. Recruitment of the guanosine exchange factors RasGRP and SOS leads to the activation of Ras which activates the MAP kinase pathway and the generation of the transcription AP-1. Entry of the transcription factors into the nucleus influences gene expression of genes encoding cytokines, cytokine receptors and antibodies in B cells

T Cell Receptor/CD3 Complex

TCR/CD3/CD4 (CD8)

Antigen/MHC association with TCR/CD3 leads to conformational changes that bring co-receptors together in close proximity. This is known as co-receptor aggregation. Immunoreceptor tyrosine based activation motifs (ITAMs) on cytoplasmic tails of TCR associated CD3 polypeptides have phosphorylation sites. There are also regulatory sites for ITAMs known as immunoreceptor tyrosine-based inhibitory motifs (ITIMs). ITAMs were first described on the lg alpha and lg beta chains associated with the B cell receptor. ITAMs consist of a motif containing tyrosines (Y) separated by 9-12 amino acids. ITAMs are phosphorylated by protein kinases of the Src family such as Lck, Blk, Lyn and Fyn. Following initial activation additional kinases (Tec kinases) are activated, leading to recruitment of phospholipase C gamma which then hydrolyzes phosphatidylinositol 4, 5 biphosphate (PIP2) leading to the generation of IP3 and DAG and calcium release → these act as second messengers. CD45 is a protein tyrosine phosphatase that dephosphorylates Lck and Fyn in order to activate them. Phosphorylation of the kinases at an inhibitory site **inactivates (Off position)** the kinase. The inhibitory phosphate needs to be removed to **activate (On position)** the kinase. Following dephosphorylation the kinases can then phosphorylate the ITAMs on the TCR/CD3 and phosphorylate ZAP-70 which is recruited and binds to zeta chain of CD3. Clustering of receptors allows the external (Ag) signals to be converted to intracellular signals leading to a change in gene expression. This is a direct result of transcription factors that enter the nucleus. Conversion of the signals leads to activation of the transcription factors. Tyrosine kinase Lck activates ZAP-70 which then activates SLP-76 and LAT (Linker of activation in T cells). LAT associates with cholesterol and lipids on the cytoplasmic site of the plasma membrane. This leads to lipid raft formation. G protein mediated signaling using the mitogen- activated protein kinase (MAP kinase) pathway leads to the activation of transcription factors like Fos/Jun in the AP-1 family.

B Cell Receptor Complex

The B cell receptor complex consists of BCR, CD19, CD21 and CD81 (TAPA-1). Syk and Src kinases together with the BCR complex (signalosome) function in the cell leading to recruitment of downstream molecules that transmit signals. CD19 on the BCR complex binds to an adaptor protein Vav that contains a guanine nucleotide exchange factor (GEF). Vav is a signaling molecule that has several functions. The activity of Vav leads to the activation of Rac, a G protein. This is followed by MAP kinase activation and the generation of transcription factors. The molecule BLNK (B cell linker protein) acts like LAT in T cells. These molecules possess multiple sites for tyrosine phosphorylation. The kinases Lyn and phosphatidylinositol 3-OH kinase (PI 3 kinase) function in B cell activation.

Cytokine/Chemokine Receptor

Signaling following cytokine binding occurs through receptor associated kinases of the Janus kinase (JAK kinase) family (Fig. 15.2). JAKs function by phosphorylating STATs (signal transducers and activators of transcription). STATs are a family of transcription factors that bind to phosphorylated tyrosine residues. STAT 1 is a well-studied example. JAKs can also be activated through phosphorylation by other JAKs. A good example is found in the interferon gamma receptor. The interferon gamma receptor consists of an alpha and beta chain, with a conserved CCCC motif. The alpha chain interacts with JAK 1 and the beta chain interacts with JAK 2. The alpha chain is involved in cytokine binding and signaling while the beta chain is also

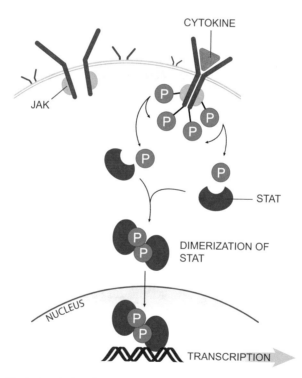

Fig. 15.2 The illustration depicts the general mechanisms of signal transduction of most class 1 and 2 cytokine receptor family members. Binding of the cytokine to the heterodimeric receptor molecule in the cell membrane leads to receptor dimerization and activation of cytoplasmic domains in the receptor by phosphorylation and recruitment of Janus kinases (JAK) and signal transducer and activation of transcription (STAT). JAK kinases phosphorylate the STATs which dimerize and translocate into the nucleus where they influence gene expression

involved in signaling with a limited role in binding. Both JAK 1 and JAK 2 become activated following phosphorylation. JAK 1 phosphorylates JAK 2 on the beta subunit while JAK 2 phosphorylates JAK 1 on the alpha subunit. As indicated above, JAKs create a docking site for STATs which bind and then becomes phosphorylated by JAKs. The STATs bind to the receptor subunits through joining of the SH2 domains on STAT with the docking site generated by JAK mediated phosphorylation.

JAKs create docking sites for STAT transcription factors. Once phosphorylated, STATs form dimers, either homodimers or heterodimers and in the dimerized state move from the docking sites into the nucleus where they influence gene expression through the transcription of specific genes. The particular combination of JAKs and STATs following receptor- mediated activation by a cytokine determines the specificity of that cytokine action. The transcriptional activity of STATs is specific, such that certain STAT dimmers recognize specific sequence motifs and therefore interact with specific gene promoters. Only the target genes expressed by a cell can be activated within a given cell. A given cytokine can induce different genes in different cells depending on the pathways that are activated within the cell.

FcεRI Receptor on Mast Cells

When IgE binds to the high affinity FcεRI, cytoplasmic signaling occurs with the use of similar signaling molecules as are found in B and T lymphocytes. The receptor consist of three subunits, an α, β and γ subunits. The ITAM is located on the cytoplasmic tail of the Fc γ. The Fc region of IgE binds to the α subunit. As with BCR and TCR signaling, Src-family tyrosine kinases phoshorylate the ITAMs and initiate signaling. The tyrosine kinase Fyn is activated in mast cells. An important difference in the calcium dependent signaling events in the mast cell, is that vesicle fusion to the cell membrane and degranulation takes place. Additionally, generation of inflammatory mediators such as prostaglandins and leukotrienes, following cleavage of phospholipids by phospholipase A2 in the membrane also occurs.

Examples of kinases associated with receptors:
Tyrosine kinases
Serine kinases
Threonine kinases
Serine/Threonine kinases
Protein kinase C (PKC)
MAP kinases

Binding sites contain src homology (SH) domains such as SH2, SH3. Binding of proteins to these sites recruits and assembles other molecules involved in signaling. Proline rich motifs on proteins recognize the SH3 domain. Other proteins involved in signaling mentioned above are adaptor proteins. The adaptor proteins function to connect the signaling events between receptors and specific pathways that use common signaling molecules. Other adaptor proteins include Shc, Grb2 and GADS. These molecules form a complex to carry out their functions. GTP binding proteins also function in signaling. These are small or large G proteins. The small G proteins are Ras and Rac. The G proteins are molecular switches (on/off). Their activation is mediated by guanine nucleotide exchange factors (GEFs). GEFs are typically bound to adaptor proteins. G proteins get activated then following their activation, they activate proteins kinases such as MAP kinases. This leads to the activation of transcription factors.

Selected References

Cantrell D (2015, 2015) Signaling in lymphocyte activation. Cold Spring Harb Perspect Biol:7, a018788

Huang L, Avery A (2015) The signaling symphony: T cell receptor tunes cytokine-mediated T cell differentiation. J Leukoc Biol 97:477–485

Liongue C, Sertori R, Ward AC (2016) Evolution of cytokine receptor signaling. J Immunol 197:11–18

Wu LC (2011) Immunoglobulin E receptor signaling and asthma. J Biol Chem 286:32,891–32,897

Chapter 16
Complement Fixation

There are over 50 complement proteins found in the serum. These are heat labile proteins involved in a cascade activity (a chain reaction of proteins) generated by a number of serine proteases among the components. The end result of the enzyme cascade in three different pathways, is the insertion of a membrane attack complex in cell membranes that results in the lysis of target cells. The initiation components of the three pathways of complement activation (complement fixation) are different. However, there are components that are shared by the three pathways, including the formation of the membrane attack complex (MAC). The proteins C1-C9 are found in the **classical pathway**, an antibody dependent pathway important in adaptive immunity. The components C2-C9, including mannose-binding lectin (MBL) and MBL-associated serine proteases (MASP) 1, 2 and 3 are found in the **lectin pathway** and the proteins C3, Factor B, Factor D and properdin (Factor P) are found in the **alternate pathway** (Fig. 16.1). Following activation of the pathways, biologically active components are generated from the C1, C2, C3, C4, C5 and Factor B. Complement activation is a highly regulated process. Complement activation through the alternative and lectin pathway act as significant effectors of inflammation in the body. The classical pathway is initiated by antibody, typically IgM binding to complement component C1. MBL binding to carbohydrate moieties on bacterial surfaces initiates the lectin pathway and for the alternate pathway, properdin or C3b generated from complement component C3 can bind to bacterial surfaces initiating the alternative pathway. Following C3b binding to microbial surfaces, Factor B binds to C3b and is then cleaved by Factor D to generate the biologically active fragments Ba and Bb. The complement proteins consist of proteins and glycoproteins, some with enzymatic activity following the cleavage of components C3 and C5.

Complement component C9 is related to the perforins contained in cytotoxic T lymphocytes and NK cells. Both groups of proteins insert complexes into the plasma membranes resulting in cell destruction. Although complement activation and lysis is nonspecific both self and non-self tissue can be recognized (see below). We will discuss the three pathways of complement fixation. The antibody dependent

© Springer Nature Switzerland AG 2021
T. Y. Sam-Yellowe, *Immunology: Overview and Laboratory Manual*,
https://doi.org/10.1007/978-3-030-64686-8_16

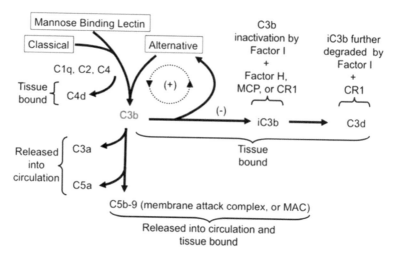

Fig. 16.1 Illustration of the three pathways of complement fixation. The classical, lectin and alternative pathways are shown. All pathways utilize complement component C3 which is cleaved to generate C3a, a soluble fragment and C3b, a tissue bound fragment. After cleavage of complement component C5 to generate C5a and C5b, assembly of the membrane attack complex (MAC) is initiated by C5b to assemble, C6, C7, C8 and multiple components of C9 to form the pore which is inserted into the cell membrane. [*Republished with permission of Elsevier publishing from Thurman, J. M. (2015) "Complement in kidney disease: Core curriculum 2015." Am J Kidney Dis, 65:156–168, Fig. 1. Conveyed through STM permission guidelines 2020*]

pathway and two antibody independent pathways, important for innate immunity. In our discussion, we want to be able to distinguish the three pathways, recognize the functions of the complement system and know how the pathways are regulated. The three pathways share three major steps. These are initiation, activation and membrane attack complex. Both initiation and activation steps possess enzymatic activity, while the membrane attack complex involves non-enzymatic assembly of complement components. The functions of the complement system comprise three major categories. Opsonization, resulting in phagocytosis, neutralization and clearance of soluble and deposited immune complexes, leukocyte activation through chemotaxins and anaphylatoxins and lysis of target cells.

Classical pathway: This pathway requires antibody for activation. The C1q component of the C1 complex binds IgM or IgG. A single molecule of IgM can activate the complement pathway. **Complement proteins:**

C1 (C1q, C1s, C1r), C2, C3, C4, C5, C6, C7, C8, C9

C3 and C5 convertase (major enzymes in the pathway)

C1q is part of a lectin family of proteins known as **collectins (collagenous lectins)**. The mannan (mannose) binding lectin MBL belongs in the same family.

Within the classical complement pathway inactive proteases (zymogens) become active and cleave and activate substrates sequentially in the pathway. Conformational changes take place in the molecules as they interact and cleavage occurs. Two new enzymes are formed in the pathway. Complement components are found in serum and can interact with antibodies in immune complexes (IC) in the case of the classical pathway or bind to microbial surfaces. Fragments released following substrate cleavage diffuse away and bind to complement receptors on phagocytic cells like macrophages. The classical pathway of complement fixation is initiated when antibody that is bound to an antigen binds to the C1 component of complement. The C1 component is a complex of proteins consisting of C1q, a large multisubunit protein with 18 polypeptides and the two copies of the serine proteases C1r and C1s (C1qr2s2). Antibody in an immune complex binds to the C1q component using the CH2 domain in the Fc region of the antibody resulting in activation of the serine protease C1r which then activates C1s. The substrate for C1s is complement component C4, which is cleaved to yield the small fragment C4a and large fragment C4b. Fragment C4b binds to C2 positioning it for cleavage by C1s to yield large fragment C2a and the small fragment of C2b. Fragment C4b combines with C2a to form the complex C4bC2a which has enzymatic activity in the C2a fragment. This complex is known as C3 convertase, the first new enzyme formed in the pathway. Once formed, C3 convertase is associated with IC and may also be on microbial or other pathogen surfaces as well as on cell membranes. C3 convertase cleaves C3 to generate the small C3a fragment and large C3b fragment. This step in the pathway is amplified due to the large number of C3b molecules that can be generated. Fragment C3b binds to C3 convertase to generate a new complex with enzymatic activity, C4b2a3b known as C5 convertase. The C3b fragment in the complex binds to C5, resulting in the cleavage of C5 to yield the small fragment C5a and the large fragment C5b. After the formation of C5 convertase, no additional enzymes are formed as downstream components C6, C7, C8 and C9 bind to the complex to form the membrane attack complex (MAC). Individual components of C6, C7 and C8 bind to the complex. However, multiple C9 components are required to form the pore that is inserted into cell membranes leading to cell lysis. The small complement fragments formed from enzymatic cleavage diffuse away from the pathway to bind receptors on cell surfaces. Fragments C3a and C5a are anaphylatoxins that can bind to complement receptors on neutrophils resulting in inflammation. In addition to participating in the pathway towards the formation of MAC, fragments C3b and C4b can also bind to complement receptors and act as opsonins to facilitate the phagocytosis of pathogens and IC.

Alternative pathway (also known as **properdin pathway; alternate pathway; tick over activation**): This pathway is important in innate immunity. C3 found in the serum is converted to C3a and C3b due to spontaneous lysis in the serum. C3b once generated can bind to antigens on bacterial (gram positive and gram negative) cell walls including lipopolysaccharide (LPS), capsule antigens, teichoic acids from bacterial cell walls or fungal cell wall antigens (zymosan), parasites and viruses. In addition, carbohydrates, polymers such as dextran sulfate and cobra venom factor can also activate this pathway.

C3 and C5 convertase are also formed in this pathway. They contain the fragment Bb unlike the enzymes of the classical pathway. The C3 convertase in this pathway is more labile than that found in the classical pathway. It decays rapidly. Factor P binds to both C3 and C5 convertase enzymes to stabilize them. Bb generated by the cleavage of factor D remains bound to C3b. The fragment C3b is generated continuously at low levels in what is referred to as the **amplification loop.** Additional proteins not found in the classical pathway are **factor B, factor D and factor P** (properdin). Although this pathway is antibody independent, immune complexes containing human IgA, IgE and IgG have been reported to activate this pathway. Aggregated globulins all high in carbohydrate also activate the alternative pathway.

Lectin pathway: This pathway is also antibody independent. Although components of the pathway have been known for some time, the understanding that the components can activate the complement pathway is fairly new. Like the alternative pathway, the lectin pathway is a significant component of the innate immune system. Following the binding of mannose binding lectins (MBL) to mannose residues on the surface of pathogens, the pathway becomes activated. MBL is structurally similar to C1q while the serine protease MBL associated serine proteases (MASP and MASP2) that interacts with MBL is similar to C1r and C1s. Typically the mannose residues are found on carbohydrates on glycoproteins. During inflammation MBL is produced (an acute phase proteins) and it can then bind to the surface of the pathogen. MASP binds to MBL leading to the cleavage of C4. C1q is able to bind directly to some microorganisms. The three pathways have in common the **activity of C3** leading to the formation of the membrane attack complex C5b6789, which includes several C9 components, which insert holes into the plasma membrane of the target cell. When we discuss the effector functions of immunity in hypersensitivities and autoimmunity we will examine functions of the complement system in disease. Opsonization of antigens and target cells for phagocytosis, participation of small fragments of complement components in inflammation (the small fragments, C4a, C3a, C5a; these fragments are also important chemotactic agents and anaphylatoxins), cell lysis and clearance of immune complexes (ICs) make up major functions of complement fixation. The most important function also seen in individuals with certain autoimmune diseases and parasitic diseases is the clearance of immune complexes. Clearance of ICs is dependent on the presence of complement receptors on macrophages. Receptors can also be found on other cell types such as neutrophils, basophils, mast cells, B and T cells, some dendritic cells.

Complement receptor proteins are expressed on cell surfaces and bind to ligands which are the complement proteins resulting in signal transduction within cells, and enhancing phagocytosis of opsonized pathogens. Inflammatory reactions are mediated by the binding of complement protein fragments to cell surface receptors. For example, C5a binding to the C5a receptor induces anaphylatoxic reactions. Other complement receptors are shown below:

CR1 (CD 35) binds C3b and C4b
CR2 (CD21) binds smaller fragments of C3 cleavage known as C3d, C3dg and iC3b
CR3 (CD11a/CD18) bind to iC3b (inactivated C3b)
C3a/C4a receptor
CR4 (CD11c/CD18) bind to iC3b (inactivated C3b)
The fragment iC3b is formed following cleavage by a regulatory component known as factor I.

Regulation of the Complement Pathway

Complement components are unstable outside of the pathway. Once the components participate in the pathway, there has to be some way of controlling their activity.

Complement components are nonspecific in their activity. Also once the MAC is formed the resulting lysis can be damaging to nearby innocent bystander cells. A number of regulatory features have developed to either inactivate complement components or block their activity once they are no longer required.

Examples of Regulatory Proteins

C1 esterase inhibitor (C1INH) permits the dissociation of C1q from C1r2S2. Deficiency of C1INH leads to uncontrolled activation of C4 and C2 resulting in the disorder Hereditary angioneurotic edema (HANE). The disease is transmitted as an autosomal dominant trait. Local edema occurs in various organs such as the gastrointestinal tract, skin and upper respiratory tract. C3 convertase regulatory proteins prevents the assembly of C3 convertase. These proteins contain short consensus repeats (SCRs) of 60 amino acid residues. The genes encoding these proteins are found in a gene cluster termed the regulators of complement activation gene cluster (RCA). In humans this gene cluster is on chromosome 1. Examples of the proteins include the following:

1. Membrane cofactor protein (CD46) (MCP)
2. Complement receptor I (CD35)
3. C4b-binding protein (C4bBP)
     The above three proteins prevent the assembly of C3 convertase which prevents the binding of C3b to factor B and the binding of C4b to C2b. C4b is cleaved to C4d and C4c
4. Decay accelerating factor (DAF) (CD55)
     Permits the dissociation of C3 convertase
5. Complement receptor 2 (CD21)
6. Factor H binds to C3b and prevents its association with factor B
7. Factor I functions with C4bBP, MCP, CRI, factor H and DAF. The additional proteins act as cofactors for factor I activity. Cleaves C3b and C4b. C3b is cleaved to generate iC3b (also written as C3bi) (bound) and C3f (soluble). The fragment iC3b is further cleaved to C3c and C3dg. C4b is cleaved to generate soluble C4c and a bound C4d.
8. Protein S (S protein) binds to C5b67 to prevent membrane insertion by preventing the binding of C9.

Additional proteins which prevent complement lysis of homologous tissue are homologous restriction factor (HRF) and membrane inhibitor of reactive lysis (MIRL (CD59). Both proteins display **homologous restriction.** They bind to C5 on C5b678 and prevent binding and assembly of C9 components. They protect innocent bystander cells from nonspecific lysis. Nucleated cells are more resistant to lysis by complement compared to erythrocytes. The nucleated cells can remove the membrane attack complex by endocytosis and exocytosis of the complement fragments from the MAC. Inhibitors of the anaphylatoxins produced from C4, C3 and CS also regulate the activity of these proteins. Anaphylatoxin activator inhibits the activity of C4a, C3a and C5a. Some of these regulatory proteins function only in the classical pathway, for example, C1INH. For the alternative pathway alone, factor H and other proteins such as DAF, CR1 and Factor I function in all three pathways.

Selected References

Mastellos DC, Reis ES, Ricklin D, Smith RJ, Lambris D (2017) Complement C3-targeting therapy: Replacing long-held assertions with evidence-based discovery. Trends Immunol 38:383–394

Murphy K, Weaver C (2017) Janeway's immunobiology, 9th edn. Garland Press, New York

Punt J, Stranford SA, Jones PP, Owen JA (2019) Kuby immunology, 8th edn. W.H. Freeman and Company, New York. Chapter 20, Antigen-antibody interactions

Ricklin D, Lambris JD (2016) Therapeutic control of complement activation at the level of the central component C3. Immunobiology 221:740–746

Thurman JM (2015) Complement in kidney disease: core curriculum 2015. Am J Kidney Dis 65:156–168

Chapter 17
Cell Mediated Immunity

Cell-Mediated Immunity (T Cell Immunity)

T cell function in adaptive immunity involves effector TH cells which provide cytokine help to B cells for antibody production against T-dependent antigens. A second T cell function involves cytotoxic T cells; CTLs in T cell immunity. CTLs mediate killing of altered host target cells infected with intracellular pathogens or **neoplastic cells**. T cell immunity mediated by CTLs involves the killing of altered host cells by apoptosis. T cell immunity is also referred to as cell-mediated immunity, and involves the activity of cytotoxic effector cells of different types. Cytotoxic T cells (Tc) also called precursor cytotoxic T lymphocytes (CTL-P) are the predominant cell in T cell immunity, aided by T helper cells, in particular TH1 cells. Cytotoxic T cells are CD8+ and have two known subsets, Tc1 and Tc2 differentiated by the cytokines they secrete and the mode of killing employed when interacting with altered host cells. Similar to TH1 and TH2 cells, Tc1 cells secrete IFNγ and Tc2 cells secrete IL-4 and IL-5. Tc1 cells kill by using both the Fas-FasL and perforin-granzyme pathways while Tc2 cell use only the perforin-granzyme pathway. The targets of CTL effects are intracellularly infected host cells, tumor cells, and cells bearing non-self MHC class I proteins (allogeneic antigens) on transplanted tissue. Other cells involved in cytotoxicity include, NK cells, NKT cells and macrophages.

Cell mediated immune reactions occurs within secondary lymphoid organs following Tc contact with antigens presented on MHC class I proteins. Generation of effector CTLs occurs in two phases. In phase 1, naïve Tc (CTL-Ps) become activated after TCR interaction with antigen on MHCI on the surface of antigen presenting cells such as dendritic cells. CD4+ TH1 cells also interacting with the DC provide cytokine help which can enhance the activity of both CTL-Ps and DCs. Dendritic cells can also cross-present antigen to CTL-Ps. Exogenous antigens expressed by intracellular pathogens and tumor cells can be endocytosed, processed in DCs and combined with MHC class I proteins for presentation to CTL-Ps.

© Springer Nature Switzerland AG 2021
T. Y. Sam-Yellowe, *Immunology: Overview and Laboratory Manual*,
https://doi.org/10.1007/978-3-030-64686-8_17

CTL-Ps lack many of the features of differentiated CTLs. CTL-Ps are immature Tc and cannot mediate cell killing. They lack the cytoplasmic granules that contain effector molecules for induction of apoptosis, they do not express the high affinity IL-2Rα chain for IL-2 binding and they also express low levels of the cell adhesion molecule LFA-1. In phase 2, CTL-Ps activated by DC interact with antigen on MHC class I on altered host cells and can secrete cytotoxins and cytokines that facilitate induction of apoptosis in target cells using Fas-FasL interaction and the release of perforins and granzymes at the point of contact between CTL and the host target cell. The cytokines IFNγ and TNF enhance activity of the CTL.

Research evidence demonstrates that three cell interactions can occur simultaneously, where the TH1 cell interacts with a DC that is also bound to a CTL-P. The TH1 interaction licenses the DC to interact with the CTL-P resulting in the activation of the cell. Individually licensed DCs can also activate CTL-Ps leading to their interaction with altered host cells. Both TH1 and CTL-P recognize the same antigen providing a layer of regulation and specificity, such that only the cell targeted for destruction is engaged by the CTL and self- tolerance is maintained. In addition, IL-2R expression after activation of CTL-Ps reduces non-specific attack and destruction of normal cells.

Similar to the activation of T helper cells, CTLs need three signals to enhance cell activation and enhance differentiation of the cells to effector and memory cells. The first signal involves binding of CTL to antigen presented on MHC class I protein by a "licensed" DC. Licensing of the DC occurs through signals generated by CD40 on the DC binding to CD40L on T helper cells. Signaling from TLRs can also mediate the cytokine and chemokine secretion by the DC to enhance activation of CTL. The signaling cascade leads to increased expression of CD80 and CD86 on the surface of DCs and the secretion of cytokines and chemokines. The signal generated by antigen specificity becomes transmitted to the CTL to initiate its activation. The second signal is obtained from ligation of CD28 on the surface of CTL-Ps with CD80 and CD86 on the DCs. This provides co-stimulatory signals. The third signal ensures that the CTL-s can bind to IL-2 produced by TH1 and CD8+ CTL, with the high affinity IL-2R. Full activation, proliferation and differentiation of CTL-P to CTL, necessary for generating effector and memory CTLs depends on IL-2.

In CTL killing by directional release of perforins and granzyme, activated CTLs release pore forming protein monomers known as perforins. They also release serine proteases called granzymes. Upon activation, microtubule organizing centers (MTOCs) also known as centromers develop at the point of synapse between the CTL and host target cell. The MTOC provides a platform for migration of secretory granules (vesicles) containing perforins and granzymes. The vesicles fuse with the membrane and release perforin and granzyme into the space between both cells. Insertion of perforin monomers into the target cell is a calcium and energy dependent process that results in polymerization of perforin into pores inserted into the target cell. Entry of granzymes into the target cell induces the activation of the programmed cell death pathway and activation of caspases resulting in apoptosis of the target cell. The CTL dissociates from the target cell and can initiate attack on another target cell. Cell adhesion molecules are important for efficient CTL attack on target cells. LFA-1 expressed on CTLs bind to ICAM-1 on the host target cell. "Inside-out signaling" in the CTL mediates conformation change on LFA-1 to enhance its binding to ICAM-1. Following interaction of CTL with the target cell, conformation change occurs to allow dissociation of CTL from the host cell. CTLs can also kill by FasL (CD95L) on the CTL interacting with Fas (CD95) on the target host cell. Ligation of FasL-Fas initiates apoptosis. Activation of initiator and executioner caspases occurs leading to cell death by apoptosis. Evidence for the necessity of IL-2 for CTL activity was demonstrated using IL-2 knock-out mice which were shown to be deficient in CTL-mediated cytotoxicity. Perforin knock-out mice were unable to eliminate lymphocytic choriomeningitis virus (LCMV) infection. Interaction of activated CTLs with LFA-1 was seen to be increased compared to CTL-P binding to LFA-1. In in vitro experiments, anti-LFA and anti-ICAM-1 antibodies inhibited CTL binding to wells coated with ICAM-1 demonstrating the requirement for both LFA-1 and ICAM-1 for effective function of CTLs.

Natural killer cells can be activated for cytotoxicity by the use of NK activating receptors expressed on the cell surface or by interaction of IgG with the FcγIII receptor (CD16) also expressed on the cell surface, leading to antibody-mediated cellular cytotoxicity (ADCC). The early activation of NK cells, within 3 days after infection provides killer activity aimed at eliminating infected host or neoplastic cells. CTLs become activated effector cells in 7 days. NK cytotoxicity by ADCC is important for elimination of intracellularly infected host cells and for elimination of tumor cells. NK cells are a heterogeneous group of cells formed from the common lymphoid progenitor cells like in B and T lymphocytes. However, NK cells do not express TCR or BCR. They are larger cells and they contain granules. They do not need prior activation to become effective killer cells and they are not MHC restricted. The cytoplasmic granules in NK cells contain perforins and granzymes. Similar to CTLs, MTOC are formed to aid exocytosis and release of cytotoxic contents at the immunological synapse between the NK cell and altered host cell. NK cells express FasL which they use to bind Fas on the target cell. Licensing of the NK cell occurs to allow cells to properly identify host cells with missing or diminished expression of MHC class I proteins, to ensure targeting and killing of altered host cells and maintaining tolerance to self by not killing normal cells. NK memory cell production has been reported but the characteristics differ from B and T cell memory cell production. NK cells participate in innate and adaptive immunity. The cytokines IFNα, IFNβ and IL-12, considered innate immunity cytokines stimulate the cytotoxicity of NK cells. These cytokines are important in viral infections and are produced early in virus infections. NK cells also secrete IFNγ which enhances macrophage activity, differentiation of T helper cells and stimulation of TH1 differentiation through IL-12 produced by macrophages and DCs. Other cytokines produced include GM-CSF which enhances the recruitment of macrophages. The cytokines produced by NK cells increase the antigen presentation function of macrophages and their phagocytic and antimicrobial activity. Natural killer T cells (NKT cells), also known as invariant NKT cells possess characteristics of NK and CTLs and can also function as helper cells. They can be CD4+ or CD4− and express invariant αβTCR on the cell surface that binds to glycolipid antigen presented on MHC-I related non-polymorphic proteins called CD1. The V region of the TCR on NKTcells is formed by the use of specific Vα, Vβ and Jα regions. Cytotoxicity of NKT cells occurs with the use of FasL-Fas interactions. Cytokine expression depends on the CD4+ or CD4− phenotype of NKT cells. Cytokines secreted include IFNγ, IL-2, IL-4 and TNFα.

Other Cytotoxicity Reactions

Macrophages may bind and destroy cells without phagocytosis. They will release cytotoxic factors. They do this by ADCC reactions. This can be slow or rapid ADCC. The cytotoxicity may be enhanced in the presence of lectins or antibodies. It could be antigen specific or nonspecific. Monocytes, eosinophils, neutrophils, B cells, NK cells can use the Fc receptor for IgG for binding to target cells. These cells will become cytotoxic by ADCC.

Cytotoxicity by macrophages requires IFN γ priming followed by antigen activation. Macrophages become activated. Once activated the cytotoxic cells take on both physiological and morphological changes. Activated macrophages secrete increased amounts of different protein, release TNF alpha, which can activate other macrophages, release increased amounts of proteases, which may activate complement components, secrete IFN gamma, IL-1, thromboplastin, prostaglandins, fibronectins, plasminogen activator, complement components C2 and B and increase MHC expression. Macrophages become enlarged and show increased membrane ruffling and pseudopod formation, increased pinocytosis, and response to chemotactic stimuli. The levels of lysosomal enzymes and respiratory burst metabolites become elevated and phagocytic activity is increased and enhanced killing of intracellular organisms or tumor cells occurs. Macrophages generate reactive nitrogen metabolites such as nitric oxide, and can destroy tumor cells and intracellular parasites. Nitrogen metabolites generated also inhibit contraction of vascular smooth muscle, aggregation and activation of platelets and macrophage protein synthesis. Macrophages express receptors for urokinase under the influence of IFN gamma and TNF alpha. Binding of urokinase to macrophages leads to tissue invasion by macrophages. Activated macrophages can destroy a wide range of normally resistant organisms and develop at the same time delayed hypersensitivity (DTH) develops.

Experimentally a homogeneous population of CTLs can be obtained. E.g. lymphocytes from mice can be sensitized with target cells sharing the same haplotype. CTLs will begin differentiating. The CTLs can then be cloned in the presence of high levels of IL-2. A homogeneous population of CTLs with identical TCRs for the target cell can then be obtained. Distribution of T cell activity in various organs can be determined using MHC-peptide tetramers. Four identical MHC I or MHC II molecules bound to peptide is incubated with fluorescent protein. The fluorescent

MHC tetramer binds to T cells with TCR specific to the peptide. The bound T cell becomes fluorescent and can be identified by flow cytometry. This provides a sensitive way to identify T cells binding to peptide. CTL mediated cytotoxicity-mechanisms can be measured using mixed lymphocyte reactions i.e. MLR (requiring TH cells for IL-2 production and macrophages). In this reaction the stimulation index is measured, by graft-vs-host (GVH) reactions where the spleen index is measured also and by CML.

Selected References

Anderson MH, Schrama D, Straten PT, Becker JC (2006) Cytotoxic T cells. J Investig Dermatol 126:32–41

Goodridge JP, Burian A, Lee N, Geraghty DE (2013) HLA-F and MHC class 1 open conformmers are ligands for NK cell Ig-like receptors. J Immunol 191:3553–3562

Murphy K, Weaver C (2017) Janeway's immunobiology, 9th edn. Garland Press, New York

Punt J, Stranford SA, Jones PP, Owen JA (2019) Kuby immunology, 8th edn. W.H. Freeman and Company, New York. Chapter 20, Antigen-antibody interactions

Wong RSY (2011) Apoptosis in cancer: From pathogenesis to treatment. J Exp Clin Cancer Res 30(87)

Chapter 18
Hypersensitivities

Hypersensitivities are a group of immune-mediated disorders caused by exaggerated immune responses to antigens. Some of the antigens known as allergens bind to IgE bound to Fc receptors on mast cells and basophils. In 1963 Gell and Coombs categorized the different types of hypersensitivity reactions into four types. Three hypersensitivity reactions involve antibody mediated reactions and the fourth is mediated by T cells. There are ongoing efforts to expand the categories to include subtypes of some of the hypersensitivities due to the presence of features that do not fit neatly into the four traditional categories. In this section we will discuss the four traditional categories to highlight how the immune system responds to particular types of antigens. Type I hypersensitivity is known as immediate or IgE-mediated hypersensitivity. Type II hypersensitivity is also known as cytotoxic or IgM/IgG mediated-hypersensitivity. Type III hypersensitivity reaction involves immune complexes formed by IgG/IgM antibodies complexed with soluble antigen. Type IV hypersensitivity is mediated primarily by CD4+ and CD8+ T cells resulting in delayed hypersensitivity reactions.

Type I hypersensitivity is known as IgE-mediated hypersensitivity or immediate type hypersensitivity. Allergens such as pollen, dust mite feces, bee venom and food allergens stimulate IgE production. IgE bound to antigen (allergen), forms cross-linked structures on mast cells and basophils. IgE binds to IgE receptors on cells. Cross-linked complexes are taken up by the cells leading to degranulation of granules within the cells. Type I hypersensitivity reactions generate responses in the skin and airways. Initial exposure to allergen results in the activation of TH2 cells and B cells leading to the production of IgE antibodies, also known as Reaginic antibodies. Upon subsequent exposure to allergen, IgE antibodies bind to the high affinity receptor, FcεRI on mast cells resulting in cell signaling, degranulation and release of pharmacologically active substances from cytoplasmic granules. The cytokines IL-4 and IL-13 secreted by TH2 cells provide the sensitization signals. Additional signals required include interaction of CD40L on TH2 cells with CD40 on B cells. Cell signaling is initiated following activation of the tyrosine kinase, Lyn which phosphorylates ITAMs on the cytoplasmic domains of FcεRI, Recruitment

© Springer Nature Switzerland AG 2021
T. Y. Sam-Yellowe, *Immunology: Overview and Laboratory Manual*,
https://doi.org/10.1007/978-3-030-64686-8_18

and activation of a second tyrosine kinase, Syk amplifies the cytoplasmic signal resulting in calcium release from calcium stores. Migration, fusion and exocytosis of cytoplasmic granules is mediated by calcium. Cleavage of phospholipids in the plasma membrane of the mast cell by phospholipase A2 results in the production of inflammatory mediators like prostaglandins and leukotrienes. Translocation of transcription factors into the nucleus leads to expression of cytokine and cytokine receptor genes and secretion of cytokines. Mediators such as histamine and heparin are secreted by mast cells. There are four histamine receptors which bind to histamine resulting in tissue damage. Binding of histamine to H1receptors on local nerve endings and H1 receptors on local blood vessels leads to dilation of blood vessels in the skin. Blood vessel dilation and resulting skin redness leads to a wheal-and-flare reaction in the skin. TH1 cell proliferation and IFNγ secretion is enhanced by H1 receptor binding to histamine. Binding of histamine to H2, H3 and H4 receptors leads to itching, sneezing and atopic dermatitis. Type I hypersensitivity reactions include anaphylactic reactions, asthma, hay fever (allergic rhinitis) and response to food allergens. Reactions can be local, targeting specific tissues and organs or systemic, involving life-threatening damage to multiple organs. Persistent release of cytokines, chemokines and inflammatory mediators as a result of sensitization to type 1 allergens can lead to late phase reactions. Atopy is an inherited condition where individuals are genetically predisposed to allergic reactions. Over 40 allergy susceptibility genes for atopic dermatitis, and allergic asthma have been identified using genome wide association studies (GWAS).

Basophils are also involved in immediate type hypersensitivity response. They are recruited to the sites of IgE-mediated allergic reactions and also express FcεRI, bind to IgE and become activated to release IL-4 and IL-13. Mast cells also express the low affinity Fc receptor for IgE, FcεRII (CD23), a C-type lectin which is also expressed on a wide variety of cells. Eosinophils are also recruited to sites of type I hypersensitivity, particularly important in responses to allergens from helminths. Eosinophils release enzymes such as eosinophil peroxidase which causes release of histamine from mast cells. Eosinophils also secrete IL-5, IL-3, TGFα, TGFβ and GM-CSF and enhance degranulation of mast cells and basophils through the release of major basic protein (MBP) from cytoplasmic granules. Eosinophils also secrete the chemokine CXCL8 (IL-8), chemokine (eotaxin) receptor CCR3 and leukotrienes C4, D4 and E4. Due to the specificity of the CC chemokines, CCL11 (eotaxin 1), CCL24 (eotaxin 2) and CCL26 (eotaxin 3) to eosinophils, they are known as eotaxins. The eotaxin receptor CCR3 also binds to other CC chemokines, CCL5, CCL7 and CCL13. Pharmacologically active substances e.g. histamine is released from the granules and combines with histamine receptors (Hl, H2, H3) on cells in different tissues of the body. Others include prostaglandins and leukotrienes from breakdown of membrane phospholipids, chemotactic factors for eosinophils, neutrophils, bradykinin, cytokines and heparin. Mouse mast cells have been shown to express FcγRIIA and FcγRIIB (inhibitory) receptors and human skin mast cells have been shown to express FcγRIIA for IgG binding leading to activation of the mast cells for allergic hypersensitivity and inflammation.

Type II hypersensitivity reactions are also known as antibody (IgG/IgM)-mediated cytotoxic reactions. The antibodies are produced in response to cell surface antigens leading to antibody dependent cellular cytotoxicity (ADCC) reactions. Cytotoxic reactions are followed by complement fixation and phagocytosis. Antibody response to erythrocyte surface antigens leads to hemolysis on erythrocytes, known as hemolytic reactions or transfusion reactions. IgM antibody response to erythrocyte surface antigens known as blood typing antigens include the A antigen (N-acetylgalactosamine) for type A, B antigen (galactose) for type B, and H antigen (fucose) for type O. IgG antibodies are produced against the Rhesus factor antigen (D antigen) in a typical primary immune response that leads to memory cell production. Individuals receiving multiple transfusions can make antibodies to surface antigens on the erythrocytes. The IgM antibodies bind to the cells and opsonize them, making the cells attractive to macrophages. The cells are phagocytized and destroyed. For example, an individual with type B blood transfused with AB or A type blood. Antibodies against the A antigen will bind to A type cells mediating antibody-dependent cell-mediated cytotoxicity (ADCC) reactions. Other blood cell antigens include Rh (also D), Kidd, Kell and Duffy. IgM-mediated complement fixation can also occur leading to damage of transfused erythrocytes. Another example is severe hemolytic disease of the newborn (HDN) also known as erythroblastosis fetalis. An Rh (−) mother pregnant with an Rh (+) fetus (from the father) will make antibodies directed against the Rh antigen. In a first pregnancy, immune cells in the mother are sensitized to make antibodies against the Rh antigen. Maternal IgG antibodies cross the placenta and destroy fetal red blood cells. In subsequent pregnancies, these same antibodies produced by memory cells can be dangerous to the fetus. Antibodies called Rhogam (anti-Rh+ IgG antibodies) can be administered to the mother 24–48 h after delivery of the first child. The antibodies bind to circulating Rh+ cells. In a second pregnancy the availability of Rhogam protects the fetus from damage.

Type III hypersensitivity reactions are also known as immune complex-mediated hypersensitivity reactions. IgG/IgM antibody-mediated damage occurs when antibody binds to antigens forming immune complexes. If the immune complexes are not cleared by macrophages following the immune response that generated the antibodies, the immune complexes become deposited on host tissue leading to complement fixation and inflammatory damage. Immune complexes bind to Fc receptors on macrophages, neutrophils and mast cells. Cell signaling in the phagocytic cells leads to the release of inflammatory mediators and cytokines and activation of the endothelium, which increases capillary permeability. Type III hypersensitivity reactions can be localized or systemic. A characteristic localized type III reaction is an Arthus reaction that occurs in the skin of individuals following an initial sensitization with antigen that results in IgG production. The reaction is observed 8–24 h after antigen introduction in a sensitized individual. For example insect bites in a previously sensitized individual can lead to an Arthus reaction. Binding of antigen introduced in the skin to antibody, forms immune complexes which bind to FcγRIII receptors on leukocytes. Cell recruitment, local inflammatory responses and increased vascular permeability result in fluid build-up.

Antibody-mediated complement fixation leads to the generation of the complement fragments C3a and C5a which bind to C3a and C5a receptors of leukocytes. Continued recruitment of cells to the site of inflammation leads to tissue injury by necrosis. A characteristic systemic reaction due to type III hypersensitivity is serum sickness. When large amounts of serum proteins are injected into an individual, such as the injection of horse serum against snake venom, IgM and IgG antibodies are made to serum proteins. Binding of the antibodies to the soluble proteins in antiserum leads to formation of immune complexes which bind to Fc receptors on mast cells. Histamine release following degranulation of mast cells results in urticaria, rash, chills and fever. Deposition of immune complexes in the joints and in the glomerular basement membrane can lead to arthritis and glomerulonephritis, respectively. Complement fixation generates C3a and C5a fragments. Antibodies produced against infectious agents, complex with the antigens and circulate in the blood. The immune complexes can deposit in various tissues in the body such as the synovial membrane of joints, glomerular basement membrane in the kidneys and choroid plexus of the brain. Immune complex deposition induces chemotactic activity recruiting neutrophils and macrophages. Complement proteins may be activated leading to tissue damage and platelet aggregation resulting in small blood clots (**microthrombi**). Generalized type III hypersensitivity reaction following passive immunization with antibodies can also occur. The recipient makes antibodies to the received antibodies leading to serum sickness. Deposition of the circulating complexes can occur in joints, glomeruli or arteries. The following diseases; systemic lupus erythematosus, rheumatoid arthritis, meningitis, malaria, trypanosomiasis or allergic reactions to drugs such as penicillin are associated with IC deposition. Farmers exposed to allergens such as hay dust, and mold spores produce IgG antibodies that complex with antigens forming immune complexes that deposit in the lungs leading to Farmer's lung.

Type IV hypersensitivity is also known as delayed type hypersensitivity (DTH) reactions also known as cell-mediated hypersensitivity. When cytotoxic T cells become sensitized to antigens, they become activated leading to memory T cell production. Subsequent T cell activation and inflammatory cytokine production lead to monocyte and macrophage recruitment occurring in 24–72 h after antigen re-exposure. T cell reactions predominate in DTH reactions. CD4$^+$ TH1 cells and CD8$^+$Tc cells participate in DTH reactions. Macrophages are recruited to sites of DTH reaction leading to the formation of granulomas. The cytokines IL-2, IFNγ, macrophage inhibitory factor (MIF), TNFβ secreted during this reaction are important in the progression and outcome of the reaction. Antigens from infectious organisms such as *Mycobacterium tuberculosis* etiological agent of tuberculosis (TB), *Mycobacterium leprae* which causes leprosy, *Leishmania* sp. which cause different forms of leishmaniasis, egg antigen of *Schistosoma mansoni* and fungal infections, result in DTH reactions. Other forms of type IV reactions occur as a result of contact dermatitis due to exposure or contact with antigens from poison oak, poison ivy, some cosmetics and metals.

These antigens are very small and are known as haptens. The haptens by themselves cannot stimulate an immune reaction but when they combine with self-proteins (carriers) the hapten-carrier complex is phagocytized by antigen presenting cells in the skin known as Langerhans cells. Presentation of the antigen to T helper cells causes their differentiation to T_{DTH} cells. These cells remain in a sensitized state until exposure to the antigen at a future time. During subsequent re-exposure to the antigen a reaction can be observed in 48–72 h. Enzymes released by macrophages act to cause swelling and redness on the skin. A characteristic DTH reaction can be observed after skin testing is performed to determine if an individual has been exposed to DTH inducing antigens. Common antigens used for skin testing include PPD-purified protein derivative (for tuberculosis), lepromin and coccidiodin (for fungal antigens), tuberculin, chromate and nickel. A DTH reaction can also be obtained when tuberculin is injected intradermally for a skin test in individuals who previously received a BCG (bacilli Calmette-Guerin) vaccine, an attenuated form of *M. bovis*. Following injection, CD4+ TH1 cells interact with APCs presenting peptides complexed to MHC class II leading to TH1 cell activation and the release of IFNγ, TNFα and lymphotoxin. Increase in local blood cell permeability leads to macrophage and blood plasma infiltration causing swelling of the injection site.

In immune-mediated allergic contact dermatitis, initial exposure to small molecules like urushiols from poison ivy or drugs like penicillin leads to binding of the molecules to host proteins creating a hapten-carrier complex. The complex is phagocytosed by Langerhans cells in the epidermis and dendritic cells in the dermis. Processing of the hapten-carrier complex and presentation of hapten and peptides to T cells in regional lymph nodes leads to T cell activation with the generation of effector and memory T cells.

Upon subsequent antigen exposure in the activation phase, antigen gets presented to memory T cells in the dermis leading to release of cytokines form T cell. Urushiols enter host cells as lipid soluble molecules that bind cytoplasmic proteins and become processed by immunoproteasomes. Peptides bind to MHCI which are recognized by CD8+ T c cells. Activated cells mediate killing or secrete inflammatory cytokines which can damage cells. The cytokines, IFNγ and IL-17 act on keratinocytes leading to release of the proinflammatory cytokines IL-1, IL-6 and TNFα. Additional cytokines released include GM-CSF, and the chemokines CXCL8 (IL-8), interferon-inducible chemokines CXCL11 (IP-9), CXCL10 (IP-10), CXCL9 (Mig, monokine induced by IFNγ).

The in vitro correlate of DTH is performed by detection of MIF production by T_{DTH} cells (CD4+TH1 cell and CD8+ Tc cells).

1. Lymphocytes are incubated with Ag plus appropriate APCs for the sensitization phase
2. Culture supernatant from #1 are incubated with macrophages in capillary tubes
3. Add tissue culture medium to cultured macrophages

Results

(+) MIF produced with no migration of macrophages

(−) MIF is not produced and macrophages migrate out of capillary tube, fanning out of capillary tube

Selected References

Descote J, Choquet-KAstylevsky G (2001) Gell and coombs classification: Is it still valid? Toxicology 158:43–49

Johansson SGO (2016) The discovery of IgE. J Allergy Clin Immunol 137:1671–1673

Jonson F, Daeron M (2012) Mast cells and company. Front Immunol 3:16. https://doi.org/10.3389/fimmu.2012.00016

Murphy K, Weaver C (2017) Janeway's immunobiology, 9th edn. Garland Press, New York

Ortiz-Garcia YM, Garcia-Iglesias T, Morales-Velazquez G et al (2019) Macrophage migration inhibitory factor levels in gingival crevicular fluid, saliva, and serum of chronic periodontitis patients. BioMed Res Intl 2019:7850392. https://doi.org/10.1155/2019/7850392

Posadas SJ, Pichler WJ (2007) Delayed drug hypersensitivity reactions-new concepts. Clin Exp Allergy 37:989–999

Punt J, Stranford SA, Jones PP, Owen JA (2019) Kuby immunology, 8th edn. W.H. Freeman and Company, New York

Rajan TV (2003) The Gell-coombs classification of hypersensitivity reactions: a re-interpretation. Trends Immunol 24:376–379

Ribatti D (2016) The discovery of IgE. Immunol Lett 171:1–4

Wesmann D, Nagler CR (2020) Origins of peanut allergy-causing antibodies. Science 367:1072–1073

Chapter 19
Parasite Immunity

Parasite Antigens

Parasites comprise protozoans, helminths (worms) and some arthropods such as fleas and lice. Endemic parasite infections occur in tropical and subtropical environments aided by geographical and climatic conditions that support parasite transmission. Diseases such as malaria, Human African Trypanosomiasis and Leishmaniasis are associated with tropical environments. Parasites also occur in temperate environments and include cosmopolitan parasites found globally such as pin worm infections, giardiasis, ascariasis and toxoplasmosis and parasites such as the trematode *Paragonimus kellikoti* that occasionally becomes the focus in infections among individuals who eat raw crayfish while camping. In each case the host mounts an immune response upon recognition of the parasite antigens. Molecules secreted by parasites or associated with cell membranes can act as PAMPs and bind to PRRs on host cells leading to innate immune responses. Parasite antigens can induce cell-mediated, humoral and tolerogenic responses. Protozoans are unicellular eukaryotic organisms that can have simple life cycles consisting of a few stages to parasites such as *Plasmodium* sp., causative agent of malaria that has multiple life cycle stages in the human and in the mosquito vector host. Each life cycle stage expresses stage specific antigens that can induce stage specific immune responses. Helminths are categorized as flat (trematodes and cestodes) or round (nematodes) worms. Flat worms include flukes and tapeworms. These are multicellular eukaryotic parasites that consist of macroscopic adult stages and microscopic juveniles and eggs. Excretory and secretory (ES) antigens as well antigens located on the tegument and cuticle of the worms stimulate humoral immune responses leading to IgE production. Some helminth antigens are allergens that induce immediate hypersensitivity responses in the host. The type of immune response generated depends on the site or location occupied by the parasite. Stage specific humoral responses are also produced to antigens associated with the juveniles and eggs.

© Springer Nature Switzerland AG 2021
T. Y. Sam-Yellowe, *Immunology: Overview and Laboratory Manual*,
https://doi.org/10.1007/978-3-030-64686-8_19

Protozoans such as *Plasmodium* sp. *Toxoplasma gondii, Trypanosoma cruzi* and *Leishmania* sp. are intracellular parasites within host cells. For example, *Plasmodium* infects hepatocytes and erythrocytes and *T. gondii* infects macrophages. Invasive extracellular stages occurring briefly in blood and other body fluids also induce immune responses such that the same parasite can induce both CMI and HI. Cell-mediated immune responses target the intracellularly infected host cell. Activated TH and B cells produce cytokines and antibodies, respectively, in response to the extracellular stages and in infections caused by *Plasmodium* sp. cytokine dysregulation occurs leading to increased inflammation and tissue damage. Allergens in helminth parasites induce TH2 responses and IgE secretion. Thymic stromal lymphopoietin (TSLP) mediates TH2 effector function that control helminth infection levels. Antibody mediated clearance of TSLP led to decreased TH2 cytokine responses. We will discuss a few examples of protozoan parasites and the helminth trematode that causes shistosomiasis.

Malaria and Leishmaniasis

In blood stage infections by *Plasmodium falciparum*, clearance of infected blood cells by the spleen is an important process, as *Plasmodium* antigens can be processed by APCs for presentation to TH cells resulting in antibody production. Intracellularly infected red blood cells are not targeted by CTLs since class I MHC is not expressed on the RBC surface. *Plasmodium falciparum* antigens synthesized within the RBC are exposed on the RBC surface and are highly immunogenic serving as the basis for vaccine candidates under investigation by research labs. An important virulence molecule synthesized by *P. falciparum* is the variant surface antigen, *P. falciparum* erythrocyte membrane antigen 1 (PfEMP1) associated with the knob proteins on the surface of infected RBC. PfEMP1 is the product of *var* genes of which there are approximately 60 variants.

The female *Anopheles* mosquito delivers infective sporozoite stages with an infectious bite, sporozoites travel to the liver where they infect liver cells (hepatocytes) and upon differentiation within the liver cells, undergo asexual division to form multinucleate schizont stages. Rupture of the schizonts, releases merozoite stages which are infective for erythrocytes. Asexual division within the erythrocyte produces schizonts that release merozoites that can reinvade erythrocyte to continue the blood stage or differentiate to form male and female gametes which are picked up by a feeding mosquito. Within the mosquito, fertilization of the female gamete by exflagellated male gametes leads to the formation of a motile zygote (ookinete) which develops into an oocyst. Sporogony within the oocyst generates sporozoites which become infective upon entering the mosquito salivary glands. Through the course of the life cycle, stage specific antigens are expressed which induce stage specific immunity. Much of the challenge to vaccine design can be found in identifying antigens that are suitable immunogenic candidates that can provide protection. The presence of zoonotic *Plasmodium* species such as *P. knowlesi* and

P. cyanomolgi in areas endemic for human *Plasmodium* sp. complicates the immune responses generated. TH1, TH2 and TH17 responses lead to CMI, humoral immunity and inflammation. Gamma/delta T cells possessing cytolytic activity against infected red blood cells have been shown to kill the infected cells. Also, increased secretion of the proinflammatory cytokines, IL-1, IL-6, TNFα, IL-12 and IFNγ occur in severe *P. falciparum* malaria. Polyclonal B cell activation leading to IgM and IgG secretion occurs in malaria infections. Fc regions of IgG subsets bind Fc receptors for antibody-dependent cellular cytotoxicity (ADCC). In contrast to *Plasmodium* sp. *Leishmania* sp. infect macrophages and consist of two life cycle stages, the promastigote and amastigote. An infected sand fly delivers the promastigote with an infective bite. The flagellated promastigote is taken up and infects the macrophage where it differentiates into an amastigote and resides within the macrophage. A feeding sand fly picks up infected macrophages and amastigote stages differentiate into promastigotes.TH1 and TH2 responses defined by antigens from each stage determine the course and severity of infection. Infections caused by *Leishmania* sp. vary from cutaneaous, mucocutaneous and visceral systemic infections. TH1 responses are protective resulting in limited infection while TH2 responses result in more parasite dissemination and disease severity.

Trypanosomiasis

Human African Trypanosomiasis (HAT) caused by *Trypanosoma brucei gambiense* or *T. b. rhodesiense* is transmitted by the Tse-tse fly which delivers the metacyclic trypomastigote (short stumpy) stage with an infective bite. Long slender trypomastigotes soon form and lie extracellularly in the blood. In *T. b.gambiense* infections, trypomastigotes can also be found in the cerebrospinal fluid (CSF). A feeding Tse-tse fly picks up slender trypomastigotes which differentiate into procyclic trypomastigotes then into epimastigote stages before differentiating into metacyclic stages for infection into a new host. Humoral immunity to trypomastigote antigens results in high titer antibodies. Complement fixation is an important means of clearing trypomastigotes. An important antigen expressed on the trypomastigote surface coat is the variable surface glycoprotein (VSG) anchored to the parasite using glycosylphosphatidylinositol (GPI). VSG is released through the flagellar reservoir to cover the entire surface of the trypomastigote. An infected host produces antibodies to the VSG protein. Recognition and binding of antibody to VSG leads to sloughing off of VSG and the expression of a new VSG coat protein, rendering the antibodies produced to the first VSG useless. Trypomastigotes also internalize anti-VSG antibodies. The parasite expresses successive VSG proteins in response to immune pressure as an effective immune evasion mechanism of antigenic variation. Approximately 1000 genes encode VSG protein making this an important mechanisms for evading host immune responses and complicating efforts to control HAT infections.

Giardiasis and Amebiasis

In comparison to the two blood infections discussed above, amebiasis caused by *Entamoeba histolytica* and giardiasis caused by *Giardia lamblia* occur in the gastro-intestinal (GI) tract resulting in dysentery and diarrhea, respectively. Both parasites have two life cycle stages, trophozoites and the cysts. The cyst which is formed in the GI tract and passed into the environment through feces can contaminate food and water, which is how individuals become infected. While trophozoite stages are confined within the GI tract, extraintestinal infection can occur with *E. histolytica* trophozoites being transported in the blood to the liver, brain and skin. Antigens from both parasites stimulate IgA production. The presence of proteases increases virulence. Lectins such as Gal/GalNAc-lectin produced by *E. histolytica* bind carbohydrates on host cells displaying the surface determinants containing galactose (Gal) or N-acetyl-D-galactosamine (GalNAc). Pore-forming proteins known as amoebapores are synthesized by *E. histolytica*, although their role in host defense is uncertain. In both infections, proinflammatory cytokines are secreted and *E. histolytica* trophozoites can activate the alternate pathway of complement.

Schistosomiasis

Helminth antigens induce TH2 activation leading to B cell synthesis of IgE. Schistosomiasis caused by the blood fluke of *Schistosoma* species affects liver, brain and bladder. Major species include *S. mansoni*, *S. hematobium* and *S. japonicum*. Multiple life cycle stages are present in the life cycle. The human host becomes infected when the cercaria stage penetrates the skin of an individual standing or swimming in water containing the snail vector host which releases the cercaria. Upon penetration of the skin the cercaria loses its tail and transforms into the schistosomule stage. Following migration of the juvenile worm through the lungs, development of the adult stages takes place in the veins that drain the large intestine (*S. mansoni*), small intestine (*S. japonicum*) and urinary bladder plexus (*S. hematobium*). Egg production commences once the trematodes mate. The eggs can be found in the tissues around the veins as they are expelled into the GI or urethra to get to the environment. Eggs become trapped in the liver and bladder tissue where granulomas form around the eggs. Cellular infiltrates containing macrophages, eosinophils and neutrophils can be found around the eggs. Secretion of fibroblast growth factor promotes development of fibrosis. In the acute phase of infection, antibodies produced combine with antigen forming immune complexes that are cleared by macrophages. Pro-inflammatory cytokines such as IL-1 and TNFα are secreted by macrophages. In chronic phase of infection cellular infiltration increases, with the formation of multinucleated giant cells, recruitment of fibroblasts and lymphocytes. Macrophage activity involving collagenase secretion can lead to less severe fibrosis. Delayed type hypersensitivity reactions, granulomas and fibrosis can obstruct blood flow leading to severe disease. Adult worms coat themselves with host proteins and also synthesize proteins expressed on the tegument that bear resemblance to host proteins in a process of molecular mimicry preventing immune recognition, binding and attack on the adult worms. Eosinophils target the adult worms and release major basic protein (MBP) from granules. Similarly, eosinophils recruited to granulomas secrete MBP and cytokines.

Selected References

Inoue S, Niikura M, Mineo S, Kobayashi F (2013) Roles of IFNγ and γδ T cells in protective immunity against blood-stage malaria. Front. Immunol 2013. https://doi.org/10.3389/fimmu.2013.00258.ecollection2013

Centers for Disease Control and Prevention (CDC) (2010) Human Paragonimiasis after eating raw or undercooked crayfish—Missouri, July 2006–September 2010. Morbidity Mortality Weekly Report 59(48):1573–1576

Murphy K, Weaver C (2017) Janeway's immunobiology, 9th edn. Garland Press, New York

Punt J, Stranford SA, Jones PP, Owen JA (2019) Kuby immunology, 8th edn. W.H. Freeman and Company, New York. Chapter 20, Antigen-antibody interactions

Roberts LS, Janovy J Jr, Nadler S (2013) Gerald D. Schmidt & Larry S. Robert's foundations of Prasitology, 9th edn. McGraw Hill, New York

Ziegler SF, Artis D (2010) Sensing the outside world: TSLP regulates barrier immunity. Nat Immunol 11:289–293

Chapter 20
Vaccines

Vaccines remain the most important tool used in public health programs to prevent infectious disease transmission. Vaccines produced against viral and bacterial pathogens have saved millions of lives globally. Due to the complex life cycles of protozoan and helminth parasites as well as fungi, development of vaccines to prevent infections by theses eukaryotic pathogens has been challenging. The presence of stage specific antigens eliciting stage specific adaptive immunity and intracellular infections caused by protozoan parasites leads to varying humoral and cellular responses to parasite antigen. The hallmark of successful vaccines is the development of long lasting memory B and T cells following administration of a vaccine, so that upon exposure to the infectious disease agent, activation of memory B and T cells leads to elimination of the pathogen. The use of adjuvants combined with vaccines provides a robust innate immune response that leads to the recruitment of antigen presenting cells such as monocytes, macrophages, dendritic cells and other cells of the innate immune response that utilize pathogen recognition receptors (PRRs) to ligate vaccine molecules leading to processing and presentation of antigen on MHC class II molecules for presentation of antigen to TH cells. Activation of APCs leads to secretion of proinflammatory cytokines which enhance the activity of T and B cells. Vaccine molecules contain B and T cell epitopes. The induced immune response is varied and spans types 1, 2 and 3 immune responses. T cell epitopes on vaccine antigens can induce activation of TH1, TH2 and TH17 cells. Epitopes from processed proteins from intracellular pathogens activate cytotoxic CD8$^+$ T cells and CD4$^+$ TH1 cells. Due to differences in the immunogenicity of vaccine antigens, the need for effective adjuvants and delivery systems is an area of intense research. Different modes of vaccine formulations are used, ranging from the use of killed whole organisms, attenuated organisms, sub-unit vaccines and recombinant proteins. The use of nucleic acids, peptides, liposomes, nanoparticles and virus like particles are under investigation for efficient vaccine delivery alone or in combination with adjuvants. These newer delivery systems will enhance uptake and processing of the vaccines by APCs for presentation to T cells. The total immune

© Springer Nature Switzerland AG 2021
T. Y. Sam-Yellowe, *Immunology: Overview and Laboratory Manual*,
https://doi.org/10.1007/978-3-030-64686-8_20

response generated in an individual is of paramount importance when evaluating the success of a vaccine and the memory response that develops.

The properties of the vaccines can be understood in the types of formulations used and in their effectiveness in preventing disease transmission and generating herd immunity. Traditional first generation (whole organism) vaccines differ from the second (recombinant protein) and third generation (nucleic acid vaccines) vaccines. The field of vaccinology has its origins in those areas of the world where individuals obtained crusts from pustules in infected individuals and " inoculated " (through scratches and cuts) immunologically naive individuals in nonvisible areas of the body to protect these individuals from serious and in some cases fatal infections. This was done with infections such as leishmaniasis and smallpox. This practice was known as **variolation.** The protection conferred to individuals following previous infection, was recognized for hundreds of years before the formal demonstration of immunity to small pox by Edward Jenner in 1798 and again by Louis Pasteur to cholera, rabies and anthrax caused by *Bacillus anthracis*, in 1881. Knowledge that a weakened pathogen **(attenuation)** or a milder strain of the pathogen could protect individuals against infection was demonstrated by these early experiments.

These discoveries changed medical practice and as we have seen with current events, vaccinology is receiving a new look as we try to understand how best to protect individuals against threats of infection by various biological agents. In 1977 small pox was eradicated through vaccination and there are indications that polio might be next. Several previously, common infections are now easily prevented by vaccines. In order for vaccines to be effective, both B and T cell (CD4 and CD8) epitopes must be present. Both antibody mediated humoral immunity and cytotoxic T cell mediated immunity are generated as a result of vaccines. When the effects of vaccines are evaluated the following types of immunity are considered; clinical immunity which is a partial immunity to an infectious agent such that re-exposure or continuous exposure to the agent results in a milder infection when compared to a non-immune/immunologically naive individual. In areas endemic for particular infectious agents, this can be useful as individuals are protected from getting severe or fatal infection. However, partially immune individuals may serve as carriers. Premunition may fall under this category and refers to immunity that develops as a result of infection with a pathogen. The immunity that develops prevents new infection in the host by the same pathogen but does not protect the host from developing disease. Sterile immunity is complete immunity, life-long immunity that provides complete protection against infection. Herd immunity is immunity of a population sufficient to block transmission of an infectious agent. Every single individual in the population does not have to be immunized to achieve this type of immunity. However, immune coverage of 60-70% may be required to stop transmission. Traditional first generation vaccines are preventative or prophylactic. The newer scope of vaccines involve changing physiology and are used in the areas of fertility, allergy and cancer. Therapeutic applications of vaccines are used in allergy, cancer and AIDS. There are two major categories of vaccines involving active stimulation of the immune system or passive administration of preformed immune products such as antibodies. Active stimulation of the immune response involve active induction of immune responses resulting in humoral and cell-mediated immune response, generating protective immunity and in some cases life-long immunity. As discussed above the first formal documentation was by Edward Jenner and Louis Pasteur. Active immune responses result in protection, elimination of pathogens and change in physiology. Examples of vaccines used to generate active immunity include live vaccines (attenuated) or killed vaccines. Passive administration of preformed immunoglobulin first described by Emil von Behring and Hidesaburo Kitasato, offers immediate protection against pathogen. They are protective but provide short-lived immunity and require multiple doses. The goal of passive immunity is to reduce reactogenicity and side effects. Considerations for effective and safe vaccines include the type of immunogen, the mode of presentation, how the vaccines are going to be used and what type of pathogen the vaccine is directed against.

Live Attenuated Vaccines

Attenuated pathogens are non-pathogenic and replicate within the vaccine recipient. They express antigens that can be recognized by the immune system leading to a robust immune response. Persistent exposure to the immunogen allows the stimulation of humoral and cell-mediated immune responses and prolonged delivery of the vaccine. In order to attenuate the pathogen for vaccine, organisms are mutated by in vitro passage or growth in increasing concentrations of bile, such as with *Mycobacterium bovis* (Bacille Calmette-Guerin, BCG). Isolation and cultivation of animal pathogens for use in humans for example, attenuated for human use can also be carried out. Reassortment viruses, growth property mutants such as temperature sensitive (ts), cold-adapted or cold sensitive (cs) strains of pathogens can be generated. Attenuation by specific deletions or modifications of genes in a viral genome or deletion of virulence or toxin genes can render the pathogen attenuated for use as a vaccine molecule. The oral polio vaccine (OPV) contains three attenuated virus strains that elicit immunity at different rates and therefore require booster administrations of the vaccine. The OPV vaccine induces secretory IgA protective for the gut mucosa as well as IgM and IgG. Attenuated vaccines are available for measles.

New vaccines being developed for *Plasmodium falciparum* include attenuated sporozoite stage of the parasite for use as whole attenuated vaccines. A single dose of a live attenuated vaccine is capable of generating a long lived immunity. Live attenuated pathogens can mutate and revert to virulent forms of the virus which can be shed in the feces aiding transmission to susceptible hosts. Post-vaccination complications such as post encephalitis after measles vaccine can occur.

Inactivated (Killed) Vaccines

Killed vaccines stimulate humoral and cell-mediated immunity. They are administered with adjuvants to enhance immunogenicity. Whole pathogens used for vaccines can be heat-killed or inactivated using formaldehyde. Unlike live attenuated vaccines, the inactivated pathogen is unable to grow or replicate within the vaccine recipient. However, antigens are still recognized by the immune system and an immune response is still mounted, and antibodies produced. Heat treatment can denature important epitopes on the immunogen, resulting in a reduced level of immune response to the vaccine. Examples of inactivated vaccines include inactivated polio vaccine (IPV), vaccines for the flu, cholera and hepatitis A. Multiple doses of inactivated vaccine may be needed to achieve immunity and memory cell development due to low immunogenicity of the inactivated vaccine.

Protein Based Vaccines

A variety of techniques are employed to generate protein-based vaccine. Genetic, immunological and biochemical techniques are used to identify an immunogen. Purified protein, recombinant protein or peptides can be used as vaccine. Peptide based vaccines can be synthetic or multivalent. Important considerations for this type of vaccine include the conformation of the peptide to ensure immunogenicity. Some questions to consider include; is the peptide conformational or linear? Immunogenicity of a peptide can be destroyed depending on the way the peptide is synthesized and the final conformation of the peptide following its synthesis and its size. Immunogenic epitopes need to be mapped on the peptide. It is important to know if the epitope is weak or strong and whether humoral or cell-mediated immunity is stimulated. The immunogenicity of a linear epitope can be increased by genetic fusion of epitopes with defined amino acid carrier proteins. The peptide can be covalently conjugated to a carrier, multimers can be synthesized and the presentation of the peptide vaccine can be enhanced. Generally peptide vaccines have not been as effective as previously expected. As indicated above this has to do with the poor immunogenicity of the peptides. The better peptide vaccines work because the T and B cell epitopes are clearly defined. However, it is still a challenge to get good peptide vaccines. Having multiple peptides in a single vaccine preparation offers improvement in immunogenicity. The humoral and cell-mediated responses generated are quite strong. Because multiple peptides are arranged on a matrix, on a carrier backbone, or incorporated into liposomes (artificial lipid vesicles) they are particulate and so they are easily phagocytosed by APCs. Examples of multivalent peptide (subunit) vaccines includes solid matrix antibody antigens (SMAA), multiple antigenic peptides (MAPS) and immunostimulating complexes (ISCOMS). Nanoparticles coated with vaccine molecules or nano delivery systems with encapsulated vaccines are being explored for delivery of vaccine molecules. Gold nanoparticles, polymeric nanoparticles and virus like particles are being investigated for vaccine delivery. Intracellular presentation of antigen for MHC I or phagocytosis for MHC II association can also increase the antigen access to T cells. There are other type of vaccines under consideration such as anti-idiotype vaccines, toxoid vaccines, recombinant protein (antigen) vaccines, recombinant vector vaccines, nucleic acid vaccines, polysaccharide based vaccines e.g. bacterial capsules from *Neisseria meningitides, Haemophilus injluenzae, Streptococcus pneumoniae* and other polymeric CHO, TD vs TI antigens.

Subunit Vaccines

The use of specific macromolecules such as protein and carbohydrate molecules from pathogens as well as the use of nucleic acids are also used as vaccines. Inactivated toxins secreted by pathogens can be used as vaccine molecules. Purified native proteins or recombinant proteins expressed from cloned genes are also used as vaccine. These types of vaccines are known as subunit vaccines. The vaccines are prepared from specific molecules obtained from pathogens instead of using whole pathogens. Inactivated exotoxins which are proteins, and known as toxoids, have been used for vaccinations against diphtheria caused by *Corynebacterium diphthereae* and tetanus caused by *Clostridium tetani*. Purified exotoxin from bacteria is inactivated using formaldehyde to form a toxoid. Vaccination with toxoid leads to development of anti-toxoid antibodies that can neutralize the exotoxin upon exposure to the bacteria. Capsular polysaccharides from bacterial capsules can also be used as subunit vaccines alone or conjugated to protein. Polysaccharide-protein conjugates elicit an immune response that activates both TH and B cells resulting in memory cell formation. Polysaccharide vaccines by themselves elicit a T-independent immune response that results in IgM production by B cells with no class switching and memory cell production. Examples of vaccines with polysaccharide antigens include capsular antigens from *Streptococcus pneumonia* causative agent for pneumococcal pneumonia and *Neisseria meningitidis* causative agent for bacterial meningitis. The vaccine against *S. pneumonia*, contains 13 antigenically distinct capsular polysaccharides.

Polysaccharide Vaccines

Capsule polysaccharides from bacteria are used as vaccines. Pneumovax 23 (Pneumococcal polysaccharide vaccine, PPSV23) which is used for *Streptococcus pneumoniae* is an inactivated vaccine prepared using 23 different capsular polysaccharides and protects against 23 types of bacteria. PV13 (Prevnar 13) is an inactivated vaccine administered with an adjuvant and also used for *S. pneumonia*. It contains 13 different capsular polysaccharides. Each of the polysaccharides is antigenically distinct. Both vaccines are used to protect individuals against bacteria that cause pneumococcal disease (CDC). As we saw in our earlier discussion of antigens polysaccharide antigens are TI antigens and so no T cell help is available for antibody production. The predominant antibodies are IgM. Some of the vaccines are conjugated to protein carriers. The Hib vaccine for *Haemophilus influenza* type b is a capsular polysaccharide vaccine covalently conjugated to tetanus toxoid which will stimulate TH activation and the formation of memory TH cells.

Nucleic Acid Vaccines

DNA vaccines: Recombinant plasmid DNA engineered to contain a gene encoding immunogen is injected into the muscle and taken up by host cells such as dendritic cells. Genetic adjuvants such as genes for cytokines may be included in the recombinant construct. CpG DNA is also added to the recombinant and is an important ligand for TLR9. DNA vaccines are being widely studied because of their potential to deliver prolonged immunogen exposure as the encoded protein is being continually expressed. Advantages of DNA vaccines include ease of purification, ease of modification and relatively inexpensive production. A cold chain is not required and the vaccine preparation can be lyophilized and stored at room temperature. No adjuvant is required during administration and the expressed protein product can be highly immunogenic leading to the stimulation of humoral and cell-mediated immunity. Immunity is potent and long-lived and can confer cross protection with single or mixed genes.

Plasmid DNA containing genes encoding specific proteins are used as vaccine molecules (naked DNA). The plasmid DNA is introduced into the host by injection (intramuscular or intradermal), gene gun using DNA coated onto microscopic gold beads, or nasal spray for antigens directed to mucosal surface. Inside host cells, the proteins is expressed thereby stimulating either a humoral or cell-mediated immune response. A "depot" is formed such that the expressed protein product is released over a long period of time. Similar to protein vaccines, memory to the antigen develops. The plasmid construct can include a variety of components aimed at enhancing immunogenicity of the expressed protein. E.g. cytokine genes can be included in the construct to direct the immune response to THI or TH2 mediated responses, or cytokines that enhance inflammation resulting in recruitment of specific cells. Several genes can also be included in a single construct-genes encoding proteins from different developmental stages of a pathogen or genes from different species. Concerns regarding DNA vaccines have been raised. Although no adverse effects have been reported, some of the concerns include integration into host cell genome, distal spread to germ cells and to next generation, autoimmunity, tolerance and DTH responses.

RNA vaccines: mRNA vaccines are novel vaccine delivery platforms being developed for use in infectious disease prevention and cancer therapy. Non-replicating mRNA and self-amplifying RNA from viral sources are under investigation for use in delivering pathogen protein coding sequences into cells. The protein is translated within host cells resulting in protein secretion and recognition of the protein by APCs for stimulation of adaptive immunity. Both humoral and cell-mediated immunity can be stimulated. The mRNA molecule is designed to contain the gene of interest in an open reading frame, flanked by 5′ and 3′ untranslated regions (UTRs) and having a 5′ cap and polyadenylation at the 3′ end (Fig. 20.1). Due to the instability of naked mRNA and vulnerability to host RNases, delivery systems are also being investigated and optimized to allow delivery in lipid nanoparticles that can protect the RNA and adsorb to host cells for delivery of the mRNA in the host cell cytoplasm. Ex vivo transfection of mRNA into dendritic cells that can be subsequently infused into vaccine recipients is undergoing investigation for cancer vaccines. The mRNA loaded DCs can be infused into autologous vaccine recipients. Injection of naked mRNA through intradermal or intranodal routes are also being explored. Naked mRNA is a PAMP and can interact with pattern recognition receptors in the host stimulating innate immunity to the nucleic acid molecule and not to the potential translated protein. In order to optimize stability and increased half-life of the mRNA vaccine, synthetic mRNA encoding the vaccine candidate delivered in a safe and non-toxic carrier is the route favored by investigators. mRNA vaccines are under investigation for influenza virus and Zika virus, with most studies showing promise in animal studies. One of the vaccine platforms under consideration for widespread administration to prevent SARS-CoV-2 infections, currently the cause of a global pandemic of COVID19 infections is mRNA vaccines. The mRNA vaccines can be co-administered with adjuvant or genes encoding adjuvant molecules that can enhance T cell activation and can be included in the transcript (Fig. 20.1), to enhance cytotoxic T cell and helper T cell activity.

Recombinant Vector Vaccines

Attenuated viruses or bacteria are used as vectors for recombinant plasmids engineered to contain the gene encoding the vaccine molecule. The recombinant vector is introduced into the host during vaccination where it replicates and expresses the immunogen. One of the most commonly used vectors is the Vaccinia virus that was used for smallpox vaccines. Humoral and cell-mediated immune responses are generated following administration of recombinant vector vaccines. The bacterium *Salmonella typhimurium* is also used as a vector for carrying and expressing genes encoding vaccine molecules. *Salmonella typhimurium* infects cells of the gut mucosa and induces the production of secretory IgA. These stimulate humoral and cell-mediated immunity. Engineered virus and bacterial vectors include Vaccinia virus, Adenovirus, Oka strain of Varicella-zoster virus, Herpes Simplex virus, attenuated poliovirus, BCG and *Salmonella* recombinant vector vaccines. The virus or bacteria is attenuated and used to deliver genes that encode proteins from virulent organisms.

Adjuvants enhance immune response by acting as immunomodulators. Adjuvant molecules activate cells of the innate immune system such as neutrophils,

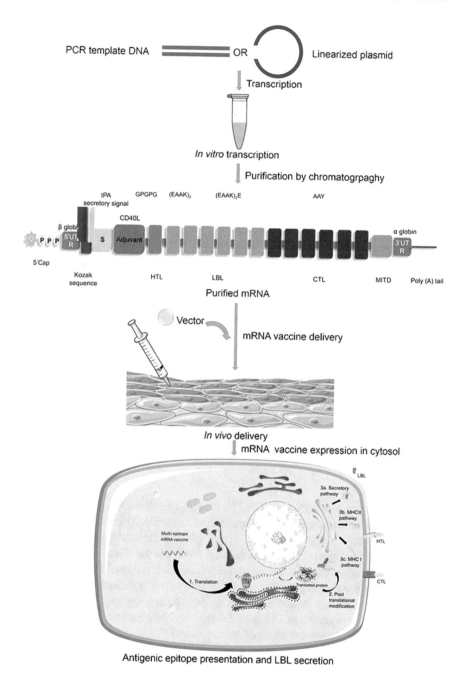

Fig. 20.1 Proposed mechanisms of synthesis, delivery and action of the mRNA vaccine against SARS-CoV-2. The PCR template DNA or linearized plasmid DNA containing the designed vaccine sequences is transcribed in vitro in a media containing RNA polymerase and nucleotide phosphates. A mixture of dsRNAs and other aberrant products are obtained. Chromatographic

(continued)

purification such as FPLC is performed to obtain the mRNA with desired content and length. After vector-mediated delivery into the body, the mRNA transits into the cytosol. In the cytosol, the cellular translation machinery synthesizes proteins which undergo post-translational modifications, resulting in properly folded, fully functional proteins. The secretory signal and MITD sequences direct the peptides to specific compartments of the endoplasmic reticulum and Golgi body for efficient secretion (linear B lymphocytes) and presentation by class I MHC for cytotoxic T lymphocytes and class II MHC for helper T cells. . [*Republished with permission of Elsevier publishing from Ahammad, I. and Sultana Lira, S. (2020) "Designing a novel mRNA vaccine against SARS-CoV-2: An immunoinformatics approach." Int J Biol Macromol, 162:820–837. Figure 7. Conveyed through STM permission guidelines 2020*]

monocytes, macrophages and dendritic cells. The only approved adjuvant for human use has been alum which enhances TH2 cells. Additional adjuvants that are used include AS04, an alum salt containing derivatives of lipopolysachcride (LPS). Virosomes consisting of virus envelope containing phospholipids and virus glycoproteins without nucleic acids can act as TLR4 agonist.

Selected References

Ahammad I, Sultana Lira S (2020) Designing a novel mRNA vaccine against SARS-CoV-2: An immunoinformatics approach. Int J Biol Macromol 162:820–837

Guimaraes LE, Baker B, Perricone C, Shoenfeld Y (2015) Vaccines, adjuvants and autoimmunity. Pharmacol Res 100:190–209

Murphy K, Weaver C (2017) Janeway's immunobiology, 9th edn. Garland Press, New York

Pardi N, Hogan MJ, Porter FW, Weissman D (2018) mRNA vacines-a new era in vaccinology. Nat Rev Drug Discov 17:261–279

Pati R, Shevtsov M, Sonawane A (2018) Nanoparticle vaccines against infectious diseases. Front Immunol 9. https://doi.org/10.3389/fimmu.2018.02224

Punt J, Stranford SA, Jones PP, Owen JA (2019) Kuby immunology, 8th edn. W.H. Freeman and Company, New York. Chapter 20, Antigen-antibody interactions

Vetter V, Denizer G, Friedland LR, Krishnan J, Shapiro M (2018) Understanding modern-day vaccines: What you need to know. Ann Med 50:110–120

Chapter 21
Transplantation

Transplantation biology has been a central area of investigation in immunology. Much of the early studies involving the induction of tolerance were based on understanding how grafted tissue (transplants) was accepted or rejected. Transplantation studies further the understanding of how the immune system works such as understanding how self-tolerance differs from acquired tolerance and indeed how both processes are similar. T cells play a significant role in tissue transplant rejection. For our discussion of transplantation we will focus on the immunological features that lead to transplant rejection and the mechanisms of rejection. Finally we will examine graft versus host disease and see how this differs from the recipient rejecting a tissue graft. There are different types of grafts and the recipient host will mount different types of responses to the grafts depending on the origin of the graft.

Types of Grafts

An **autograft** is tissue grafted within the same individual e.g. skin excised from one part of the body and used in a different location i.e. after serious burns. No rejection occurs.
  Syngeneic grafts or isografts are types of tissue transplanted between individuals that are genetically identical. The tissue is accepted. An **allograft** is tissue grafted between unrelated individuals of the same species. The individuals are termed allogeneic. There are allelic variants of specific genes present on the allograft. Alloantigens will be expressed on the transplanted tissue. These will be seen as foreign by the cells of the recipient (the basis for histoincompatibility) and an immune response will be made. In this case the graft is accepted for a few days and then it is rejected. This is known as first-set rejection. If tissue from the same individual is grafted again the recipient rejects the graft in a rapid manner, known as second-set rejection. The rejection is dependent on T cells and can be transferred by adoptive means i.e. if cells from the recipient are transferred to a naive individual a

© Springer Nature Switzerland AG 2021
T. Y. Sam-Yellowe, *Immunology: Overview and Laboratory Manual*,
https://doi.org/10.1007/978-3-030-64686-8_21

similar rejection mediated by the adoptively transferred cells will occur. The allograft is the most common type of tissue transplant used clinically. Rejection or acceptance of tissue and organs is dependent on the effectiveness of immunosuppressive therapy to reduce the effects of T cells (both CD8 and CD4 positive) and as a result prolong the acceptance (the retention) of the graft. **Xenografts** is transplantation of tissue from individuals of different species. The genetic differences between the individuals are pronounced. For example, a transplant from a pig to human is a xenograft. Rejection of the tissue is rapid. T cells as well as antibodies can mediate rejection.

Major histocompatibility antigens play a very significant role in graft acceptance or rejection. The more similar the MHC antigens the more likely the tissue graft will be accepted. The more different the MHC antigens, the higher the chance that tissue will be rejected. This is known as the **alloreactive response** and is the result of the recipient recognizing the foreign or non-self alloantigens on the graft. This is because the recipient and the donor have differences in the histocompatibility antigens or MHC. Both major and minor MHC antigens are responsible for the response to foreign alloantigens. Recall from our discussions of the MHC antigens that an individual inherits MHC haplotypes from both parents and these are co-dominantly expressed. In addition, the MHC are highly polymorphic along the ~20–40 gene loci. Therefore when tissue typing is performed, ABO typing alone is not sufficient to identify a histocompatible match. The MHC loci have to be matched as closely as is possible for an outbred human population.

Alloantigens on grafted tissue can be seen by the host response in different ways. First of all the region bearing the graft needs to be in direct route of lymphatic drainage, for the most serious consequence of rejection to occur. Note that the grafted tissue may have with it T cells or antigen presenting cells (of donor origin)-these are called passenger leukocytes. The APCs can migrate to lymphoid tissue and stimulate recipient T cells.

APCs from the recipient can also recognize and process alloantigens from the graft.

Cytotoxic T cells (CD8) from the recipient can also mediate direct attack on the alloantigens. Cytokines can induce cell activation reactivity to alloantigens. Macrophages can also be nonspecifically activated leading to inflammation and tissue damage.

Antibody in combination with complement fixation can also mediate hyperacute rejection of tissue. This is particularly important when there might have been previous exposure to alloantigens from blood transfusions, individuals that have had multiple pregnancies, or individuals that have had a previous transplant. Rejection can occur within minutes of organ transplant-In this case because the organs transplanted are vascularized cells, antibodies and complement will have direct and immediate access to the graft.

Graft-Versus Host Disease

Unlike host versus-graft rejection, graft-versus host disease (GVHD) occurs when cells from the donor contained within the graft, attack recipient tissue. The donor cells recognize alloantigens on host tissue. Mature T cells play a significant role. This is very important in bone marrow transplants (most of the T cells are contaminants). The effects of GVHD are intense inflammation, severe damage to the skin, rashes, intestinal damage, diarrhea and pneumonitis. Very careful MHC typing for histocompatibility is necessary. Depletion of mature T cells and treating transplant patients with immunosuppressive drugs generally leads to improved outcomes.

The mixed lymphocyte response (MLR) is generally carried out to identify alloreactive T cells. Both major and minor MHC antigens are important in GVHD. A more reliable assay where the alloreactive T cells are enumerated is also used. The types of tissue rejection that can occur include hyperacute rejection that can occur within minutes of grafting the donor tissue. Acute rejection can occur within 6-8 days and chronic rejection can occur within a few months to years. Over time a variety of causes will lead to damage of the graft. Toxicity to immunosuppressive drugs such as cyclosporin A may develop. Thickening of the walls of blood vessels in the graft, blocking of the blood vessels, scar tissue, deposition of immune complexes, cell-mediated immune responses, cytokines such as TGF beta, IFN gamma may also mediate chronic rejection. Experimentally, TNF alpha, RANTES, and MCP play a role. Viral infections notably CMV infections can also accelerate rejection of a graft.

Regarding the tolerance of the fetus (technically an allograft), a number of explanations have been proposed. However, there is still much that is unclear about the repeated tolerance that develops. This is particularly significant in cases where a woman has several children. Each time the fetus expresses paternally derived alloantigens or nonself MHC proteins that are tolerated. The fetus occupies a protective or privileged site and so due to immunosuppressive factors is not recognized by maternal immune responses. Placental sequesteration of the fetus from maternally reactive T cells protects the fetus.

Cyokine production by the uterine endothelium and trophoblast leads to a suppression of THI responses. Fetal blood cells do make their way into maternal circulation providing the opportunity for alloantigens to be detected. Immunosuppression of the recipient immune system can allow acceptance and retention of allografts. Plasmapheresis can be performed to remove antibodies that may cause acute rejection. Plasma is removed ex vivo and the washed cells returned to the body. Tolerance can be induced to allografts by exposure of the recipient to alloantigens in blood transfusions to tolerize the recipient to B and T cells. T cell activation can be inhibited by immunosuppressive treatment or by lysis. Corticosteroids lyse T cells through endogenous activation nucleases that cleave DNA. This is most effective for immature T cells (thymocytes). Cytokine gene transcription and cytokine secretion can be blocked. Cytokines such as IL-1, IL-6, TNF and chemokines can be blocked to prevent inflammation and to remove costimulators of T cell activation.

Cyclosporin A is important clinically for immunosuppression. It is a cyclic peptide produced as a natural metabolite of fungus. The major action of cyclosporine A is to inhibit transcription of specific T cell genes especially IL-2. Cyclosporin A binds to the active site of a ubiquitous cellular protein known as cyclophilin that functions as an enzyme. This molecule may be involved in the proper folding of a transcription factor. No IL-2 is produced resulting in a profound effect on CMI activities as well as the activity of T helper cells. Other cytokines are affected, and genes for c-myc for example are inhibited. The result is that there is a lack of T cell growth, effector T cell activation, and a loss in specific immunity. Side effects or toxicity can occur affecting the kidneys. Other immunosuppressive drugs include FK506 (tacrolimus) or OKT3. Inhibition of CD80/86 signaling by the binding to the drug CTLA4-Ig (belatacept) inhibits T cell activation by rendering the T cells anergic when otherwise the cells would be targeting transplanted tissue, targeting the tissue for rejection.

Selected References

Ferrara JLM, Levine JE, Reddy P, Holler E (2009) Graft-versus-host-disease. Lancet 373:1550–1561
Murphy K, Weaver C (2017) Janeway's immunobiology, 9th edn. Garland Press, New York
Punt J, Stranford SA, Jones PP, Owen JA (2019) Kuby immunology, 8th edn. W.H. Freeman and Company, New York. Chapter 20, Antigen-antibody interactions

Chapter 22
Immune Regulation and Autoimmunity

When the immune response is generated against self-antigens (autoantigens), the resulting response is an autoimmune response. Response to self-antigens can occur due to failure of central tolerance in primary lymphoid organs and failure of peripheral tolerance in secondary lymphoid organs and other peripheral tissues after migration of lymphocytes into peripheral tissues. During B and T cell development in the bone marrow and thymus, central tolerance mechanisms render cells tolerant to host antigens. The development of tolerance to self-antigens is the regulatory mechanism that allows host cells to ignore self-antigens so that T and B cells do not become activated following encounter with antigen. For suppression, MHC-antigen engagement leads to suppression or anergy rather than activation. Instead of immunogenicity the response is tolerogenicity. An immunogen that can elicit an immune response can also act as a tolerogen. Various factors can lead to tolerance. Antigen exposure during fetal development can lead to tolerance. Lack of co-stimulatory molecules such as CD40-CD40L engagement or CD28-CD80/86 engagement can lead to anergy. Inhibitory surface molecules and cytokines can also render cells tolerant. For example CTLA4-CD80/86 interaction is inhibitory instead of activating T cells. High doses of antigen, long term persistence of antigen in the host, intravenous (iv) or oral administration of antigen can also lead to tolerance. The elimination of high affinity self-reactive cells by apoptosis during negative selection of B and T cells in the bone marrow and thymus respectively, ensures those cells will not encounter host antigen leading to cell activation. During T cell development, self-antigens on privileged host tissue is not exposed to T cells in the thymus medulla. Tissues of the eyes, testes and brain are considered immune privileged and antigens from these tissues are not exposed to developing T lymphocytes. While self-reactive lymphocytes may be found in sites considered immuneprivileged, regulatory mechanisms that include suppression of T cell activation may function to prevent host cell attack and the release of proinflammatory cytokines that mediate host tissue damage.

Central tolerance occurs in the bone marrow and thymus. Self-reactive lymphocytes with high affinity to self-antigen can be eliminated by negative selection

© Springer Nature Switzerland AG 2021
T. Y. Sam-Yellowe, *Immunology: Overview and Laboratory Manual*,
https://doi.org/10.1007/978-3-030-64686-8_22

through apoptosis. Self-reactive T lymphocytes can also be rendered anergic through the lack of co-stimulatory signals. Within the thymic medulla, medullary epithelial cells express tissue specific self-antigens which when recognized by self-reactive T cells leads to their deletion. Expression of self-antigens from peripheral tissues and their presentation to developing T cells in the thymus is mediated by the transcription factor AIRE (autoimmune regulator). AIRE turns on peripheral genes in the thymus. Inability to express peripheral self-antigens in the thymus leads to autoimmune disease. Not all self-antigens are expressed in the thymus during T cell development. In developing B cells, receptor editing can occur following initial rearrangements for V-J recombination. Binding of unmethylated CpG to B cell receptors followed by internalization and binding to TLR9 leads to anti-chromatin auto antibodies. Ribonucleoprotein complexes activate naïve B cells by binding to TLR7 or TLR8. Self-reactive B cells are also found in the germinal centers. Peripheral tolerance occurs after T cells have emigrated from the thymus. They can be induced to become regulatory T cells (TREG). Self-reactive lymphocytes from the thymus can be found in the periphery.

Regulatory T cells (TREG) are self-reactive FoxP3 expressing T cells. They suppress autoimmune responses to self-antigens in the periphery. They suppress self-reactive lymphocytes that recognize antigens recognized by the TREG and also those antigens different from those recognized by the TREG, as long as the antigens are presented by the same antigen presenting cell. In peripheral immune tissue, induced TREG also express FoxP3 in response to antigens recognized in the presence of TGFβ in the absence of proinflammatory cytokines. TREG also express CTLA4 and IL-2Rα (CD25). TREG interact with APCs leading to inhibition of APC function, blocking the expression of proinflammatory cytokines such as IL-6, and TNFα as well as blocked expression of CD80/86. TREG also secrete the inhibitory cytokines IL-10, TGFβ and IL-35. In addition to TREGs, regulatory cells from other leukocytes have been described. These include regulatory macrophages, dendritic cells and B cells. Regulatory B cells (B10 cells) secreting IL-10 have been reported to suppress inflammatory activity. Other cells described to be important regulatory cells in tumor environments are myeloid-derived suppressor cells (MDSCs). These cells suppress antigen specific T cell response in tumor environments and secrete IL-10, indoleamine 2, 3-dioxygenase (IDO), arginase-1 and inducible nitric oxide synthase (iNOS). MDSCs also express inhibitory surface molecules like PD-L1.

Autoimmunity

Immune response to self, or autoimmunity was described as "horror autotoxicus" by Paul Ehrlich. Destruction of self-tolerance leads to autoimmune reactions, where the host immune system attacks host tissue. The consequences can be mild, minimal, severe or lifethreatening. The attack can be antibody-mediated or cell-mediated. Autoimmunity is a dysregulation of the immune response, where the host immune response targets self-antigens leading to activation, cytokine release and tissue damage. Tissue damage can release intracellular antigens which then activate T and B cells resulting in autoimmunity. In addition to T and B cells, NK cells are also implicated in the events that lead to alterations in the development of peripheral tolerance such that autoantigen induced cytotoxicity can occur. This is due to the effector functions of NK cells that involve ADCC responses and interactions that take place among DCs, CTLs and TH1 cells. NK activity can be detrimental or beneficial in the development of different autoimmune diseases. Immune complexes formed after antibody response to antigen are cleared by phagocytic cells. Anti-IgG autoantibodies generated against the constant region of IgG produced as a result of immunization or infection known as rheumatoid factor is found in rheumatoid arthritis. In the absence of danger signals from damaged tissue, normal cell activity continues and there is no exposure of self-reactive T cells to damage associated molecular patterns (DAMPs). Autoimmune diseases can be organ specific or systemic, with wide spread tissue damage occurring in systemic disease. Failure of tolerance to self-reactive T and B cells that recognize and engage with specific antigen in different tissue leads to autoimmune disease. In organ specific autoimmunity, immune response targets specific organ and reacts with specific antigens unique to the organ. Both humoral and cell-mediated responses develop to self-antigens. Anti-self-antibodies may overstimulate or block the normal function of the target organ. Examples of autoimmune diseases that are organ specific include Hashimoto's disease, type 1 diabetes and Myasthenia gravis.

Systemic autoimmune disease occurs when autoantibodies to specific antigen on different host tissues results in immune complex formation and cell mediated immunity. If antigen is not cleared and if immune complexes are not cleared by phagocytes reducing complement fixation and the generation of inflammatory mediators, tissue damage may occur. Examples of systemic autoimmune diseases include, systemic lupus erythematosus, multiple sclerosis, rheumatoid arthritis, ankylosing spondylitis, scleroderma and Sjogren's syndrome. The development of autoimmune disease can be influenced by genetic and environmental factors. Major histocompatibility complex genes can influence susceptibility to autoimmune diseases. Ankylosing spondylitis has been shown to be strongly associated with the HLA-B27 allele. Non-MHC genes such as genes encoding cytokines, co-stimulatory molecules and adhesion proteins can also influence disease development. Environmental factors that influence autoimmune disease include infection, smoking, obesity and the microbiome. Infections by different pathogens can cause tissue damage that exposes sequestered antigens that can stimulate the reactivity of self-reactive B and T cells.

Landmark observations and experiments were performed by Ray Owen in 1945 where he observed dizygotic cattle which were twins. They shared a common vascular supply and were erythrocyte chimeras that developed due to intrauterine anastomosis. Skin grafts from either twin were tolerated from one another. The Nobel Prize was awarded to Peter Medawar for the reproduction of natural tolerance in the laboratory. Neonatal mice of strain A were injected with viable spleen cells from another histocompatible strain B mouse. The mice grew to adulthood and received grafted skin from strain B. The graft was accepted. A skin graft from strain C mice onto strain A mice was rejected in a normal way. The findings showed that neonatal mice injected with strain B cells were interacting with immature antigen specific cells. They recognized the antigens as self and switched off resulting in long-lasting tolerance. Tolerance occurred during the presence of immunocompetent cells. Injection of syngeneic lymphoid cells abolished tolerance.

Acquired tolerance can occur in mature animals. It is easier to induce tolerance in embryonic or neonatal animals, generally in immature animals. In adults tolerance can be induced in individuals with non-functional immune systems due to irradiation, immunosuppressive drug treatment such as methothrexate, cyclophosphamide and 6-mercaptopurine. The immunogenicity of the antigen is important. For example in experimental antigens BCG-bovine gamma globulin is weakly immunogenic, while HEA (hen egg albumin) or diphtheria toxoid are strong immunogens. The form of the antigen is also important. For example soluble antigens are tolerogenic while particulate antigens are immunogenic. Adjuvants plus antigen or antigens aggregated by heating are immunogenic. Dosage may be critical.

Opposite extremes of dosage such as very small doses or very large doses of antigen may lead to tolerance rather than an immune response. Substances that are not easily metabolized are tolerogenic: For example pneumococcal polysaccharides, unnatural D isomers of amino acids (D-polypeptides) in low doses (0.5–1 μg) are immunogenic while in high doses (10–500 μg) are tolerogenic.

Antigen presenting cells are central to the outcome of immune responses. APCs will determine whether antigen is processed or by-passed. Accessory molecules on APCs are also important for providing the additional signals necessary to either activate a T cell or induce anergy. Chiller and Weigle experiments demonstrated the kinetics of B and T cell tolerance and showed that both B and T cells are susceptible to tolerance induction. They showed that susceptibility differs with respect to dose of antigen and time required for induction. The duration of tolerance is shorter in B cells than in T cells. The immunological status of the animal reflects the population of T cells for T dependent antigens. The transfer of cells to irradiated mice showed that T cells tolerized rapidly after antigen injection by 24 h. Tolerance was maintained for about 100 days. B cells were tolerized by 10–11 days and tolerance maintained for 49–50 days. Tolerance in normal animals paralleled T cell pattern. B cell recovery in animals still immunologically unresponsive i.e. no antigen specific T cells. Ontogenic origins of T and B cells are responsible for the different recovery times i.e. whether the cells are from the bone marrow or thymus. T cells become tolerant to lower doses of antigen. With high doses of antigen both B and T cells become tolerized. The mechanisms of B and T cell tolerance are similar. **B cell tolerance can occur due to c**lonal anergy and clonal deletion of both bone marrow and peripheral B cells. Clonal exhaustion may also occur. T cell tolerance can occur due to clonal deletion in thymus and also extrathymically. Clonal anergy can also occur due to absence of costimulatory and/or progression signals.

Mechanisms Leading to the Development of Autoimmunity

Both genetic (MHC genotype) and environmental factors are partly responsible for the development of autoimmunity. Reaction to self-antigens in this case is the result of acquired immune response to self-antigens. This response is a specific T cell response. Self-tolerance is lost and so the autoimmune reaction is a sustained reaction to self. This potential for the host to turn the immune response against itself is known as *horror autotoxicus,* a term coined by Paul Ehrlich, and is responsible for severe self-reaction to host tissue and extensive tissue damage in some individuals. During development both B and T cells develop open repertoires that allow them to recognize antigens from any pathogen or foreign substance as well as self-antigens. Clones recognizing self-antigens are eliminated in a clonal deletion mechanism. However, some self-reactive clones remain. There is a lot of speculation regarding the nature of the self-reactive T cells and those T cells that regulate their activity in the body. This speculation gave rise to the ideas concerning the presence of a subset of T cells known as suppressor T cells which we now recognize as TREG cells. Some $CD4^+$ and $CD8^+$ TREGs may carry out this role.

The question is how to differentiate these cells from non-regulatory effector helper and cytotoxic T cells. In mouse and rat studies, regulatory effector $CD4^+$ T cells bearing the CD25 marker (CD25 = alpha chain of the IL-2 receptor) ($CD4^+$, $CD25^+$) are recognized as important for preventing autoimmunity whereas $CD4^+CD25^-$ T cells are self-reactive in the animals and account for the development of different autoimmune conditions. The former cell type is anergic to antigenic stimulation in vitro and expresses CTLA-4 constitutively. CTLA-4 interacts with CD80 and CD86 (B7-1 and B7-2) on APCs.

Binding of CTLA-4 by specific antibodies leads to the loss of the suppressive function of these cells.

In our discussion of T cell activation, we talked about CTLA-4 being expressed on activated T cells, generating a negative signal to the activated T cell. With the regulatory effector T cell ($CD4^+$, $CD25^+$), CTLA-4 sends an activating signal to the cells. In the absence of regulatory effector T cells self-reactive T cells become activated, differentiate and may function with B cells to produce self-reactive antibodies as well as function with self-reactive $CD8^+$ cells. **Note** the two different ways that CTLA-4 can control the immune response. In other mouse studies there have been conflicting reports of the effects of CTLA-4 in enhancing autoimmune disease- this is a wide open field with much still to be learned regarding the mechanisms responsible for autoimmunity.

Clearly other factors may contribute to autoimmune disease development. In order for tolerance to be maintained the immunological process that underlies that tolerance has to be continuously sustained by cells whose role it is to regulate the activity of self-reactive cells. Some loss of self-tolerance and development of autoimmunity results from host infection by infectious disease organisms. So we have at least two major routes for the development of autoimmunity. In the first instance the defective regulation is not associated with pathogens. Some of the difficulty in studying autoimmunity is related to the observation that all individuals predisposed to autoimmune risk factors will develop autoimmune disease, Some conditions are more common such as in rheumatoid arthritis while others are fairly rare in their occurrence. Several studies have looked at the association of specific autoimmune diseases with specific HLA antigens and relative risk values have been calculated. E.g. Individuals with the HLA-B27 allele have a relative risk value of 87% of the development of ankylosing spondylitis, while individuals with the HLA-DR3 allele have a relative risk value of 6% for developing systemic lupus erythematosus (SLE).

The presence of the DR3 allele is also associated with other autoimmune conditions such as Graves' disease. The presence of other HLA alleles confers protection for the development of some autoimmune diseases. For example HLA-DR2 confers protection for type I insulin dependent diabetes whereas the same allele is associated with multiple sclerosis. Some of the polymorphisms associated with the different alleles are the result of single amino acid changes and these are also found to differ among racial groups. There is also an observed gender predisposition for some of the diseases. MHC genotyping is used to detect these associations. Note that MHC antigens are important in T cell development and in the presentation of self-antigens as well as foreign antigens. It is thought that in the case of some self-reactive T cells that do not get deleted in the thymus i.e. they are positively selected, they interact poorly with self-MHC molecules and so the signals are not strong enough to induce apoptosis in these cells.

Autoimmunity can result from tissue destruction by T cells as well as antibodies. Serological detection of self-reacting antibodies is typically a clue that self-antigens have triggered a specific immune response. Different antibody isotypes have been implicated in autoimmunity; lgM, IgG and lgE. Where lgE responses are noted the response is reminiscent of type I hypersensitivities/immediate hypersensitivity response. While lgM and IgG responses to cell surface molecules reflect type II and type III hypersensitivities (immune complex disease). These responses (IgG and lgM) may be accompanied by classical complement fixation, massive release of cytokines and chemokines and can lead to severe inflammation and tissue destruction.

Mechanisms for induction of autoimmunity include **molecular mimicry**. Pathogens may express protein antigens with sequences resembling those found in host proteins. Immune responses to epitopes on those antigens may activate self-reactive B and T cells Molecular mimicry leading to autoimmunity after infection can occur following viral, bacterial and parasitic infection. Inappropriate expression of class II MHC molecules on tissue cells in IDDM and on beta cells. In Graves' disease on thyroid acinar cells. Induced antigen expression e.g. phytohemagglutinin on thyroid cells, interferon gamma by beta cells of the pancreas. Cytokine imbalance by TH subsets secreting IFN gamma and IL-2 occurs. Dysfunction of the idiotype network. Dysfunction of T cell mediated immune regulation also occurs.

Examples of Autoimmune Diseases

Myasthenia Gravis (Blocking Autoantibodies)

The target of the disease is the acetylcholine receptor at neuromuscular junctions. The reaction of receptors with antibodies specific to the receptors blocks the reception of nerve impulses normally transmitted by the acetylcholine molecules. Muscle weakness develops, difficulty in chewing, swallowing and breathing. Death can occur from respiratory failure. This is linked with the thymus resulting in the development of thymoma. Hypertrophy or removal of the thymus leads to regression of the disease. The disease can be experimentally induced in animals. Injection of purified acetylcholine receptors obtained from torpedo fish or electric eels leads to development of significant cross-reactivity with mammalian receptors. The antibody to the fish receptors binds to the mammalian receptor and mimics the natural disease. The antibodies can also be passively transferred.

Graves' Disease (Stimulating Antibodies)

This is a multisystem disease that manifests as a hyperactive thyroid gland (hyperthyroidism). Autoantibodies produced are directed against a hormone receptor. The antibodies may activate the receptor rather than block its activity. The autoantibodies are specifically directed against thyroid cell surface receptors for the thyroid stimulating hormone (TSH). Interaction of the antibody with the receptor activates the cells in a manner similar to TSH activation, leading to continuous cell stimulation and activation of the cell leading to hyperthyroidism.

Systemic Lupus (Red Wolf) Erythematosus (SLE)

SLE is an immune complex mediated autoimmune disease. It is a systemic disease with multiple organ involvement causing fever, joint pain, and damage to the central nervous system, heart and kidneys. Death results typically from kidney damage. A characteristic reddish rash develops on the cheeks and bridge of the nose. SLE patients produce autoantibodies directed against several nuclear components of the body including chromatin. Autoreactive anti-nuclear antibodies (ANA) are produced against native ds DNA, denatured ssDNA and nucleohistones. Clinically the presence of the anti-dsDNA antibodies correlates best with pathology of renal involvement in SLE. In the past, DNA was not thought to be immunogenic and so the development of DNA reactive antibodies was a mystery. Experimentally it was very difficult to induce antibodies to DNA by immunization. Recent studies have shown that it is not unusual to develop anti-DNA antibodies. Immunogenicity of the

DNA differs depending on the source of the DNA. The auto antibodies to DNA bind to DNA and the circulating immune complexes are filtered out of the blood into the kidneys and the ICs get trapped against the basement membranes of the glomeruli. ICs also get deposited in the arteriolar walls, joint synovial spaces (lumpy-bumpy deposits), complement gets activated resulting in inflammation and the recruitment of granulocytes occurs into sites of inflammation. Glomerulonephritis (inflammation of the glomeruli), proteinuria (protein leakage) and hematuria (hemorrhage) develop. The severity of the symptoms is dependent on the extent of IC formation. There are instances where no circulating ICs are found. In these cases the DNA may be trapped as antibodies react with the DNA and similar sequence of events are observed. Infection by some strains of *Klebsiella* sp. induce DNA reactive antibodies. The common antigenic epitopes of the DNA is believed to be the phosphate backbone of the DNA as well as the polysaccharide moieties.

Rheumatoid Arthritis, RA (IC Mediated Disease)

Inflammation resulting from deposited immune complexes leads to the disease, rheumatoid arthritis. Abnormally produced autoantibodies react with rheumatoid factor (IgM) forming immune complexes. The Fc portion of the patient's self-IgG complexes with the rheumatoid factor and the complexes become deposited in the synovia of the joint spaces. Complement activation, release of chemotactic factors and recruitment of granulocytes occur. Inflammation develops leading to increased vascular permeability, joint swelling and pain. Exudate also accumulates. Hydrolytic enzymes released by neutrophils break down collagen and cartilage in the joints. Damage to the sliding surfaces of the joints occurs. Fibrin deposits can be found, cartilage is replaced by fibrous tissue, and joints fuse (ankyloses) leading to immobility of the joint.

Antibody and T Cell Mediated Autoimmune Disease

Hashimotos's Thyroiditis

This is a disease of the thyroid, most common in middle-aged women and resulting in Goiter formation. Hypothyroidism is seen as a result of destruction of thyroid function. Autoreaction is against several antigens including thyroglobulin, a major hormone made by the thyroid and microsomal antigens from thyroid epithelial cells. In the thyroid follicles mononuclear cell infiltrates are seen, among them effector T cells, B cells, and macrophages. Local antibody production leads to follicle destruction. Efforts to regenerate the gland leads to enlargement with resultant decline in thyroid hormone production. Symptoms of hypothyroidism are dry skin, puffy face, brittle hair and nails, a constant feeling of being cold. In experimentally induced disease T cell involvement is seen. Animals are immunized with thyroglobulin in complete Freund's adjuvant (CFA). T cell clones specific for thyroglobulin can be passively transferred. In the experimental disease, acute non-recurring symptoms are observed while in the natural disease, chronic recurrent ongoing processes are seen. Development of disease depends on multiple "immunizing" events.

Multiple Sclerosis (T Cell Mediated Autoimmune Disease)

Demyelination of central nervous system tissue leads to progressive paralysis. Lesions that develop have the same cellular infiltrate seen in DTH reactions. In experimental animals induced allergic encephalomyelitis (EAE) is observed. Myelin emulsified in CFA is used for immunization and a T cell mediated response is obtained. A deficiency in complement components may enhance autoimmunity due to impaired removal of immune complexes.

Other Examples

Goodpasture's syndrome
    Autoantibodies are made to the basement membrane antigens of the kidneys and lungs.
    Insulin Dependent Diabetes Mellitus (IDDM)
    Cell mediated DTH response and autoantibodies to beta cells of the pancreas.

Experimental Animals Used

F1 from NZB × NZW mice used to study SLE
    Nonobese diabetic (NOD) mice used as a model for human IDDM

Selected References

Brent L (1997) The discovery of immune tolerance. Human Immunol 52:75–81

Chiller JM, Habicht GS, Weigle WO (1971) Kinetic differences in unresponsiveness of thymus and bone marrow cells. Science 171:813–815

Gianchecchi E, Delfino DV, Fierabracci A (2018) NK cell in autoimmune diseases: Linking innate and adaptive immune responses. Autoimmunity Rev 17:142–154

Guimaraes LE, Baker B, Perricone C, Shoenfeld Y (2015) Vaccines, adjuvants and autoimmunity. Pharmacol Res 100:190–209

Murphy K, Weaver C (2017) Janeway's immunobiology, 9th edn. Garland Press, New York
Punt J, Stranford SA, Jones PP, Owen JA (2019) Kuby immunology, 8th edn. W.H. Freeman and
    Company, New York. Chapter 20, Antigen-antibody interactions
Ribatti D (2009) Sir Frank MacFarlane Burnet and the clonal selection theory of antibody forma-
    tion. Clin Exp Med 9:253–258

Chapter 23
Immunodeficiencies

Immunodeficiency Diseases

These are immune system defects that lead to the inability of an individual to mount an effective innate, humoral (HI) or cell-mediated immune (CMI) response. When host immune responses fail to occur due to the absence of specific molecules or cells required for mounting host defenses, this is known as immunodeficiency. The consequence of immunodeficiencies is that the host becomes vulnerable to infections that are normally kept in check by a competent immune system. Immunodeficiencies that occur due to inherited genetic mutations are known as congenital or primary immunodeficiencies. **Primary immunodeficiencies** are seen in infants and young children. Recurrent infections occur frequently and are typically very severe. Infections or other external factors that affect an already established competent immune system lead to deficiencies known as **acquired or secondary immunodeficiencies**. Acquired immunodeficiencies are caused by known agents such as viruses or immunosuppressive drug treatments. They can occur in children and adults and are also recognized clinically by recurrent and severe infections as well as increased susceptibility to cancers.

Immunodeficiencies can affect the function of both innate and adaptive immune responses. Both effector and regulatory functions of the immune system can be affected. Genetic mutations can lead to loss of expression of specific molecules or the loss of function of the expressed molecule. The genetic mutation of different genes may produce the same effect on the immune system and affect the same branch of the immune system. If the genetic mutation affects developing cells in the bone marrow during hematopoiesis, the resulting immunodeficiency results in the absence of specific cells in the periphery leading to profound deleterious effects on the host. Immunodeficiency can be due to hematopoietic abnormalities such as the absence of cells, development of abnormal cells or persistence of immature cells. Various cells can be affected, including macrophages, dendritic cells, neutrophils or lymphocytes. The deficiency can be as a result of non- production of antibodies,

© Springer Nature Switzerland AG 2021
T. Y. Sam-Yellowe, *Immunology: Overview and Laboratory Manual*,
https://doi.org/10.1007/978-3-030-64686-8_23

complement proteins, cytokines, cytokine receptors, non-expression or reduced expression of Ig and T cell receptors, MHC antigens or cell surface adhesion molecules. The deficiencies can also be due to a lack or non-functional enzymes in the signaling pathways leading to the secretion of various immune products. Below, we discuss examples of deficiencies that affect individual cells and molecules and the resulting effect of the deficiencies on the function of the innate and adaptive branches of the immune system.

Primary Immunodeficiencies

Adaptive Immunity (B and T Cells)

An absence or reduced number of T and B cells results in a condition known as severe combined immunodeficiency (SCID). While the condition occurs due to a lack of functional T cells, B cells require T cell help to secrete antibodies of different isotypes from isotype switching. Without T cells, B cell function will also be impaired. The development of SCID also affects the development of the thymus. A combination of a small and dysplastic thymus, low to no T and B cell detection and evaluation of cell function are used as diagnostic features for SCID. Severe combined immunodeficiency disease (SCID) results from a mutation in the RAG 1 and RAG 2 genes leading to a severe depression in B and T cell counts. RAG 1 and 2 genes are required for VJ and VDJ recombination in B and T cells. Mutations in genes encoding proteins required for DNA repair during gene recombination can also lead to SCID. For example, Artemis is activated by DNA-PKCs to open up the hairpin formed following DNA cleavage by RAG 1. A defect in Artemis results in the accumulation of hairpin-sealed coding ends which interferes with the progression of the recombination process. A defect in DNA-PKC will affect the function of Artemis. A defect in the Ku70/80 complex required for signal and coding joint repair in both B and T cells will also interfere with the VJ and VDJ recombination process. The Ku70/80 complex facilitates the alignment of DNA ends before repair. Adenosine deaminase (ADA) deficiency results in the accumulation of adenosine metabolites which are toxic to B, T and NK cells. A defective common γ (γc) (CD132) chain required by cytokine receptors also leads to SCID. Cytokine signals required for lymphocyte maturation and proliferation are absent in γc deficiency. The following cytokine receptors; IL-2R, IL-4R, IL-7R, IL-9R, IL-15R and IL-21R in which the γc associates with JAK3 required for intracellular signaling in cells, fail to function in the absence of functional γc. JAK3 is a tyrosine kinase required for intracellular signaling. A deficiency in JAK3 can also be detrimental to cell signaling within cells. A deficiency in CD3 subunits due to mutations in the gene encoding the subunits leads to impairment of T cell function. Interaction of the TCR with CD3 is required for the pre-T cell receptor as well as for the intracellular signaling that occurs following antigen binding to the TCR and subsequent activation of the T cell.

T Cells

T cells are affected when thymus development is impaired resulting in DiGeorge syndrome, or when there is a deficiency in CD3 (δ, ε or ζ) subunits. Mutations in the gene encoding the WASP protein affects T cells and platelets resulting in Wiscott-Aldrich syndrome (WAS). Bare lymphocyte syndrome (BLS) resulting from MHCI and MHCII deficiencies affects the development of CD8$^+$ T cells and CD4$^+$ T cells, respectively. MHCI deficiencies occur due to mutations in the genes encoding β2-microglobulin which interacts with the alpha chain of MHCI and required for proper functioning of the MHCI molecule. Mutations in the gene encoding the TAP protein required for transportation of processed peptides from the proteasome to the ER also affect MHCI function and presentation of peptides to CD8$^+$ T cells. Mutations in the gene encoding the chaperone protein tapasin interfere with peptide loading into the peptide binding groove and also affect peptide presentation to CD8$^+$ cytotoxic T cells. Mutations in the genes encoding transcription factors necessary for expression of the α and β chains of the MHCII proteins results in a lack of MHCII proteins. In the absence of MHCI molecules, the number of CD8$^+$ T cells is severely reduced. In the absence of MHCII proteins, there is a deficiency in CD4$^+$ T cells.

B Cells

B cells are affected when there are mutations in Bruton's tyrosine kinase (Btk), leading to X-linked agammaglobulinemia. Mature B cells are not formed. Common variable immunodeficiency results in low IgG, IgA and variable IgM levels. Activation-induced cytidine deaminase (AID) is required for somatic hypermutation and isotype switching in B cell. Mutations in AID lead to the absence or reduced levels of IgG, IgA and IgE. IgM levels may remain normal or become elevated. Mutations in the co-stimulatory molecules CD40L and CD40 results in Hyper-IgM syndrome, with increased levels of IgM production and impaired activation of APCs and reduced T cell response to intracellular pathogens.

Natural Killer Cells

In Chediak-Higashi syndrome, cytotoxic activity of CTLs and NK cells are decreased due to defects in lysosomal trafficking regulator protein (LYST). Enlarged cytoplasmic organelles are observed in NK and CTLs, and transport of organelles is impaired. The defect also affects melanosomes leading to loss of pigmentation. Neutropenia, a lack of neutrophils is also characterized by this syndrome. Phagocytes with enlarged organelles are impaired and cannot kill phagocytized pathogens.

Innate and Adaptive Immunity

Cell adhesion protein deficiency affects the migration (chemotaxis) and diapedesis of leukocytes. In leukocyte adhesion deficiency (LAD), mutations occur in the gene encoding the common β chain required for expression of integrins in LFA-1 (CD11a), Mca-1 (CD11b) and gp150/95 (CD11c). Lack of integrins, impairs cell-cell adhesion between APCs and T cells and results in impaired recruitment of cells to sites of inflammation. Deficiencies in complement proteins can affect the three pathways of complement fixation. Deficiencies in the early proteins of the complement pathway, such as C1, C2, C3 and C4 leads to recurrent bacterial infections caused by gram positive and gram negative bacteria. Infections by pus forming (pyogenic) bacterial species of *Staphylococcus* and *Streptococcus* also occur. C3 deficiencies can be severe, as this affects the three pathways of complement fixation. Impaired clearance of immune complexes can lead to immune complex diseases. Mannose binding lectin (MBL) deficiency affects the lectin pathway of complement fixation. Pyrogenic (fever-inducing) bacterial infections occur in babies and children. As well recurring upper respiratory tract infections occurs in children due to MBL deficiency. Deficiencies in the regulatory components of the complement pathway can also result in impaired function of the complement pathways. The C1 inhibitor (C1INH) inhibits the activity of C1. Specifically, in the presence of the plasma protein C1INH, persistent association of the C1q component with C1r2s2 is reduced to prevent excessive activation of C4 and C2 by C1. This prevents continuous activation of the classical and lectin pathways. C1INH also inhibits MASP-2 protease in the lectin pathway. A deficiency in C1INH leads to continuous activation of the classical and lectin pathways of complement and development of the condition, hereditary angioedema (HANE). Excessive production of vasoactive mediators leads to edema as a result of extracellular fluid accumulation. Edema occurs in the face, gastrointestinal tract and upper respiratory tract. Airway obstruction can become severe and lead to death.

Regulatory T Cells

Mutations in the genes encoding the transcription factors AIRE and FoxP3 affects negative selection of T cells and development of TREGs. This leads to decreases in cell numbers and the development of autoimmunity. Mutations in the AIRE gene, results in a condition known as autoimmune polyendocrinopathy with candidiasis and ectodermal dystrophy (APECED). Negative selection of T cells in the thymus is impaired and development of TREGs is impaired. Mutation in the FoxP3 gene results in an absence of TREGs and development of the condition known as immune dysregulation, polyendocrinopathy, enteropathy, X-linked (IPEX) syndrome.

Secondary Immunodeficiencies

Immunocompetent individuals may experience loss of immune function due to exposure to environmental factors, exposure to ionizing radiation, treatment with immunosuppressive drugs, being infected by infectious disease agents, presence of metabolic or chronic diseases and malnutrition. Tissue injury following surgery or trauma to tissues can also result in reduced immune responses. This type of loss of immune function is known as secondary or acquired immunodeficiency. The two major causes of secondary immunodeficiencies are malnutrition and HIV infection leading to AIDS.

Radiation treatments for cancer, damage actively dividing cells in the body including hematopoietic cells in the bone marrow. The bone marrow can become depleted of hematopoietic cells. Damage to B and T lymphocytes can also occur leading to impaired immune responses to antigen. Individuals receiving cytotoxic drugs may also experience secondary immunodeficiencies as a result of damage to hematopoietic cells. Drugs such as cyclophosphamide, methotrexate, sulfasalazine and hydroxychloroquine can inhibit B and T cell proliferation that can dampen responses to pathogens and render individuals susceptible to viral, bacterial, fungal and parasitic infections. Cytotoxic drug treatment cause cytopenias that can affect different organs such as the gastrointestinal tract and skin leading to secondary immunodeficiencies and susceptibility to infections. DNA synthesis is impaired, cell cycle arrest occurs and apoptosis is induced in cells. The gut barrier mucosa becomes weak leading to breaches of the barrier by opportunistic organisms leading to infection. Immunosuppresssive drugs used for treatments of transplant rejection, allergic disorders and autoimmune diseases can also decrease immune function causing susceptibility to infections. Cyclosporin (Cyclosporin A) and tacrolimus interact with immunophilins in the T cell cytosol, leading to inhibition of the phosphatase calcineurin with resultant inhibition of the transcription factor NFAT and decreased T cell activity. Corticosteroid treatments can lead to decreased cytokine production, cell adhesion and leukocyte chemotaxis. Interleukin-2 mediated responses become inhibited and effector T and B cell functions affected. Inflammatory responses as a result of tissue injury following surgery or as a result of trauma to tissues can lead to DAMPs binding to PRRs such as TLRs leading to cytoplasmic signaling and the secretion of proinflammatory cytokines. Splenectomy patients experience increased infections by capsule producing bacteria like *Streptococcus pneumonia*.

Immature immune systems and waning responses in adult immunity as seen in neonates and the elderly, respectively, can lead to increased susceptibility to viral and bacterial infections. In neonates, the secondary and tertiary lymphoid tissue is immature and may compromise specific recognition and response to antigen by B cells. Premature infants may not have circulating maternal IgG and will be susceptible to infections. In the elderly, chronic diseases, metabolic diseases and malignancies render individuals susceptible to viral and bacterial infections. Involution of the thymus leads to reduced T cell production and T cell oligoclonality. Impaired T cell function can lead to low B cell diversity.

On a global scale, malnutrition due to macronutrient and micronutrient deficiency is the most important cause of secondary immunodeficiencies. In particular, chronic low protein calorie malnutrition can manifest in low protein availability for leukocyte development and the production of the protein products needed for immune function such as antibodies and cytokines. T cell numbers and effector T cell function are affected. Both innate and adaptive immunity are affected by malnutrition. Micronutrient deficiencies of vitamins C and D are also important contributors to the effects of malnutrition to secondary immunodeficiencies. Infectious disease agents play an important role in the development of secondary immunodeficienceis.

One of the most important cases of secondary immunodeficiency is caused by the HIV virus in AIDS patients. Acquired immunodeficiency syndrome (AIDS) is caused by the human immunodeficiency virus (HIV; HIV-I and HIV-II). HIV is a retrovirus i.e. it has an RNA genome, a single stranded RNA. HIV consists of T cell tropic strains that infect CD4+ T helper cells and monocyte/macrophage tropic strains that infect macrophages also expressing some CD4. The CD4 molecule is used as the receptor for cell binding but for cell entry additional proteins known as chemokine receptors are required. The chemokine receptor CCR5 expressed on T cells and CXCR4 expressed on monocytes and macrophages provide the additional entry receptors. These latter proteins are co-receptors and are transmembrane proteins spanning the membrane seven times. Transmission of the virus is by body fluid contact through the exchange of bodily fluids. Sexual contact, shared needles from intravenous drug use, use of shared contaminated needles for multiple treatment injections among individuals that are infected with HIV, mother-fetus transfer of HIV and transfer of virus during breast feeding.

Life Cycle of HIV

1. HIV attachment through gp120 glycoprotein to CD4 and chemokine receptor on host cell and entry of viral nucleocapsid into cell.
2. Viral genome and enzymes released into host cell cytoplasm.
3. Viral reverse transcriptase reverse transcribes the RNA into cDNA, RNA is degraded by ribonuclease H and second strand DNA is synthesized.
4. DNA is integrated into host cell genome by viral integrase enzyme, activation of viral transcription factors and transcription of viral mRNA for virus protein translation.
5. Virus mRNA translocates to cytoplasm associates with host cell ribosomes and synthesis of viral proteins (precursor proteins) occurs. Proteins are cleaved by viral proteases.
6. The viral proteins assemble beneath the host cell plasma membrane, the virions are assembled and gp 120 and gp 41 are inserted into the virions.
7. The virions bud out of the host cell enclosed by membrane lipid.

HIV infects cells expressing CD4 and coreceptor molecules CCR5 and CXCR4. T helper cells mostly express CD4. However, cells of the monocyte/ macrophage lineage also express CD4; including glial cells in the brain. Also, megakaryocytes express CD4. Following infection of CD4⁺ T helper cells with the HIV virus, infected cells migrate to the lymph nodes where viral replication and reinfection of TH cells occurs. The infection spreads to the GI tract where memory TH cells become infected. Infection of cells in the gut associated lymphoid tissue (GALT) and their subsequent destruction leads to depletion of cells in the GALT. A decrease in T helper cell populations of 200–400 cells/μL, decreases TH cell function and impairs the effectiveness of CD8⁺ Tc cells in cell mediated immunity required for clearance of infected cells. As infection progresses other cell functions dependent on TH cells also become impaired. The deficiency of TH cells makes AIDS patients susceptible to a number of opportunistic infections caused by fungi, parasites, bacteria and other viruses. Infections that define AIDS include, pneumonia caused by *Pneumocyctis jirovecii* (formerly *P. carinii*), cryptosporidiosis resulting in diarrhea caused by *Cryptosporidium parvum*, toxoplasmosis, candidiasis and malignancies such as Kaposi's sarcoma. Other infectious disease agents that can lead to secondary immunodeficiencies include, Epstein-Barr virus which infects B lymphocytes causing infectious mononucleosis. CD8⁺ Tc cells activated by the infection induce apoptosis in the B cells leading to their destruction and suppression of the adaptive immune responses. Toxic shock syndrome-1 superantigen produced by strains of *Staphylococcus aureus* bind to the TCR on T cells, at particular Vβ chains leading to T cell activation and production of large amounts of cytokines. The resulting T cell anergy leads to suppression of adaptive immune responses.

Selected References

Geha R, Notarangelo L Case studies in immunology: A clinical companion, 6th edn. Garland Sciences, London

Murphy K, Weaver C (2017) Janeway's immunobiology, 9th edn. Garland Press, New York

Punt J, Stranford SA, Jones PP, Owen JA (2019) Kuby immunology, 8th edn. W.H. Freeman and Company, New York. Chapter 20, Antigen-antibody interactions

Chapter 24
Cancers

Cancer cells are host cells that have become transformed with resultant dysregulated cell cycles leading to **neoplastic** growth. This is due to a mutation(s) that occurs in the cell resulting in abnormal growth. Continued survival and growth of the abnormal cell will result in cell division that produces progeny with the same mutation and cell cycle dysregulation. A local accumulation of the neoplastic cells will result in a **tumor**. If the tumor remains localized and does not spread, it is known as a **benign tumor**. A benign tumor cell does not invade the surrounding healthy tissue. If the neoplastic cells become invasive and enter the blood stream, where they become transported to other tissue sites, the invasive tumors are known as **metastatic** or **malignant tumor** cells. Malignant tumor cells become increasingly more invasive and spread to surrounding or distant tissue sites. **Cancer cells** are neoplastic or abnormal cell growth leading to uncontrollable cell proliferation. Normal cells become transformed due to inherited genetic mutations or extrinsically induced mutations. This leads to autonomous growth of the transformed cells. The growth is of **monoclonal origin**. A single abnormal cell enters into the cell division cycle resulting in all progeny containing the same defect. This type of growth represents the basis for benign or malignant growth.

Since cells from each of the four basic tissue types can become cancerous, cancers are categorized according to the embryonic tissue of origin. Epithelial tissue cancers are known as carcinomas. Cancers can develop in the mucosal linings and skin. Connective tissue cancers can originate from mesodermal connective tissue such as bone, cartilage and adipose tissue. Connective tissue cancers also occur in blood cells and from cells developing in the bone marrow during hematopoiesis. Cancers developing during hematopoiesis are known as leukemias. After blood cells leave the bone marrow and migrate to the peripheral tissues, cancers that develop in those cells are known as lymphomas and myelomas.

Classification of Cancers
- Skin cancers: Non-melanoma (basal cell carcinomas from epidermal basal cells, and squamous cell carcinomas also in the epidermis from epithelial cells derived from basal cells) and Melanomas.

© Springer Nature Switzerland AG 2021
T. Y. Sam-Yellowe, *Immunology: Overview and Laboratory Manual*,
https://doi.org/10.1007/978-3-030-64686-8_24

Carcinomas: most common type; epithelial tissue cancers
Sarcomas: connective (supporting) tissue cancers such as bone
Lymphoma: lymphoid tissue cancers, solid tumors (masses)
Leukemias: Hematopoietic tissue cancers affecting single cells e.g. bone marrow cancers
Brain and nervous system cancers

Transformed cells are neoplastic with increased cell proliferation. A change in the expression of antigens on cancer cells and a suppression in apoptosis characterize cancer cells. The immune system targets cancer cells, with CTLs recognizing antigen presented on MHC class I proteins on neoplastic cell. However, cancer cells escape CTL cytotoxicity and continue to proliferate. When the cell cycle in cells is no longer being regulated, cells will begin to grow uncontrollably and this type of cell growth will produce tumors or cancer cells. Cells can become transformed due to exposure to ionizing radiation, chemicals, viruses or other infectious agents such as parasites. For example, among viruses, hepatitis B (HBV) and C (HCV) viruses, which are DNA viruses, cause liver carcinoma. Epstein-Barr virus (EBV), a DNA virus causes Burkitt's lymphoma and nasopharyngeal carcinoma. Burkitt's lymphoma develops when the transcription factor gene c-myc is translocated from chromosome 8 to the immunoglobulin (Ig) heavy chain enhancer region on chromosome 14. The RNA virus HTLV-1 (human T cell leukemia virus-1), causes adult T-cell leukemia or lymphoma. Infection by the parasitic fluke, *Schistosoma hematobium* is associated with the development of squamous cell carcinoma of the bladder. Additional parasitic flukes associated with cholangiocarcinoma include *Clonorchis sinensis* and *Opistorchis viverrini*. The gram negative bacterium *Helicobacter pylori* is associated with gastric adenocarcinoma and mucosa associated lymphoid tissue lymphoma.

Example of Carcinogenic Agents:

1. Chemical agents
2. Radiation exposure
3. Physical agents
4. Parasites and infectious agents
5. Gene rearrangements
6. Random mutations in the genes
7. Dietary components, e.g. aflatoxin

Genes important during the cell cycle include, proto-oncogenes, tumor suppressor genes and genes that regulate programmed cell death or apoptosis. **Proto-oncogenes** are present in normal host cells and encode growth factors and growth factor receptors. Mutations in proto-oncogenes as a result of cell exposure to carcinogens leads to aberrant gene expression, loss of control in gene expression and increase in cell proliferation, leading to cell transformation and development of cancer cells. For example, the growth factor gene *neu* encodes HER2 a protein related to epidermal growth factor (EGF) receptor. Mutations in *neu* are associated with breast cancer. Mutated proto-oncogenes are known as **oncogenes**. Proto-oncogenes also encode transcription factors and cell signaling molecules. Mutations in the genes encoding the tyrosine kinases, src, abl, and ras are also associated with cancer cell development. Overexpression of *src, abl, ras* and *neu* lead to uncontrolled cell proliferation. Similarly, mutations in the genes encoding the proteins jun and fos, components of the AP1 transcription factor are also associated with neoplastic growth. The increased secretion of growth factors, cytokine and transcription factors leads to increased cell proliferation. Apoptosis of cancer cells prevents proliferation and accumulation of neoplastic cells. Expression of pro-apoptotic genes such as Bax, Bim and Puma will lead to apoptosis in transformed cells, as well engagement of CTLs with neoplastic cells will lead to cytotoxicity and apoptosis. Expression of the anti-apoptotic genes, bcl-2 and Bcl-XL leads to suppression of apoptosis and cancer cell survival.

Proteins encoded by **tumor suppressor genes** inhibit uncontrolled cell proliferation. Non-functional tumor suppressor genes allow excessive cell proliferation. Mutations in TP53 a gene that encodes the nuclear phosphoprotein p53, is found in more than 60% of cancers. The TP53 gene product is involved in diverse cellular activities including growth arrest, DNA repair and apoptosis. Mutations in the retinoblastoma gene leads to hereditary rare childhood cancer. Cytotoxic cells of the immune system such as CTLs, NK, NKT and macrophages attack cancer cells under the influence of cytokines released by CD4+ helper T cells. The cytokines IFNα, IFNβ, IFNγ and IL-12 are important for recruiting NK, NKT, M1/M2 macrophages and myeloid derived suppressor (MDSCs) cells. The environment of chronic inflammation developed as a result of the proliferating cancer cells, generation of the inflammatory mediators and cell recruitment becomes an ideal environment for the recruitment of MDSCs. Macrophages also secrete TNFα which has anti-tumor activity. With the progression and persistence of the cancer cells, TREGs and other regulatory cells secrete immunosuppressive cytokines like IL-10, TGF-β and indoleamine-2,3-dioxygenase (IDO). Cancer cells can evade attack by CTLs. Mutations in MHC class I gene can result in decreased MHCI expression leading to tumor cell growth.

Cancer cells may express antigens that are unique to the cancer cells and not expressed on normal cells. These antigens known as **tumor specific antigens (TSA)** can be recognized by CTLs and by B cells. The unique antigens may contain unique amino acid sequences defining new epitopes. The unique antigens may also result from mutations in the genes present in normal cells and encode antigens resulting in variants on the cancer cells. Lineage specific antigens normally expressed during hematopoiesis or in fetal tissue may become expressed in differentiated cells. Particular antigens may also become overexpressed in some cancer cells. The proteins found on normal cells that have differential expression on cancer cells are known as **tumor associated antigens (TAA)**. Oncofetal tumor antigens such as **carcinoembryonic antigen (CEA)** are normally expressed in the GI and liver of 2–6 month old fetuses in utero. This antigen can be expressed on some cancer cells. Epidermal growth factor receptor is overexpressed in some cancer cells.

Molecular Mechanisms for the Expression of Tumor Antigens

1. Biosynthesis of new molecules
2. Angiogenesis i.e. formation of new blood vessels
3. Unique degradation products of abnormal cell proteins

4. Alteration in the structure of normal molecules
5. Uncovering of normally protected proteins
6. Incorrect assembly of multimeric antigens
7. Aberrant expression of fetal or differentiation antigens

A lack of T cells results in an increase in cancers. CTLs recognize antigens on cancers in association with MHCI and target the cell for destruction and elimination. In the microenvironment of the cancer, tumor infiltrating lymphocytes (TILs) are recruited and infiltrate the tumor environment. The lymphocytes include NK and NKT cells. Mutations in the perforin gene affect the activity of CTLs, NK and NKT cells which use perforin to induce apoptosis in target cancer cells. Interferon-γ produced by CD4+ TH1 cells is important for CTL, NK and NKT activation and elimination of cancer cells. The cytokine IL-12 is important for recruiting dendritic cells (DCs) which can activate TH1 and CTLs. Mutation of the genes for Fas and the TNF-related apoptosis-inducing ligand (TRAIL), leads to upregulation of anti-apoptotic mediators and results in increased cell proliferation and decreased apoptosis. Mutations in the genes encoding co-stimulatory molecules such as CD80/86 and CD 28 leads to T cell anergy and development of immune tolerance to cancer cells. Immunosupression in the tumor microenvironment by secretion of TGFβ, IL-10 and IDO prevents apoptosis. Chronic inflammation increases angiogenesis. With increase blood cell development, there is increased invasion of tissue by cancer cells and increased production of cellular stress signals. Genotoxic stress leads to increases in mutation rates. Checkpoint inhibitors are among the many immunotherapeutic agents used to treat cancers. The molecules CTLA-4 and PDL1 are targets of checkpoint inhibitors. Antibodies to CTLA-4 block interaction with CD80. B cells also produce antibodies to antigens expressed on the surface of cancer cells. The antibodies target the cancer cells expressing the antigens; either TSA or TAA. Immunotherapies directed at tumors cells utilize monoclonal antibodies (Mab) alone or complexed with toxic molecules. Monoclonal antibodies to CD20 are used for non-Hodgkins lymphoma and HER2 receptor for breast cancer. Anti-idiotype antibodies are used for treating B cell lymphoma.

Terms to Know

Proto-oncogenes: Normal regulatory genes whose products are involved in the cell cycle, cell growth, division and differentiation.

Oncogenes: Proto-oncogenes with mutations. Oncogenes (oncogenic) can cause transformation in cells.

Oncogenesis: Transformation of normal cells to neoplastic (cancer) cells.

Oncology: The study of cancer

Oncologist: A scientist or physician that studies or treats cancers

Tumor suppressor genes: Cell cycle regulatory genes that prevent abnormal cell growth, e.g. p53 gene

Malignant: Invasive cancerous growth

Metastatic (metastasis): Secondary growth of tumor at a new site in the body

Benign: Non-invasive cancerous growth

Neoplastic (neoplasm): New or abnormal cell growth.

Appendix

Practice Questions

Part I

1. Define or explain the following terms: Be specific and brief.
   Innate immunity
   Intron
   Hematopoiesis
   Phagocytosis
   Exogenous antigen
   Syngeneic mice
   Restriction endonuclease
   Antibody
   Stem cell
   Immunogen
2. Northern blotting detects the presence of _____ while western blotting detects the presence of _____.
3. What is the difference between a cDNA library and a genomic library?
4. Name two primary lymphoid organs.
5. Name two secondary lymphoid organs.
6. What cells express the following cell surface markers: CD4, CD8, CD16, CD19, CD40L, mIgM?
7. Which of the cells in # 6 secrete antibodies?
8. Which is the correct order for gene expression? Circle the correct choice and name the events in each section (of the correct choice only) e.g. translation, replication, etc.

   (a) DNA<------->DNA ---- >RNA----->PROTETN
   (b) RNA<------- > RNA---- >DNA----->PROTEIN
   (c) PROTEIN<-------- > PROTETN ----- > DNA----->RNA

9. What is the clonal selection theory?
10. Name the five features of specific immunity.
11. What is the difference between a hybrid lymphoid cell line and a cloned lymphoid cell line?

Part II

1. Define or explain the following terms:
   Cluster of differentiation antigen
   Colony stimulating factors
   Progenitor cells
   Hapten

Epitope
Antigenic shift
Antigenic drift
High endothelial venule
Apoptosis
Cell adhesion molecule
Germinal centers
M cells

2. Very briefly i.e. in two to three sentences, what is the function of primary and secondary lymphoid organs?
3. Name two biological functions each for IgG and IgA.
4. List three properties each for B and T cell epitopes.
5. What do the following immunologic properties of an antigen mean?
   Immunogenicity:
   Antigenicity:
6. List five factors that influence immunogenicity.
7. Name three families of cell adhesion molecules.
8. Give two conclusions about the origins of blood cells derived from the experiments of Ernest A. McCulloch and James E. Till.

Part III

1. Outline the antigen processing pathways for an endogenous antigen and exogenous antigen.
2. The HLA-A genes on human chromosome _____ encoded class _____ proteins.
   The equivalent histocompatibility genes on mouse chromosome _____ are
3. What is antibody diversity? How is antibody diversity generated in B cells? What features are employed in the process of generating the antibody molecule?
4. Illustrate the arrangement of the Ig transcript in (a) a pre-B cell and (b) a mature B cell.
5. Define or explain the following:
   Congenic mice
   Isotype switching
   Recombination activation genes (RAG-l/RAG-2)
   12/23 Joining rule
6. Diversity genes encode the hypervariable regions of light chains. T or F.
7. To what region of the MHC class I and class II proteins does peptide bind? What are the following proteins: beta-2-microglobulin, and Ii chain? Where are they found?

Part IV

1. How does antigen processing and presentation differ in a class I and class II MHC pathway for an MHC restricted T cell?
2. What does positive and negative selection in T cell development mean?
3. What is the primary signal required for T cell activation? What is the secondary signal? What happens if the signaling sequence is impaired?
4. What cells express or secrete the following co-stimulatory molecules?
   CD40
   CD40L
   CD80
   CD86
   CTLA-4
   CD28
   CD45 IL-I
   IL-6
   In general why are co-stimulatory molecules necessary?
5. Name the cells that express the following cell surface markers.
   IgM
   CD8
   CD4
   CD2
   CD3
   CD45
   CD19
   CD22
   CD5
   CD18/11a
6. What are cytokines? How are cytokines used to differentiate TH1 and TH2 cells? How are the cytokine receptors grouped? List the cytokines required for optimal T cell-B cell interaction to occur. What is the role of each cytokine in this process?

Part V

1. Describe the kinetics of the immune response.
2. Name the fragments of an IgG molecule generated following treatment with:
   Papain
   Pepsin
   2-mercaptoethanol
3. What are the differences between the following: Be specific and brief.
   Synthetic peptide vaccine, anti-idiotype vaccine, attenuated vaccine and multi-subunit vaccine.
4. In general why is it more difficult to prepare vaccines against bacterial and parasitic infections as compared to viral infections?

5. Correct the following processing and presentation pathways:
   Intracellular Ag → phagosome → proteosome → peptides → MHC class II/beta 2 microglobulin → CD4$^+$ cells. This is an example of an exogenous antigen. T or F
   Extracellular Ag → proteosome → endocytic vesicles → MHC class II/Ii chain → CD8$^+$ cells.
   This is an example of an endogenous antigen. T or F
6. Define or explain the following:
   Antigen
   Carrier protein
   Immunogen
   Toxoid
   Vaccine
   Active immunization
   Passive immunization
   Affinity maturation of antibody
   Somatic mutation
   Carrier effect
   Allogeneic effect
   Germinal centers
   Variolation
   Cell homing
   Transgenic mice
   Targeted gene-knock-out mice
   Allelic exclusion
   Positive T cell selection
   Negative T cell selection
   Tolerance

Part VI

1. An antibody molecule can have either a kappa or lambda light chain but never both. Discuss why two types of light chains are required by the body.
2. What are mitogens? What are superantigens? Name specific B and T cell mitogens. How does mitogenic stimulation differ from antigenic stimulation of lymphocytes?
3. What is the difference between the following assays, and when is it appropriate to use them?
   Enzyme-linked immunosorbent assay
   Western blotting
   Immunofluorescence
   Immunoelectron microscopy

4. Diagram a typical lgG molecule and include immunoglobulin domains, hinge region, H and L chains, inter- and intradisulfide bonds, antigen binding sites, Fab and Fc domains. How would you modify the diagram to depict secretory lgM?
5. Diagram the alpha/beta T cell receptor complex. Label the transmembrane regions and the regions that have the immunoglobulin fold.
6. What role do helper T cells play in an antibody response? Briefly describe distinguishing features of the alpha/beta, and gamma/delta receptor complexes. Outline the biochemical consequences of triggering a TCR/CD3 with the appropriately presented antigen.
7. What is the significance of MHC polymorphism in infectious diseases? Is the polymorphic feature always an advantage to the host? How is MHC polymorphism generated?
8. What are the major features of cell mediated immunity and humoral immunity?
9. Describe three assays used for detecting cell mediated immune reactions. (Cellular cytotoxicity or delayed type hypersensitivity reactions).
10. Diagram the interaction of antigen with macrophages to show the following events:

   (a) Antigen presentation to MHC class II restricted T cells leading to antibody production and isotype switching to IgE.
   (b) Antigen presentation to MHC class I restricted T cells leading to cytolysis.
   (c) If an inflammatory response develops as a result of T cell activation and cytokine secretion leading to DTH response, what cell types would be involved? Show these events in your diagram. Indicate the cytokines involved, and the cell surface markers depicting the major cell types in each case.
   (d) Briefly describe the expected course of events if the B and T cells are functionally inactivated. What are some of the causes of cell inactivation or anergy?
   (e) What does the clonal selection theory have to do with a-d?

11. Describe the classical and alternate pathways of complement activation.
12. If C3 and C5 convertase are detected in the serum but the membrane attack complex is not formed, what genes might be affected in this individual?

Study Guide Immunology Examination 1

Define or explain the following terms:

Innate immunity
Adaptive immunity
Passive immunity
Herd immunity

Afferent branch of the immune system
Efferent branch of the immune system
Lymphoid organs
Stem cells
Inflammation

What are the benefits of the inflammatory response?

Humoral immunity
Cell-mediated immunity
Antigen

Know the difference between antigenic shift and antigenic drift and how different antigens can be used for serotyping of bacteria.

Cluster of differentiation antigens
Phagocytosis
Endocytosis
Immunogen
Hapten

Know the significance of the Landsteiner experiments with haptens.

Epitope
Know the characteristics of B and T cell epitopes

Adjuvant
Antibody
Immunoglobulin superfamily

What characteristics define an antigen?
What are the five features of the adaptive immune response?

Cells
Know the function of the different leukocytes.
How is hematopoiesis regulated?
What is leukocyte homing? Extravasation?
Why do leukocytes migrate/recirculate?
How do lymphocytes migrate?
What are stem cells? What do the terms totipotent, pluripotent and multipotent stem cells mean? How can the cells be manipulated to differentiate?

Antibody structure:

Know the experiments of Rodney Porter, Gerald Edelman and Alfred Nisonoff.
Be able to illustrate a typical antibody molecule. Know the structural differences between the five isotypes, functions of each isotype, the significance of dimerization/polymerization of IgA and IgM.
Know which of the isotypes have subisotypes. Be able to explain the difference between allotypic, idiotypic and isotypic determinants.

Know the parts of an antibody molecule i.e. constant region domains-know function of domains, variable region, hypervariable region, framework regions, hinge region etc.

Know which parts of the antibody contribute to antigen binding and biological activity. Be able to name examples and explain biological activities of antibodies e.g. precipitation, opsonization etc.

Know the difference between polyclonal and monoclonal antibodies. How are monoclonal antibodies prepared? What are the uses of monoclonal antibodies?

Immunoglobulin rearrangement:

What is the clonal selection theory?
What is the Dryer and Bennet two gene model? How was this model verified?
Know Susumu Tonegawa experiments
Know the features that contribute to the development of lg structure and lg diversity.
Multiple immunoglobin genes in the germ line
Know location of genes, organization of genes,
Heavy and light chain rearrangements
Know mechanisms of variable gene rearrangements for H and L chain
Expression and combination of the heavy and light chains
Allelic exclusion
Isotype switching
Somatic hypermutation
Expression of membrane or secreted immunoglobulin
Regulation of immunoglobulin rearrangement

Antibody-antigen interaction

What is affinity?
What is avidity?
What types of interactions occur between an antigen (epitope) and the antigen binding site on an antibody?
What is the difference between primary and secondary binding assays? Name some examples of primary and secondary binding assays.

Worksheet 1

Vocabulary: Define or explain the following terms

Immune system
Lymphatic system
Innate immunity
LPS binding protein
C-reactive protein
Mannose binding lectin

Complement proteins
Antigen
Non-pathogeneic antigen
Pathogenic antigen
Microbe
Bacteria
Virus
Cell
Molecule
Lymph nodes
White blood cells
Macrophages
Dendritic cells
Spleen
Lymphocytes
Antibody
Vaccine
Toxoid
Inflammation
Pattern-recognition receptors
Toll-like receptors
Scavenger receptors
Active immunity
Passive immunity
Variolation
Attenuation

Worksheet 2

Multiple Choice Questions

1. The two branches of specific immunity are:

   (a) Humoral immunity and innate immunity
   (b) Humoral immunity and specific immunity
   (c) Cell mediated immunity and humoral immunity
   (d) None of the above

2. In addition to T and B cells there is a third distinct type of lymphocyte called:

   (a) Dendritic cells
   (b) Langerhans cells
   (c) MHC cells
   (d) Natural Killer cells

3. High endothelial venules of lymph nodes are important for:

(a) antigen trapping
(b) antigen presentation
(c) lymphocyte emigration from blood to lymph node
(d) production of plasma cells

4. High endothelial venules of lymph nodes are:

(a) highly developed in germ free animals
(b) are required for neutrophil extravasation
(c) all of the above
(d) none of the above

5. Lymph nodes perform the following functions except:

(a) trapping antigen on dendritic cell processes
(b) pumping returning lymph
(c) exposing trapped material to macrophages
(d) filtering lymph

6. B lymphocytes in the spleen are largely found in:

(a) the marginal zone
(b) the red pulp
(c) the periarteriolar lymphoid sheath
(d) the follicular areas

7. The thymus is:

(a) a primary lymphoid organ
(b) a secondary lymphoid organ
(c) a reticuloendothelial organ
(d) a lymphoreticular organ

8. In which areas of the lymph nodes are T cells mainly found?

(a) subcapsular
(b) sinusoids
(c) germinal center
(d) paracortex

9. Germinal centers of lymphoid tissues largely contain:

(a) macrophages
(b) neutrophils
(c) T cells
(d) B cells

10. Individuals lacking adhesion molecules will:

    (a) experience recurrent bacterial infections
    (b) have no extravasation of cells
    (c) all of the above
    (d) none of the above

Adaptive Immunity

11. Explain the significance of each of the following features in adaptive immunity:

    Self/nonself recognition Specificity
    Diversity Regulation
    Immunological memory

Innate Immunity

12. How do recognition receptors differ in innate and adaptive immunity? How is self/non-self-recognition achieved?

Worksheet 3

1. Consider the general overview of the immune system that we have discussed. Why do we continue to suffer from infectious diseases if the immune system is so efficient at recognizing and reacting with antigens?
2. What is the clonal selection theory? Name and briefly describe five features of specific immunity that support this theory.
3. Define or explain the following terms:

    Adjuvant
    Passive immunization
    Active immunization
    Intron
    Exon
    Hapten
    Epitope
    Immunogen
    Allergen
    Restriction mapping
    Northern blotting
    Southern blotting
    Western blotting
    Plasmid
    cDNA library
    Secondary lymphoid organs
    Primary lymphoid organs

Tertiary lymphoid organs
Cell homing
Hematopoiesis
Pluripotent stem cells
Apoptosis
Cluster of differentiation antigens
High endothelial venules
Immunoglobin
Transgenic mice
Polymerase chain reaction
Flow cytometry
SDS-PAGE gels

4. Assuming that you have the antibodies for interferon gamma, outline how you will clone a gene for interferon gamma from a cDNA expression library.
5. Outline the similarities and differences between viral and bacterial antigens.
6. Describe three properties of B and T cell epitopes.

Worksheet 4

1. What are mitogens?
2. What are phorbol esters?
3. What are superantigens?
4. Name specific B cell and T cell mitogens.
5. How does mitogenic stimulation differ from antigenic stimulation of lymphocytes?
6. Define or explain the following terms:

   (a) Immunoglobulin superfamily
   (b) Myeloma protein
   (c) Null cells
   (d) Dendritic cells
   (e) Lymphoid follicles
   (f) Extravasation
   (g) M cells
   (h) Polyclonal antibodies
   (i) Monoclonal antibodies
   (j) Hybridoma
   (k) Clonotypic monoclonal antibodies
   (l) J chain
   (m) Secretory component
   (n) Transcytosis
   (o) Antibody-dependent cell-mediated cytotoxicity

(p) Abzymes
(q) Immunotoxins
(r) B cell receptor

7. How is hematopoiesis regulated?
8. What are the differences between the following immunoassays?

(a) Enzyme-linked immunosorbent assays, enzyme linked-immunospot assay (ELISA, ELISPOT)
(b) Western blotting
(c) Immuofluorescence
(d) Immunoelectron microscopy

Worksheet 5

1. Diagram a typical IgG molecule and include immunoglobulin domains. Label the following structures: hinge region, H and L chains, inter- and intradisulfide bonds, antigen binding sites, CHO binding regions, pepsin cleavage site, papain cleavage site, VL, VH, CL, CH2, CH3, Fab, Fe, and F(ab')$_2$.
How would you modify the diagram to depict IgE?
2. Define the following terms:

(a) idiotype
(b) isotype
(c) allotype
(d) immunoglobulin fold
(e) complementarity determining regions
(f) framework regions
(g) constant regions

3. Describe the process of preparing monoclonal antibodies.
4. What type of antibody will be produced following the immunization of a goat with the F(ab')2 fragment of rabbit IgG? Specify the components (heavy, light, Fab, Fc, CHI, CH2, CH3 etc.) of the IgG molecule that will be recognized by the goat immune system and the components that will not be recognized.

Worksheet 6

1. What are the functions of the following features in B cell gene rearrangement and generation of antibody diversity?

(a) recombination activating genes
(b) recombination signal sequences

  (c) nonamer-heptamer sequences
  (d) multigene segments
  (e) non-germline nucleotide additions
  (f) allelic exclusion
  (g) nonproductive and productive joining
  (h) somatic mutation
  (i) DNA binding proteins
  (j) Isotype switching

2. Describe how B cells can first produce lgM alone, IgM and lgD together and then lgM alone again. What molecular features determine if IgM will be membrane bound or secreted?

3. Draw diagrams illustrating the general structure, including domains, of class I MHC molecules, class II MHC molecules, CDI, membrane bound antibodies and B cell receptor complex, T cell receptor-CD3 complex; include molecules that are associated with the proteins. Label each chain and the domains within the chains. Label antigen binding regions, transmembrane domains and regions that have the immunoglobulin fold structure.

4. Name the major antigen binding molecules of the immune system.

5. What is the significance of MHC polymorphism in infectious diseases? Is the polymorphic feature always an advantage to the host? How is MHC polymorphism generated?

6. Define the following terms:

  (a) Major histocompatibility complex antigens
  (b) Human leukocyte antigens
  (c) Haplotype
  (d) Clonotypic
  (e) Congenic mouse
  (f) Syngeneic mouse
  (g) Transgenic mouse
  (h) Invariant chain
  (i) Self-MHC restriction
  (j) Bi-specific antibodies
  (k) Humanized antibodies
  (l) Relative risk
  (m) Nonameric peptide
  (n) Anchor residues
  (o) Beta-2 microglobulin
  (p) Linkage disequilibrium

Worksheet 7

1. What is the subtractive hybridization technique? How was this technique used to identify and isolate the T cell receptor?
2. Describe the gene transfection experiments performed to demonstrate that alpha/beta TCR alone recognizes both antigen and MHC molecules.
3. Compare and contrast T and B cell gene rearrangement to produce the T cell receptor and B cell receptor, respectively.
4. Outline the events that take place during T cell and B cell activation following antigen contact.
5. Diagram the interaction of antigen with macrophage to show the following events:

   (a) Antigen presentation to MHC class II restricted T cells leading to antibody production and isotype switching to IgE.
   (b) Antigen presentation to MHC class I restricted cell leading to cytolysis.
   (c) If an inflammatory response develops as a result of T cell activation and cytokine secretion leading to a DTH response, what cell types will be involved? Show these events in your diagram. Indicate the cytokines involved and the cell surface markers depicting the major cell types in each case.
   (d) Briefly describe the expected course of events if the B and T cells are functionally inactivated. What are some of the causes of cell inactivation (anergy)?
   (e) What does the clonal selection theory have to do with questions a-d above?

Study Guide Immunology Examination 2

1. Be able to identify explain or define the following terms:
   Major histocompatibility complex antigens
   Congenic mice
   Syngeneic mice
   Haplotype
   T dependent antigen
   Transporter of antigenic peptides (TAP-1 and TAP-2)
   Recombination signal sequence
   Affinity maturation
   Agretope
   Positive T cell selection
   Mixed lymphocyte response
   Carrier priming

Carrier effect

Proteosome

Allogeneic effect

Proteosome

Centrocytes

Iccosomes

Tingible body macrophages

2. Know the cells that express the following markers, what they bind to and know their function.

   Sca-1, IgD, CD3, CD4, CD8, CO2, CD45, CD40/CD40L, CD80/CD86, CD28, CTLA-4,

   ICAM-1, LFA-1 and others that we talked about.

3. Be able to illustrate and correctly label MHC class I and II proteins and TCR/CD3 complex showing globular domains and antigen binding sites. Know the difference in the characteristics of both molecules, the appearance of the antigen binding pockets for MHC I and II and whether they interact with exogenously or endogenously derived peptides. What is the advantage of polymorphism in the function of the MHC antigens? Know pathways of antigen processing and presentation.

4. Be able to illustrate, fill in blanks or tables or correctly label interacting molecules between APC/T helper cells and T helper cell/B cell conjugate. What are competence signals, progression signals and differentiation signals?

5. Know the differences and similarities between Ig and TCR rearrangements leading to the interaction of the antigen binding receptors with diverse antigens. What are the differences and similarities between the alpha/beta and gamma/delta TCR? What would happen if there were deficiencies?

6. Know the following experiments:

   (i) Binding of thymocytes to class I or MHC class II molecules leads to positive selection of MHC-restricted cells.

   (ii) Binding of thymocytes to class I or class II MHC molecules leads to positive selection of MHC-restricted cells

   (iii) T cells recognizing self-antigens are clonally deleted.

   (iv) Alpha/beta TCR alone binds to antigen and MHC II proteins.

7. How are membrane bound and secreted Ig generated? How can a B cell express IgM alone, co-express membrane IgM and IgD and then secrete IgM alone?

8. Know the biochemical pathways involved in signal transduction during T cell and B cell activation. What are the consequences of B and T cell activation? Indicate if activation occurs in a primary or secondary lymphoid organ. What takes place in the germinal centers within spleen and lymph nodes? Where does cyclosporine A act? What are the co-stimulatory signals required for effective T cell activation?

9. Draw and label a graph showing the kinetics of primary and secondary immune responses for the following immunization schedules:

   (a) Primary immunization with DNP-BSA and secondary immunization with DNP-BSA

   (b) Primary immunization with DNP-BSA and secondary immunization DNP-HGG

   (c) Primary immunization with DNP-BSA +OVA and secondary immunization with DNP-OVA

10. What are cytokines? How are cytokines and cytokine receptors categorized? (What features are used for categorization?) Are cytokines always beneficial? Can they be harmful? How do cytokines mediate signaling within lymphocytes? How is lymphocyte proliferation induced and regulated by cytokines? How are cytokines used to differentiate T helper subsets?

11. What is cell-mediated immunity? What cells are involved in cell-mediated immunity? Briefly describe the evidence for T helper cell involvement in cytotoxic T cell activation and in specific CTL haplotype involvement for effective CTL activity. What is apoptisis? Know inducers and inhibitors of apoptosis. How do cells migrate and home to lymphoid organs? How does extravasation differ in neutrophils and lymphocytes? What are the different types of cell adhesion molecules? During inflammation, what role do chemokines play?

12. Know how complement is activated in the alternate, lectin and classical pathways. What are the triggers? How is the pathway regulated? What is the function of complement proteins?

Worksheet 8

1. Define or explain the following terms:

   (a) Fas ligand
   (b) Idiotypic determinant
   (c) Herd immunity
   (d) Adjuvant
   (e) Germinal centers
   (f) Mitogen
   (g) Superantigen
   (h) **WSXWS** amino acid motif
   (i) Class I receptor family (hematopoietin receptor family)
   (j) Signal transducers and activators of transcription (STATS)
   (k) Janus kinases
   (l) Chemokines
  (m) Membrane attack complex (MAC)
   (n) C3 convertase

   (o) Anaphylatoxins
   (p) Perforins
   (q) Granzymes
   (r) Caspase
   (s) Mixed lymphocyte reaction
   (t) Cell-mediated lympholysis

2. What are the major differences between lymphocyte and neutrophil extravasation?
3. Describe the role of chemokines and lipids in inflammatory responses. How are the chemokines and chemokine receptors differentiated functionally and structurally?
4. Explain how chemokine signaling differs from cytokine signaling.
5. Corticostroids are powerful anti-inflammatory agents. What is the mechanism of action of corticosteroids?
6. Compare and contrast the four types of hypersensitivity reactions.

Multiple Choice Questions:

7. The following are features of the acquired immune response:

   (a) C-reactive proteins
   (b) Release of reactive oxygen intermediates
   (c) Secretion of lactic acid
   (d) Complement activation by the alternative pathway
   (e) None of the above

8. Which of the following statements are **true?**

   (a) specific immunity occurs independently of innate immunity
   (b) in an innate response there is specific discrimination in the response to macromolecules
   (c) innate responses are not intrinsically affected by previous antigen contact
   (d) acquired immunity is highly specific for distinct macromolecules

9. Individuals lacking adhesion molecules will:

   (a) experience recurrent bacterial infections
   (b) have no extravasation of leukocytes
   (c) all of the above

10. B cell epitopes tend to be:

   (a) accessible amino acid residues that can interact with the B cell receptor
   (b) amphiphilic residues that can associate with MHC class II antigens
   (c) hydrophobic residues that are processed by macrophages
   (d) none of the above

11. The mixed lymphocyte reaction is used to evaluate:

   (a) T helper activity
   (b) T cytotoxic cell activity

(c) Natural killer cell activity
(d) B cell activity

12. Perforins and granzymes are produced by:

(a) T helper cells
(b) Cytotoxic T cells

13. The accessory molecule CD3 is found on:

(a) CD4⁺ T cells
(b) CD8⁺ T cells
(c) Both CD4 and CD8 positive cells
(d) None of the above

14. An effective vaccine molecule must contain:

(a) only B cell epitopes
(b) only T cell epitopes
(c) both B and T cell epitopes

15. Which of the following is not a biological function of complement?

(a) opsonization
(b) anaphylaxis
(c) inflammation
(d) immune complex clearance
(e) antigen recognition

16. The insertion of one or more additional bases at a given gene splice site is called:

(a) N-region addition
(b) Somatic mutation
(c) Looping out

17. Thy lytic activity of complement is destroyed by heating sera at _____ for 30 min.

(a) 37 °C
(b) 25 °C
(c) 56 °C
(d) 40 °C

18. All antibodies secreted by a single plasma cell have the same idiotype and isotype.

(a) True
(b) False

19. The H2-A and H2-E genes of the MHC complex encode class II proteins in humans.

(a) True
(b) False

20. Indirect immunofluorescence assay can be performed using F(ab′)$_2$ as the initial nonlabeled antibody because:

    (a) this fragment is easier for the body to make
    (b) only this fragment can be used in IFAs
    (c) the antigen binding regions are located in this region

21. Calculate the potential number of antibody molecules that can be generated from germ-line DNA containing 600 VL and 5JL gene segments and 300 VH, 20 DH and 5 JH gene segments.
22. How does apoptosis differ from necrosis?
23. Cytotoxic T lymphocytes are very efficient in the destruction of target cells. Explain why we still need to have a humoral response as part of the immune response.
24. Explain the process of gene recombination for the alpha/beta T cell receptor (TCR), from embryonic DNA to translated protein.

Study Guide for Final Exam

1. The following terms will be used for definitions, matching or multiple choice questions.
   Toxoid
   Pattern recognition receptors
   Variolation
   Attenuation
   Active immunity
   Passive immunity
   Adoptive transfer
   C-reactive protein
   Immuogen
   Allergen
   Cluster of differentiation antigens
   Polyclonal antibodies
   M cells
   Tingible body macrophages
   Abzymes
   Immunotoxins
   Idiotype
   Allotype
   Somatic mutation
   Herd immunity
   Sterile immunity
   Syngeneic mice

Humanized antibodies
Nonameric peptides
Anchor residues
Linkage disequilibrium
Signal transducers and activators of transcription (STATS)
Superantigen
Mitogens
Granzymes
Adjuvant
Affinity
Avidity

2. Know the following markers. Know the cells that express the markers, know what they bind to and know their function.
CD2, CD3, CD4, CD8, CDI la,b,c, CD14, CD16, CD19, CD21, CD25, CD28, CD45, CD64, CD40, CD40L (CD 154), CD80, CD81, CD86, CD94, CD95, CDl15, LFA-1, ICAM-1, CTLA4 and CD209.

3. Know the functions of the following cytokines, the cells that secrete them, the receptor families they belong to and the amino acid motifs of the receptor families: IL-1, IL-2, IL-3, IL-4, 1 L-5, L-8, IL-10, IL-12, IFNa, IFNp, IFNy, MIF, TNFa, TNFP, GM-CSF and RANTES.

4. Know how to illustrate and label an antibody molecule and an MHC class II protein. Be able to explain biological activities of antibodies e.g. precipitation, opsonization, antibody dependent cellular cytotoxicity (ADCC), etc.

5. Know the names and functions of the major antigen binding molecules of the immune system and know the professional antigen presenting cells of the immune system.

6. Know the lymphoid organs and their functions. What is the function of cell adhesion molecules in leukocyte migration? What is the role of negative and positive selection in T and B cell development?

7. Know the features of an inflammatory response. What are the functions of the following components during inflammation (acute or chronic): bradykinin, prostaglandins, cyclooxegenase, thromboxanes, leukotrienes, TNFα, IFNγ, IL-I, MIP-la, MIP-IP and IL-6. How does an inflammatory response contribute to the development of the adaptive immune response?

8. Know the properties of antigens and know the differences between Band T cell epitopes and T dependent and T independent antigens. Know the differences between antigen processing for endogenous and exogenous antigens. What are the differences between antigen interaction with MHC class I and MHC class II antigens?

9. Know the mechanisms of immunoglobulin and T cell receptor rearrangements and the features contributing to specificity and diversity of lg and TCR.

10. **Know the following assays:**
Radioimmunoassay (RIA), Enzyme-linked immunosorbent assays, enzyme linked-immunospot assay (ELISA, ELISPOT), radioimmunosorbent test (RIST), Radioallergosorbent test (RAST), Western blotting, Immuofluorescence and Immunoelectron microscopy and graft versus host response.

11. How are monoclonal antibodies (the steps for immunization, fusion, selection and expansion) prepared? What are the uses of monoclonal antibodies?
12. What is the clonal selection theory? Name and briefly describe the five features of adaptive immunity that support this theory.
13. Know the lectin and alternate complement pathways. How are these two pathways regulated? What are the triggers for both pathways?
14. Know the four types of hypersensitivities. What are the functions of the following cells in immune responses: natural killer cells, cytotoxic T lymphocytes, delayed type hypersensitivity T cells, eosinophils, basophils, macrophages and neutrophils.
15. **Signal transduction:** Know the common features of signal transduction events, including the triggers, the process of cell activation i.e. enzyme cascades, G proteins etc. and the consequences of the activation process to the specific cell.

    (a) Be able to compare signal transduction following chemokine and cytokine receptor binding on cells.
    (b) Be able to compare FcεRl receptor and Toll-like receptor signaling.
    (c) Be able to compare BCR and TCR signaling following antigen binding. Know the competence, progression and differentiation signals required for cell activation. How does isotype switching take place? Be able to describe, identify or answer questions related to what happens in the germinal center and answer questions related to properties of memory cells. What are immunophilins? What is their importance in immunosuppressive therapy?

16. Be able to diagram or label a graph showing the kinetics of an antibody response during a primary and secondary response. Know the effects of tolerance and anergy on the expected response.
17. **Know the following diseases:**
    Hemolytic disease of the newborn (HDN)
    Myasthenia Gravis
    Systemic Lupus erythematosus
    Hashimoto's thyroditis
    Multiple sclerosis
    X-linked agammaglobulinemia
    Severe combined immunodeficiency disease (SCID)
    DiGeorge syndrome
    Acquired immunodeficiency syndrome
    Be able to identify the contributions of the following individuals to the field of immunology:
    Rosalyn Yalow
    Karl Landsteiner
    Rodney Porter and Gerald Edelman
    Cesar Milstein and Georges Kohler
    Susumu Tonegawa
    Peter Doherty and Rolf Zinkernegel

Quizzes Covering Chapter Material

Quiz 1

1. The two interconnected branches of vertebrate immunity are _____ and _____ .

2. Any substance that elicits a specific response by B and T cells is an _____ .

3. The fundamental theory of modern immunology is known as _____ _____ .

4. The production of one's own immunity or the response obtained by vaccinations:

    (a) Humoral immunity
    (b) Active immunity
    (c) Adoptive immunity
    (d) Passive immunity

5. Organisms causing disease are known as _____ .

6. Which of the following molecules are found on host cell surfaces?

    (a) PAMPs
    (b) DAMPs
    (c) PRRs
    (d) AGs

7. The differences observed in the primary and secondary responses of adaptive immunity is due to:

    (a) Natural killer cells
    (b) Antigen presenting cells
    (c) Memory cells
    (d) Neutrophils

8. The hematopoietic stem cell is defined by the following marker designations:

    (a) $Lin^-Sca-1^+c-Kit^+$
    (b) $Lin^+Sca-1^+c-Kit^-$
    (c) $Sca-1^+CD34^+IL-7R^+$
    (d) $Sca-1^+cKit^+Rag1/2^+$

9. Granulocytes consist of the following cells listed below except:

    (a) Monocytes
    (b) Neutrophils
    (c) Basophils
    (d) Eosinophils

10. The following cell surface molecules; CD19, CD20, CD21, CD40 are expressed on :

    (a) NK cells
    (b) B lymphocytes
    (c) T lymphocytes
    (d) Dendritic cells

11. The following cell surface molecules, CD2, CD3, CD28 are expressed on:

    (a) NK cells
    (b) B lymphocytes
    (c) T lymphocytes
    (d) Dendritic cells

12. The major antigen presenting cells are:

    (a) T lymphocytes, B lymphocytes, macrophages
    (b) B lymphocytes, macrophages, neutrophils
    (c) B lymphocytes, macrophages, dendritic cells
    (d) Plasma cells, B lymphocytes, T lymphocytes

13. Which of the following is not associated with the white pulp of the spleen?

    (a) Central artery
    (b) Marginal zone
    (c) Pariarteriolar lymphoid sheath
    (d) Paracortex

14. The thymic medulla is defined by the presence of :

    (a) Afferent lymphatics
    (b) Hassal's corpuscles
    (c) Thymocytes
    (d) Thymic epithelia cells

15. Lymphocytes entering the spleen pass through high endothelial venules (HEVs).

    (a) True
    (b) False

16. An antigen peptide bound to MHC class II protein is presented to _____ lymphocytes by antigen presenting cells.

    (a) Cytotoxic T
    (b) Helper T
    (c) B
    (d) None of the above

17. Which of the following sites within secondary lymphoid organs are T cell zones?

    (a) Marginal zone and subcapsular sinus
    (b) PALs and hilum
    (c) Germinal center and follicle
    (d) Paracortex and PALS

18. An early lymphoid progenitor (ELP) is defined by the expression of:

    (a) RAG1/2
    (b) C-Kit
    (c) IL-7R
    (d) GATA-1

19. The medullary cavity of the bone marrow is divided into two compartments; the
    _____ niche and _____ niche.

20. A group of cells derived from the common lymphoid progenitor, lacking antigen-specific receptors:

    (a) Innate lymphoid cells
    (b) Mast cells
    (c) B lymphocytes
    (d) Monocytes

21. What are cytokines?

Quiz 2

A. PU.1/ GATA-1	B. Panning	C. hypervariable regions	D. Ligand for CD28
E. LSK cells	F. Ikaros/ GATA-3	G. Leukocytosis	H. Ligand for MHCII
I. Pleiotropic	J. δε/γε/ζζ/ζη	K. hapten	L. γ, α and β fractions of serum proteins
M. Igα/Igβ	N. Ligand for MHCI	O. αβ	P. γcβα
Q. Redundant	R. JAK kinases	S. Western blotting	T. Diapedesis

Use the word bank above to fill in the blanks in questions 1–14. Place the correct letter in the blank space.

1. _____ Aminobenzene in Landsteiner experiments
2. _____ CD 86
3. _____ Hematopoietic stem cells
4. _____ The process in which mature bone marrow cells were separated from Lin- hematopoietic stems cells

5. _____ Complementarity determining regions on an antibody molecule
6. _____ transcription factors for myeloid lineage
7. _____Co-receptor molecules for TCR
8. _____ a cytokine that induces different biological effects on multiple cell targets
9. _____ transcription factors for lymphoid lineage
10. _____ Co-receptor molecules for BCR
11. _____ CD8
12. _____ cytokine signaling
13. _____ Transient increase in the number of circulating neutrophils
14. _____ Antibodies in serum
15. _____ high affinity IL-2 receptor
16. List the major cytokine families. Which family is the largest? Which family is the most recently identified?
17. List the antibody isotypes found in human serum. Which 2 are expressed on mature, unstimulated B cells?
18. A defect in the common γc-chain gene leads to X-linked severe combined immunodeficiency (X-SCID). Which cytokine required for lymphoid development is affected? Why is this cytokine critical?
19. The following marker designation: Sca-1$^+$c-kit$^+$fl-3$^+$CD34$^-$IL-7R$^{+/-}$RAG1/2$^+$Tdt$^+$ represents _____.

   (a) MPP
   (b) LMPP
   (c) ELP
   (d) CLP

20. Diagram a general model (flow chart) of typical events that occur during signal transduction in lymphocyte signaling.

Quiz 3

1. Many γδ TCRs recognize lipids and glycopilids.

   (a) True
   (b) False

2. The alpha gene encoding the alpha subunit of TCRs is equivalent to the heavy chain gene of Ig.

   (a) True
   (b) False

3. The substrate for the RAG1/2 recombinases is:

   (a) MHCI
   (b) dsDNA
   (c) Artemis
   (d) ssRNA
   (e) mRNA

4. Deficiencies in RAG1/2 will lead to loss of:

   (a) B lymphocytes
   (b) T lymphocytes
   (c) Dendritic cells and B lymphocytes
   (d) B and T lymphocytes
   (e) Natural killer cells and T lymphocytes

5. In early B cell development, heavy chain gene rearrangement occurs, resulting in the expression of :

   (a) Surrogate light chain consisting of VpreB and κ5
   (b) Surrogate light chain consisting of VpreB and λ5

6. The proposal that two genes encoded the heavy and light chains of antibody molecules were made by:

   (a) Hozumi and Tonegawa
   (b) Dryer and Bennet

7. TCR and BCR gene rearrangements occur:

   (a) Before antigen exposure
   (b) After antigen exposure
   (c) After T and B cell activation

8. Three gene segments recombine to generate the variable region of the heavy chain of the Ig molecule.

   (a) True
   (b) False

9. The cleavage and rearrangement of DNA segments to produce BCR and TCR occurs in _____cells.

   (a) Gametes
   (b) Somatic cells

10. Upon activation, _____cells secrete product with the same specificity as the receptor.

    (a) T cells
    (b) B cells

11. V and J segments encode:

   (a) K and λ variable regions
   (b) α and γ variable regions
   (c) all of the above
   (d) none of the above

12. Lymphoid specific proteins involved in V(D)J recombination:

   (a) Artemis
   (b) High mobility group B proteins 1 and 2
   (c) Terminal deoxyribonucleotidyl transferase
   (d) DNA ligase
   (e) Ku70/80

13. Protein that opens up hairpin at coding end joint:

   (a) Artemis
   (b) DNA-PKc
   (c) RAG ½
   (d) Tdt
   (e) Ku70/80

14. J chain is associated with:

   (a) IgM
   (b) IgG
   (c) IgD
   (d) IgE

15. Stabilizes the binding of RAG1/2 to recombination signal sequences:

   (a) Artemis
   (b) HMGB1/2
   (c) Tdt
   (d) DNA Pol μ
   (e) ATM

16. Which of the following is incorrect regarding the antigen binding pocket of MHC class I:

   (a) Consists of α1 and α2 domains
   (b) Consists of α1 and β2 domains
   (c) Peptides of 8–10 amino acids can bind
   (d) Conserved hydrophobic anchor residues bind peptide

17. MHC class II binds _____ peptides in a binding pocket _____ at the ends:

   (a) Hydrophilic, closed
   (b) Hydrophobic, open
   (c) Hydrophilic, open
   (d) Hydrophobic, closed

18. MHC class I and II proteins are:

 (a) Secreted proteins
 (b) Transmembrane protein
 (c) Peripheral membrane proteins

19. Mouse H2-K is the equivalent of human:

 (a) MHC class I
 (b) MHC class II
 (c) MHC class III

20. Human HLA-D is the equivalent of mouse:

 (a) H2-D
 (b) H2-L
 (c) H2-A
 (d) None of the above

21. In humans, HLA-A, HLA-B and HLA-C molecules can present peptides to:

 (a) $CD8^+$ T cells
 (b) $CD4^+$ T cells

22. MHC genes contribute to diversity because they are highly polymorphic.

 (a) True
 (b) False

Quiz 4

1. Name the cells expressing the listed surface molecules and provide the ligands for each molecule.

 CD2, CD4, CD28, LFA-1, CD154, CD152, MHCII, MHCI, TCR, CD8, CD40, ICAM-1

2. List 4 molecules each (apart from TCR and BCR), specific for B and T cells, that are part of the activation and signaling pathways following binding of the BCR and TCR to antigen.

3. Name the effector cytokines and master gene regulators for the following T helper cell subsets:

 TREG, TH17, TH1, TH2, TH9, and TFH

4. For TH1 and TH2 cells in #3, what are the polarizing cytokines required for differentiation?

Quiz 5

A. Cytokines	B. TI-2Ag	C. ICOS/CD28/ PDL-1	D. Bcl-6
E. SHM	F. Follicular dendritic cells	G. B-10 B cells	H. Centrocytes
I. AID	J. Long-lived plasma cells	K. Nude mice	L. FoxP3
M. Granzymes and perforin	N. CD3	O. IgM/IgD	P. GATA-3
Q. TI-1 Ag	R. MHC class II S. Centroblasts		

Fill in the blanks with the correct letters on the question sheet.

1. ____ B cells in the dark zone of the germinal centers
2. ____ Generated late in the primary immune response, long survival in the bone marrow
3. ____ Foxn1 mutation
4. ____ TH2
5. ____ Mature B cells
6. ____ Reduce inflammatory response during ongoing immune response
7. ____ Treg
8. ____ Required for CSR and SHM
9. ____ Ligands for B7 family member receptors
10. ____ TFH
11. ____ Light zone of germinal center
12. ____ Capsular bacterial polysaccharide
13. ____ T cells
14. ____ Dark zone of germinal center
15. ____ Signal 3 for T cell activation
16. ____ Lipopolysaccharide
17. ____ CTLs
18. ____ Exogenous antigen presentation to TH cells
19. Your lab has purchased IL-12 deficient mice for use in CMI studies. The mice possess cytotoxic T cells and are able to mount humoral immune responses producing IgG1, IgA, IgE, IgG2b but no IgG3, or IgG2a. The mice can clear helminth infections but are unable to clear virus infections. You set out to identify what cells and molecules are missing in the mice. You suspect the absence of IL-12 is involved in the lack of antiviral immunity. Your supervisor asks you to use 4 mice for your investigations and provides you with **recombinant IL-12, anti CD4 antibodies, anti CD8 antibodies** and **anti IFNγ antibodies**. You are also asked to obtain spleen cells from 2 mice and mouse blood for collection of serum from the remaining 2 mice. Explain how you would use the 4 mice to determine what may be responsible for the lack of antiviral immunity. What cells and molecules would you look for and why? Explain.

20. The following sentences are incorrect. Identify the error and provide the correct explanation.

(a) PU.1 and RORγt are effector cytokines.

(b) Th17 and TFH cell subsets are the major sources of B cell help in secondary lymphoid organs

(c) Toxic shock syndrome is an example of an autoimmune disease

(d) CD4$^+$ T cells interact with MHC class I on CD8$^+$ T cells.

21. List the following intracellular signaling molecules in the <u>correct order</u> of involvement/activity after TCR engagement: LAT, LcK, Ca^{2+}, ZAP-70, NFAT.

22. In what major way is an NK cell different from B and T lymphocytes?

Quiz 6

Circle the correct choice.

1. The most abundant antibody isotype in the mucosal environment is IgA.

(a) True
(b) False

2. Immune cells, blood and lymphatic vessels are located in the lamina propria underlying the epithelium in mucosal environments.

(a) True
(b) False

3. All of these are ways in which antigen can be captured from the GI lumen for delivery to APCs: M cells capture antigen, Goblet cells capture antigens, APCs extend dendrites into lumen and FcR bind antibodies which have bound antigen.

(a) True
(b) False

4. The first antibody produced in an immune response is IgG

(a) True
(b) False

5. Immediate type hypersensitivity is IgE mediated.

(a) True
(b) False

6. Delayed type hypersensitivity is also known as type IV hypersensitivity and is a T cell mediated hypersensitivity.

(a) True
(b) False

7. Hemolytic disease of the newborn resulting from immune response to the rhesus antigen on cells of the child in utero leading to red blood cell hemolysis is an example of a type III hypersensitivity.

   (a) True
   (b) False

8. The ligand for the T cell receptor is an antigen.

   (a) True
   (b) False

9. Paneth, goblet, tuft and M cells are located in the GI mucosa.

   (a) True
   (b) False

10. The ILC3 subset of innate lymphoid cells plays an important role in maintaining gut homeostasis.

    (a) True
    (b) False

11. Eosinophils and basophils are particularly important in helminth infections in the gut.

    (a) True
    (b) False

12. Class switching of antibody involves a switch of the constant region while retaining the variable region of the antibody.

    (a) True
    (b) False

13. ILC2 subsets of innate lymphoid cells secrete the trio of cytokines; IL-4, IL-5 and IL-13 that are important in type 2 responses to worms.

    (a) True
    (b) False

14. Pathogen recognition receptors recognize PAMPs and DAMPs. This is an example of adaptive immunity.

    (a) True
    (b) False

15. The cytokines IL-10 and TGFβ regulate immune responses by suppressing responses or providing anti-inflammatory responses.

    (a) True
    (b) False

16. Briefly describe how immune homeostasis is maintained in the mucosal environment. Give examples of specific cells and molecules involved. How are pathogens recognized and eliminated?

Quiz 7

1. Name the human equivalent major histocompatibility genes for the following mouse genes:

    (a) H-2K
    (b) H-2I
    (c) H-2L

2. Which of the following MHC proteins, MHC I or MHC II has a closed binding pocket? What domains make up the binding pocket?
3. When thymocytes arrive in the thymus they already have T cell receptors expressed with CD3, they are also CD4$^+$ and they enter the medulla of the thymus. Once they acquire the CD8 antigen, all thymocytes leave through the cortex to enter the periphery.

    What are the errors in the above statements?
4. What is the difference between the determinant-selection model and the holes-in-the-repertoire model?
5. Name the 3 major APCs and the cell that produces antibodies.
6. Name cells expressing CD3, CD19, MHC I, MHC II, CD8

Quiz 8

1. What is the deficiency in X-linked lymphoproliferative (XLP) syndrome? What cells are affected?
2. How is the diagnosis of XLP confirmed?
3. In familial hemophagocytic lymphohistiocytosis (FHL), different aspects of intracellular trafficking within NK cells are affected. In FHL2 _____ is deficient or impaired. In FHL4 _____ does not occur.
4. In hemophagocytic lymphohistiocytosis (HLH) what cytokine is associated with the "cytokine storm"?
5. A child is diagnosed with a clinical condition where examination of peripheral blood cells shows abnormal clustering of giant lysosome-like vesicles around the nucleus. The child has recurrent bacterial infections and partial absence of pigmentation of skin, hair and eyes.

    (a) What is the possible diagnosis?
    (b) What is cause of pigmentation defect?
    (c) In one sentence what is the underlying problem within cells of patients with this condition?

6. In this clinical condition, examination of lymphocytes by scanning electron microscopy showed a loss of microvilli on T lymphocytes. Also examination of a spleen section from the patient showed a very reduced marginal zone (MZ). A failure to produce IgG2 against capsular polysaccharide antigens and blood group antigens was also noted.

   (a) What is the clinical condition?
   (b) What is the underlying defect in this condition?

Quiz 9

1. Name four T cell types and four B cell types
2. Name the five antigen binding molecules of the immune system
3. Name the three major antigen presenting cells of the immune system
4. What is the antibody secreting cell of the immune system?
5. What are the major identifying surface molecules (CD marker) for B cells, T helper cells, cytotoxic T cells and NK cells
6. List the five antibody isotypes

Quiz 10

1. Define the following terms:
   Antigens
   Haptens
   Immunogens
   Mitogens
   Polyclonal activators
   Superantigens
   Epitope
   Immunoglobulin
   Avidity
   Affinity
   Antigen binding site
2. What are the factors that influence immunogenicity?
3. In the absence of TdT can cells still rearrange the V (D) J genes?
4. What are some of the factors that can affect the generation of the potentially large numbers of antibodies possible in mice and humans?

Quiz 11

1. How do the following features function in the generation of antibody diversity?

   Recombination signal sequences

   Recombination activation genes

   Somatic hypermutation

   Isotype switching (class switch recombination)

Selected References

Murphy K, Weaver C (2017) Janeway's immunobiology, 9th edn. Garland Press, New York

Pennock GK, Chow LQM (2015) The evolving role of immune checkpoint inhibitors in cancer treatment. The Oncologist 20:812–822

Punt J, Stranford SA, Jones PP, Owen JA (2019) Kuby immunology, 8th edn. W.H. Freeman and Company, New York. Chapter 20, antigen-antibody interactions

Trapani JA, Darcy PK (2017) Immunotherapy of cancer. Australian Family Physician 46:194–199

Part II
Immunology Laboratory Manual

1.1 Immunology Laboratory Policies

1. There will be no make-ups for missed laboratory exercises.
2. Eating, Drinking, or Smoking is not allowed in the laboratory.—All safety rules must be observed.
3. Mouth pipetting is not allowed.
4. All students must have laboratory coats. Coats must be worn during all laboratory exercises. No exceptions will be made.
5. All students must work with gloves on.
6. Items contaminated with blood, serum etc. must be disposed of properly.
7. Do not throw away anything—tubes, samples, etc. until you have been instructed to do so.
8. Always label your samples properly with your name, the date, and type of sample—for easy identification.
9. Read the laboratory manual and any handouts related to the exercise before coming to the laboratory. Prepare a flow chart of the experiment to be performed. The laboratory exercise will be a lot easier to perform.
10. Record all your work in a **BOUND AND NUMBERED** laboratory notebook (not hand printed numbers). Loose leaf notebooks or ring binders will not be accepted.
    All graphs should be plotted on graph paper and not on notebook paper. All notebooks are due on the last day of class. There will be no exceptions.
11. Most of the experiments require preparatory work and follow-up observations outside the regularly scheduled laboratory period. Arrangements should be made by members of a group or pair, so that samples, buffers, injections etc., are prepared, processed or performed, and that results will be properly recorded and shared with lab partners.
12. All students are responsible for recording changes to laboratory protocols. Changes resulting from non-availability of reagents, poor performance of

reagents when tested before laboratory meetings etc. will be announced in the lecture or laboratory meeting.

1.2   Laboratory Safety Guidelines

Performing exercises in immunology lab provides an opportunity to experience the concepts discussed in lectures at a practical level and to gain a deeper understanding of the experimental approaches discussed in the various topics. Safety in the lab is of paramount importance when working with reagents, chemicals, cells and lab equipment. Students will be working in groups or in pairs, therefore safe lab practices will need to be observed when working in close proximity at the lab bench and as students move around lab benches and lab equipment. When students work with cell cultures, we will use the laminar flow hood to maintain a sterile environment for the cells. Media, sterile plastic and glassware and the cultures will be placed in the laminar flow hood for diluting and feeding cells. Media to be used for culture will be prepared under the laminar flow hood and used for feeding cells. Left over media will be stored at 4 °C. Preparation of solutions and buffers containing acids, acetone or other caustic material will be carried out under a chemical hood.

In order to work safely in the lab, lab coats, gloves and goggles offer protection from cells, laboratory animals, microorganisms, spills and splashes as students perform exercises in the lab. Some exercises will not require protective gear. However, developing a habit of wearing a lab coat and gloves ensures that students are prepared to handle different types of materials and reagents and to work safely with the materials. Lab benches will be wiped with 70% ethanol and bench paper will be placed on benches before exercises are performed. Students will pay attention to chemical hazard or biohazard labels placed on chemicals, reagents and cultures.

Biohazard bags and waste containers will be provided in the laboratory for disposal of items marked as biohazardous waste. Needles, contaminated glass items, including slides, scalpels, and sharp objects that can pierce skin should be placed in a designated sharps container.

Biosafety levels (https://www.cdc.gov/labs/pdf/CDC-BiosafetyMicrobiological BiomedicalLaboratories-2009-P.PDF); (https://www.fss.txstate.edu/ehsrm/safety-manual/biologic/cdcnihlev.html), Biosafety in Microbiological and Biomedical Laboratories, 5th edition (2009) and handling small lab animals

Biosafety level 1 (BSL-1): Microorganisms in BSL-1 do not cause infections in healthy individuals and can be handled using standard microbiological practices without protective lab gear. Examples, *Bacillus subtillis, Escherichia coli.*

Biosafety level 2 (BSL-2): When working with human bodily fluids and tissues, such as blood, cells and other specimens that may contain infectious agents (known or unknown). In addition to standard microbiological practices, a laminar flow hood or biological safety cabinet should be used when working with specimens. Pathogens in this category may cause human infections for which treatments are available. Exposure risk for BSL-2 pathogens is through injection or exposure to sharp objects such as needles that can pierce the skin, ingestion or inhalation or aerosols generated from spilled or splashed fluids. Examples, *Plasmodium falciparum, Toxoplasma, Salmonella enterica.*

Biosafety level 3 (BSL-3): Microorganisms categorized under BSL-3 are local or exotic infectious agents that can be transmitted by inhalation of aerosols, ingested and injected. Infections may be lethal. All exercises and experiments with BSL-3 organisms should be performed using laminar flow hoods with special ventilation systems, biosafety cabinets or other appropriate containment that prevents transmission of organisms outside the lab area. Laboratory access should be restricted to individuals trained to work with BSL-3 organisms. *Mycobacterium tuberculosis, Bacillus anthracis.*

Biosafety level 4 (BSL-4): Infectious agents categorized under BSL-4 pose life-threatening infections with no known treatments and should be performed by highly trained individuals. Laboratories are isolated from other buildings with ventilation systems specially designed to prevent transmission aerosols into the environment and surrounding areas. Individuals working with BSL-4 agents will be required to wear air-supplied, positive pressure, full-body body suits. They will also use class III biosafety cabinets which are completely sealed and accessible by specialized arm-length gloves worn by individuals handling specimens. Examples, Ebola and Marburg virus,

Institutional Animal Care and Use Committee (IACUC): This committee provides oversight for the use of animals in research and teaching. IACUC reviews and approves protocols that involve the use of animals. When planning exercises that will involve animals, the protocols completed according to institutional guidelines need to be submitted early and ahead of the semester to allow enough time for any revisions requested by the committee and upon approval to have enough time to purchase the animals. (Cdc.gov)

1.3   Instructions for Notebook Entries

1. Notebooks should be **bound and commercially numbered**. Spiral notebooks should not be used. Do not tear out pages from your notebook and do not use white-out on the notebook pages. Cross-out mistakes by ruling a line across an entry or page and continue on the next page.
2. Save the first two pages of the notebook for table of contents.
3. Have a title or heading for each exercise that is performed and include 4–5 paragraphs of an introduction or explanation for the exercise. This will include materials from notes provided by your TA on the board, as handouts or PowerPoint slides.
4. Write down your lab partner's name for each exercise performed.
5. Write down the reagents, cell lines, kits, materials and equipment used for the exercises and prepare a flow chart or scheme to help you understand the protocol for each exercise. This should be shown in the notebook. Know what step of

the protocol you will start in class and indicate this in your notebook. If an exercise has multiple parts or sections and only one section is performed in class, note which section you will perform. If a reagent is changed for a particular step of the protocol, write the change in your notebook.

6. Record information for each lab exercises in your notebook, i.e. purpose of the exercise, procedures, results, calculations and interpretations of lab exercises.

7. Illustrate and label images viewed on slides, noting morphology, structures and their functions.

8. After each exercise, summarize your data succinctly but completely in 1–2 pages. Prepare tables or graphs and include pictures of gels or other figures obtained. This will help in the preparation of lab reports and experimental plans. No information is trivial. The more information you have in your notes the easier it will be to prepare for quizzes, prepare lab reports and complete experimental plans.

9. Answer questions related to each exercise in the notebook (these are questions for each exercise, either from the protocols, handouts, research articles/cases, PowerPoints or textbooks). If any research articles, case studies, videos etc. were used, these should be mentioned and referenced correctly.

10. Provide conclusions obtained from the exercise performed and at least two follow up questions or experiments that will provide a better understanding of the exercise performed or provide a better understanding of the concept covered in the exercise. **Notebook entries should reflect activities performed during each lab meeting. When notebooks are collected, there should be no blank spaces/pages for exercises that have already been completed.**

1.4   Instructions for Writing Laboratory Reports

Lab reports should be typed double spaced in Times New Roman Font, 12 point. Pages should be numbered. Use the Council of Science Editors (CSE) name year citation style for citations within the report and for listing references. Pay attention to the headings and the content required in each section. **Your grades will be determined by the accuracy of the report, the contents, your understanding of the exercise and the style and organization of the report.** The key is not whether an experiment works or not but whether the concept underlying the exercise(s) is understood.

1.4.1   Points: 100 Points for Each Report

Each lab report should include the following sections:

1.4.1.1   Cover Page: (1 Page)

Each lab report should have a cover page that includes the course number, your name, your lab partner's name or group members' names, title of the report and a date.

1.4.1.2   Abstract: (On a Separate Page; About ½ Page)

The lab report should have an abstract. The abstract is a short summary of what was done, what the exercises were about, the purpose of the exercises, the methods used, results obtained and conclusions.

1.4.1.3   Introduction: (Approx. 1 Page)

Provide a general background for the exercises that were performed. If the report covers two or more exercises, clearly state what the exercises have in common. What principles or concepts were being evaluated? What were the objectives of the exercises? Was there a hypothesis (or hypotheses) being tested? Use sources from the lab protocols and handouts, as well as the immunology textbooks. Cite your references correctly.

1.4.1.4   Purpose: (½ Page)

Clearly state the purpose of the lab exercise (or exercises)

1.4.1.5   Methods: (1–3 Pages Depending on the Exercise(s))

What was done in the exercise (or exercises)? If methods were used exactly as written in the lab manual, briefly summarize what was done and refer to the methods, citing the exercise number and page number where the details can be found. Note any changes that were made to the protocol. Include subheadings to indicate types of methods or protocols used. If exercise kits were used and you were given a handout, briefly summarize what was done and refer to the handout where details can be found. Be specific in terms of measurements performed, volumes used, length and times of incubation, types of equipment used, correct order of the procedures on the protocols and who you worked with. If a demonstration was performed as part of the exercise, indicate who performed the demonstration. If groups or pairs of students performed different parts of an exercise, indicate this in your methods. Methods should be written in past tense. Be clear that the methods that you have listed are the methods that were performed in the exercise(s). Cite references correctly.

1.4.1.6   Results: (1–4 Pages Depending on the Exercise(s))

Report your results (data) succinctly. Do not discuss the results. Use subheadings to indicate the results reported. Use tables, graphs, charts or other types of illustrations to summarize your results. Each figure shown should include a number and should be reported in chronological order (e.g. items in Table 1 should be reported before items in Table 2 etc.). Each figure should contain a legend describing what is contained in the figure. Graphs prepared using Excel may be embedded in the text. If large tables, graphs, other illustrations or lab data are included (gels, nitrocellulose paper) these should be attached to the report as appendices.

1.4.1.7   Discussion: (1–3 Pages Depending on the Exercise(s))

The data should be discussed to demonstrate an integrated understanding of the exercise or exercises that were performed. The exercises aim to highlight particular immunological principles, concepts or techniques. It should be clear from your discussion that you can identify these aims. First, restate what was done in the exercise and why, then use the following questions as guides to write the discussion: What do the results mean? Were the objectives of the exercise(s) met? Was a proposed hypothesis supported or not? Did the results clarify concepts or principles that underlie the exercise(s) performed? Did a particular technique convey an understanding of the concept studied? Can the results be easily interpreted? Were there any limitations to the techniques used? What connections can be made from the data obtained to class discussions or textbook readings? If more than one exercise is being discussed, indicate if the exercises are related and specify how they are related and provide the concept (s) underlying the exercises. If there are any question to be answered for the exercise, provide your responses in the discussion section. If a research article or case study was used as part of the exercise, then the study or case should be discussed and the article or case properly cited and referenced. What are your impressions of the data? Identify two modifications (these can be alternate exercises or experiments) that can be applied to the protocol used, to enhance understanding of the concept that is the subject of the exercise(s). Identify a clinical (medical), research or epidemiological application for the exercise(s) performed. Journal research articles used should be cited correctly, using the CSE style.

1.4.1.8   Conclusions: (1–2 Paragraphs)

Highlight the major (significant) features of the exercise(s) and the major lesson learned from the exercise.

1.4.1.9   Acknowledgements

Acknowledge students that provided or shared data for the whole class, specific demonstrations by student pairs or any contributions from classmates or TA for help with discussions or organizing report.

1.4.1.10   References

List references using CSE citation style. This is a good style to know for biology students. Do not use internet site (i.e. sites for comments, advertising, medical reports or opinions) references.

1.5   Laboratory Report Topics

Transgenic mouse models
Severe combined immunodeficiency mouse models
Nude mouse models
Major histocompatibility antigen test systems
Immune mechanisms of acquired immunodeficiency syndrome
Immune complex disorders-rheumatoid arthritis
Immune complex disorders-Schistosomiasis
Immune mechanisms of complement related disorders
Immune mechanisms of B cell deficiencies
Immune mechanisms of inflammatory responses
Immune mechanisms of neutrophil deficiency
Immune mechanisms of B cell tolerance
Immune mechanisms of T cell tolerance

Chapter 25
Exercise 1: Using a Compound Microscope

The compound microscope is one of the most important instruments found in laboratories engaged in the examination of cells and microorganisms. We will examine mouse blood stained with Giemsa stain to identify red blood cells (erythrocytes), white blood cells (leukocytes) and platelets (thrombocytes). Some of the red cells are infected with *Plasmodium yoelii* and *P. berghei*, intracellular parasites within the red cells, and causative agents of rodent malaria. The parasites are protozoans, eukaryotic cells and therefore the nucleus and cytoplasm will be stained. Uninfected erythrocytes lack a nucleus and will be stained red/pink. The **objectives** of the introductory exercise are to: (1) Review parts and function of a compound microscope; (2) Review calculation of magnification and (3) Identify uninfected erythrocytes, *Plasmodium* infected erythrocytes, leukocytes and platelets. A differential count of the leukocytes will be performed to determine the percentage of each leukocyte in the blood smear.

Materials and Reagents (Per Pair)

Microscope
Giemsa stained mouse blood cells
Differential laboratory counter
Oil immersion
Kimwipes
Lens paper
Bench paper

Parts and function of a compound microscope (Fig. 25.1):
Ocular lens (eyepiece): (10× or 15×) magnifies the specimen on the slide together with objective lenses; magnifies the image with the objective lens. The eyepiece has an eyepiece focus used for adjusting the ocular magnification.

© Springer Nature Switzerland AG 2021
T. Y. Sam-Yellowe, *Immunology: Overview and Laboratory Manual*,
https://doi.org/10.1007/978-3-030-64686-8_25

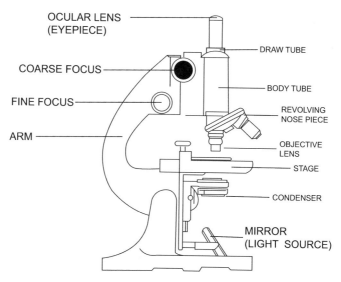

Fig. 25.1 Compound microscope showing labeled parts

Diopter adjustment: used to adjust the differences for each eye when viewing image with both eyes using binocular eyepieces.

Head or Body tube (depending on whether binocular or monocular eyepiece): connects ocular lenses to body of microscope and maintains the proper distance between the ocular and objective lenses.

Objective lenses (objectives): (4×, 10×, 40× and 100×) magnifies the image together with ocular lens. The objectives are color-coded.

Revolving nosepiece (Turret): Rotates the objective lenses, allowing changes from one objective to the next; from low to high power magnification

Arm (frame): Support for the upper part of the microscope grasped along with the base of the microscope for handling and moving the microscope. The arm connects the tube or head with the base of the microscope

Mechanical stage: A platform on which the slide is placed and supported when viewing specimens. The stage is moved with knobs from left to right and from top to bottom. The slide to be viewed is supported so that it does not slide off the stage and is held steady while specimens are viewed.

Stage clips: One or two clips may be present on the stage. Secures and supports the slide on the stage.

Stage control: moves the stage left to right and top to bottom.

Coarse adjustment knob: This is used to bring the image into initial view.

Fine adjustment knob: This knob is used to clarify or sharpen the focus of the image to show more detail.

Condenser lens: focuses the light from the illuminator onto the specimen on the slide. The lens is non-magnifying.

Iris diaphragm with lever: This is used to regulate the amount and intensity of the light reaching the slide. The lever is used to make adjustments for the amount of light.

Illuminator (light source): The light source is built into the microscope (internal feature of the microscope) in the newer microscopes. The light illumines the specimen and directs the light towards the ocular lens (in some older microscopes the light source is external to the microscope and a mirror present on the microscope reflects the light towards the specimen and ocular lens).

Light switch: turns light source on and off.

Rheostat knob: increases or decreases (dims) the amount of light directed to the slide.

When viewing slides, start with the lowest power objective. Lower the objective close to the slide. Do not touch the slide with the objective lens. In some microscopes a **rack stop** is present and pre-set to prevent the objective lens from hitting the slide. Since the microscope you are using may not be pre-set, it is important to lower the objective gently. Look through the ocular lens to see the image of the specimen using the coarse knob to adjust the focus until the image comes sharply into view. Lower the stage, shift the objective to the next power, and then adjust the focus with the fine focus adjustment knob, until the image is sharp.

An image viewed with the 4× objective can be switched to 10× or 40×. Similarly, an image viewed with the 10× objective initially can be changed to the 40× objective. For greater magnification, oil immersion can be used **ONLY with the 100× objective lens.** To use the 100× objective lens, a drop of immersion oil is placed on the slide after the slide has been viewed with the lower power objectives. The 100× objective is then lowered gently into the drop of oil, and then using the fine focus adjustment, the image is brought into sharp view with a minor adjustment of the fine adjustment knob. The total magnification of the image viewed is obtained by multiplying the power of the ocular lens by the power of the objective lens used. The product is the total magnification of the viewed specimen. For example, a specimen viewed using the 10× ocular lens and 10× objective lens results in a 100× total magnification.

10× ocular lens × 10× objective lens = 100× total magnification (see table below).

Ocular lens	Objective lens	Total magnification
10×	4×	40×
10×	10×	100×
10×	40×	400×
10×	100× (oil)	1000×

When viewing slides, the following features of the microscope and the slides need to be taken into consideration: **Working distance, thickness of specimen, diameter of magnification field** and **resolution.** We will be viewing stained smears and tissue sections so these features are important in ensuring successful study of the prepared slides that will be viewed in lab. These features include the thickness of the smear or tissue section, which will determine what power objective to use and thereby indicate the diameter of the magnification field and the level of resolution achieved. The ability to distinguish cells or structures clearly and distinctly under the microscope define the resolving power of the microscope. For example, two cells next to each other in a magnification field should be seen as two distinct cells. The lowest power objective has the greatest diameter of magnification field and the longest working distance. The 4× objective lens has a greater working distance in contrast to the 100× which has the least working distance. The intensity of light illuminating the specimen on the slide is greater with the low power objective compared to higher power objectives. The rheostat control knob can be used to adjust the amount of light illuminating the specimen.

Examination of Mouse Blood Using Giemsa Stained Slides with the Oil Immersion Lens

Students will be assigned microscopes for the semester. The following steps will serve as a guide for slide examination.

Procedure

1. Retrieve the microscope from the cabinet by holding the arm and base of the microscope to provide support.
2. Take the microscope to your bench and plug it into the outlet on the side of the bench (some lab benches will have the plugs in the center of the bench).
3. Switch on the microscope.
4. Obtain a slide from the slide box provided; wipe the bottom of the slide with kimwipes to remove any oil that might be on the back of the slide. This is the side of the slide without the smear. Be careful not to wipe the top of the slide, which is where the smear is located. Record the information written on the frosted edge of the slide.
5. Place the slide on the mechanical stage and secure the slide with the stage clip, then raise the stage bringing it closer to the objective lens
6. Adjust the mechanical stage by moving it left to right or top to bottom and use the coarse adjustment knob to bring the specimen into focus. Sharpen the focus by turning the fine adjustment knob.
7. Check the stage from the side to ensure that the objective does not hit the slide.
8. Raise the condenser lens close to the slide (this may require just a minor adjustment as previous users of the microscope may have already raised the condenser).

9. Lower the stage and turn the revolving nosepiece to move to a higher magnification (10× or 40×) objective lens, then raise the stage and make minor adjustments to the focus using the fine adjustment knob to sharpen the focus and show more detail in the specimen. At this point, cells should be obvious on the slide.

10. Lower the stage and move the low power objective away from the slide, so as not to get oil on the low power objective. Add a drop of immersion oil to the slide, then rotate the 100× objective lens till it is above the oil. Gently lower the objective lens into the oil, touching the oil with the lens immersed in the oil. Adjust the focus first with the coarse knob then using the fine adjustment knob sharpen the focus. Move the stage with the stage control from side to side or top to bottom to find a good viewing field. Identify uninfected red cells, infected red cells, platelets, neutrophils, basophils, eosinophils, lymphocytes and monocytes.

11. Use the differential cell counter to count the leukocytes (white blood cells). Move the slide to different fields counting 100 white blood cells and keeping track of each type of white cell with the red and white buttons on the cell counter. Your TA will demonstrate how to use the counter.

12. Prepare a table showing the distribution of the different leukocytes.

13. After recording and or illustrating the image, lower the stage, remove the slide from the stage clip and place the slide on the lab bench. Gently blot the oil off the smear using kimwipes. If there are no more slides to view, gently wipe off the oil from the 100× objective lens using lens paper.

14. Rotate the nosepiece and position the 4× objective above the condenser lens.

15. Switch off the microscope, unplug the cord by pulling the plug NOT the cord. Wrap the cord around the base of the microscope and return the microscope to the cabinet by supporting the microscope at the base and grasping the arm of the microscope.

Questions
1. What is the resolving power of a microscope?
2. Is the resolving power greater when using the 10× objective or 100× objective lens?
3. How does the resolution differ when viewing an image with 4×, 40× or 100× objective lenses?
4. An image viewed using an ocular lens of 15× magnification with a 40× objective lens has a total magnification of _____×.
5. How does the condenser lens contribute to the total magnification of images viewed under the microscope?
6. What is the advantage of first using the low power objective to view a specimen before switching to a high-powered objective lens?

Chapter 26
Exercise 2: Pipetting and Dilution Techniques, Identification of Mouse Lymphoid Organs

Pipetting Techniques

Introduction

Pipettes are essential laboratory tools used to transfer and dispense measured liquids between tubes, flasks, microtiter wells and various other vessels. Pipettes range from large serological pipettes used in tissue culture, capable of measuring 50 milliliters (mL) of media to Gilson pipets (micropipets) that are used to transfer very small volumes; as little as 0.5 microliter (μL) (Fig. 26.1). Knowing how to measure volumes of liquids accurately using pipets, is an important skill that can be applied to experiments in tissue culture, molecular and cell biology and immunology labs. Plastic pipets ("squeezers"), calibrated to 1 or 2 mL are also used to transfer small volumes of liquids. The 10 mL serological pipet is one of the most commonly used pipets. The pipet is graduated with measurements in increments of 0.1 mL intervals. Two scales are displayed on the pipet; on one side the scale increases in volume from 0 to 9 with the last 1 mL towards the tapered end of the pipet for the total volume of 10 mL. On the other side, graduations increase from the bottom to the top of the pipet. Some pipets are marked at the top with the letters **"TD"** (to deliver) or **"TC"** (to contain), with a double or single band, respectively at the top of the pipet to indicate each type. The "TD" pipets are also known as blow-out pipets because the entire measured volume must be completely dispensed. The pipets are filled using a **pipet pump**, **tri-valve bulb** or **automatic pipet dispenser**. Pipet pumps are color coded for the different sizes of pipets.

When working with serological pipets, avoid touching the tips, i. e. tapered ends, even with gloved hands. In particular, when working with sterile pipets, this is important to prevent contamination of the pipet tip. Serological pipets may have a cotton plug at the top of the pipet to prevent the solution being filled to enter and

© Springer Nature Switzerland AG 2021
T. Y. Sam-Yellowe, *Immunology: Overview and Laboratory Manual*,
https://doi.org/10.1007/978-3-030-64686-8_26

Fig. 26.1 Pipet pump with serological pipet, pipettor and transfer pipet (squeezer)

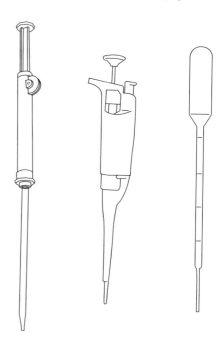

contaminate the pump, bulb or automatic pipet dispenser. Tri-valve bulbs have three settings; A (air valve), S (suction, to fill) and E (Empty, exhaust) that are used to remove air from the bulb, fill liquid and dispense the liquid.

<u>**DO NOT MOUTH PIPET**</u>.

Using pipets with a bulb or pump

Bulb

Attach the serological pipet to the bulb without pushing the pipet too far into the bulb. The bulb is squeezed to remove air by pressing "A". With the tip, i. e. the tapered end of the pipet inserted into the liquid to be measured, the suction "S" is pressed to fill the pipet to the desired volume. For example, if measuring 6 mL of liquid, fill till the 4 mL mark. Transfer the pipet to the vessel or container for dispensing the liquid and press "E" to empty the pipet.

Pipet Pump

If using a pump, attach the pipet to the pump gasket, exhaust any air that may be in the pump by pushing the plunger or piston all the way down, place the pipet tip in the container with the liquid to be dispensed (submerge the tip just underneath the liquid to be filled), roll the dial (*thumb wheel*) at the side of the pipet downward to fill the pipet. Transfer the pipet to the vessel or container to be filled. Roll the dial (*thumb wheel*) upward to dispense the liquid. Push the plunger down to dispense all the liquid in the pipet.

Micropipets

For micropipets, always know what volume you will need to pipet so that the correct micropipette (s) is selected for the experiment. The most commonly used micropipettes are the **P-10, P-20, P-200 and P-1000** used for volumes up to 1 mL (1000 µL). The numbers indicate the maximum volumes that can be filled using each type of pipet. Commonly used tips for the P-20 and P-200 are yellow tips. For the P-10, small white tips and for the P-1000 blue tips. An additional micropipette used in immunology and molecular biology labs is the **P-2** pipet. The volume of liquid to be transferred is pre-set before filling the tip. Always use the micropipette with a tip. Each pipet has an adjustment knob used to set the volume. Never set the volume above or below the maximum volume set for each pipet. Each pipet has a control plunger that has two stops. The **first stop** is for the calibrated pre-set volume. The **second stop** is the maximum volume that can be dispensed at the calibrated setting. There is also an **ejector button** for discarding pipet tips. To use the micropipette, set the volume to the desired amount (see Table 26.1 for settings), attach the correct size tip and holding the pipet vertically, and immerse the tip just below the surface of the liquid. Do not submerge the tip too far into the liquid to avoid contaminating the pipet. Depress the control plunger to the **FIRST STOP**. Do not press to the second stop to fill. Doing so will result in filling the pipet tip with more volume than the preset measurement. Transfer the tip still attached to the pipet, to the vessel, tube or well to be filled. Depress the control plunger to the **SECOND STOP** to dispense the liquid. After dispensing the liquid, use the ejector button to eject the pipet tip into a waste basket or biohazard waste basket provided at your bench. The **major objective** of this exercise is to learn how to accurately measure and transfer volumes of liquids between tubes.

Table 26.1 Pipet settings for measured volumes

P-1000 (200–1000 µL)	P-200 (20–200 µL)	P-20 (2–20 µL)	P-10 (1–10 µL)	P-2 (1–2 µL)
0	0	0	0	1
5	5	5	5	0
0	0	0	0	0
500 µL	50 µL	5 µL	5 µL	1 µL
Blue tip	Yellow tip	Yellow tip	White tip	White tip

Materials and Reagents (Per Pair)

Pipets (P-1000, P-200, P-20)
  Pipet tips (white, yellow, blue)
  Eppendorf tubes (Microcentrifuge tubes) 1.5 mL, 200 µL
  Tube rack
  Vortex
  0.05% Methylene blue dye in distilled water
  Distilled water in 50 mL flasks
  Sharpie

1. Select eight 1.5 mL and four 200 µL microcentrifuge tubes. Label the 1.5 mL tubes 1A, 1B; 2A, 2B; 3A, 3B; 4A, 4B; 5A, 5B and label the 200 µL tubes 6A, 6B; 7A, 7B.
2. Using the P-200 pipet with a yellow tip, add 200 µL distilled water to tubes 1A and 1B. Add 150 µL distilled water to tubes 2A and 2B. Add 75 µL distilled water to tubes 3A and 3B.
3. Using a P-1000 with a blue tip, add 300 µL of blue dye to tubes 1A and 1B. Check both tubes visually to see that both volumes are approximately 500 µL. Look at the graduation marks on the tubes for 500 µL.
4. Using the P-1000, add 400 µL of blue dye to tubes 2A and 2B. Check both tubes visually to see that both volumes are approximately 550 µL.
5. Using the P-1000, add 250 µL of blue dye to tubes 3A and 3B. Check both tubes visually to see that both volumes are approximately 325 µL.
6. Using the P-1000, set the pipet to 500 µL and transfer the total volume of 500 µL to tubes 4A and 4B. Use a different tip for each tube.
7. Set the P-1000 to 550 µL and transfer the total volume of 550 µL to tubes 5A and 5B. Use a different tip for each tube.
8. Set the P-20 pipet to 7.5 µL. Transfer 7.5 µL of the solution from tubes 3A and 3B into tubes 6A and 6B. Adjust the P-20 to 12.5 µL. Add 12.5 µL of distilled water to tubes 6A and 6B for a total volume of 20 µL in each tube. Adjust the P-20 to 20 µL and transfer the 20 µL volume to tubes 7A and 7B. Use a different tip for each tube.

Questions

1. Did you transfer the same total volume each time for each set of tubes in steps 5, 6 and 8?
2. Were you accurate in your pipetting at each step? Explain how you know you were accurate
3. What is the difference between accuracy and precision?
4. Did you fill your pipet tip with more or less volume of liquid than the preset volume in your pipet?

Dilution Techniques

Introduction

In this experiment, you will become familiar with dilution techniques and the anatomical arrangement of mouse lymphoid organs. Many serologic assays performed in clinical and research laboratories involve dilutions of concentrated solutions of antibodies, antigens, and other commonly used solutions and reagents. Antibody is often diluted or titrated to obtain a titer or working concentration of the antibody solution. The type of dilutions frequently performed in serological assays are referred to as serial dilutions. Serial 1:2 dilutions are the most common type of dilutions performed when diluting antibodies and antigens. Serial 1:10 dilutions are also performed, and are used when diluting cells.

When performing dilutions, a known volume of the concentrated solution, such as an antibody, is added to a fixed volume of the diluting solution or diluent. The diluent is usually physiological saline or any other buffered solution. A given number of cells such as lymphocytes from the spleen, thymus, lymph nodes or from cell culture can also be diluted into a fixed volume of saline or culture medium.

Serial dilutions involve the transfer of a concentrated solution (cells, antibody, antigen etc.) through a series of tubes with each transfer of solution resulting in a less concentrated solution. In serial 1:10 dilutions (1:10, 1:100, 1:1000), also known as ten-fold dilutions, each dilution is 1/10th as concentrated as the preceding dilution. In serial 1:2 dilutions (1:2, 1:4, 1:8, 1:16 or written ½, ¼, 1/8, 1/16), also referred to as two-fold dilutions, each dilution is 1/2 as concentrated as the preceding dilution.

When a serial 1:2 dilution of an antibody is performed and mixed with a given concentration of antigen, the titer of the antibody solution can be obtained. The titer is the reciprocal of the highest dilution of antibody that results in a visible end point reaction. In this exercise, we will perform serial 1:2 and 1:10 dilutions. Students will dilute a known number of mouse erythrocytes after determining cell counts using a hemocytometer. The diluted erythrocytes will be hypotonically lysed in ice-cold distilled water and the amount of hemoglobin released measured using a spectrophotometer at 690 nm wavelength. In the second exercise, you will serially dilute a concentrated dye solution and observe the change in the dye color intensity by visual examination and spectrophotometric measurement of the solution in the tubes.

The dilution factor of a solution can be obtained as follows:

$$\text{Dilution factor} = \frac{\text{volume of concentrate transferred}}{\text{volume of concentrate} + \text{volume of diluent}}$$

The total dilution factor is the product of all the individual dilution factors in a dilution scheme. For example, if 1 mL of an antibody solution is transferred to a test tube containing 9 mL of diluent, the dilution factor is 1/1 + 9 or 1/10 or 10^{-1}. If a serial 1:10 dilution procedure is carried out by transferring 1 mL into 9 mL, 0.1 mL into 9.9 mL, and 0.5 mL into 4.5 mL, the final dilution factor for this scheme is 1/10,000 or 10^{-4}. If the dilution factor is known, the concentration of solutions can be calculated. The **first objective** of this exercise is to learn dilution techniques. The **second objective** is to learn how to use the spectrophotometer and hemocytometer, the **third objective** is to learn to identify mouse lymphoid organs and the **fourth objective** is to learn to separate mononuclear cells and to differentiate T and B lymphocytes.

Materials and Reagents (Per Pair)

1 tube of 5% mouse erythrocyte suspension in PBS (Phosphate buffered saline)
Ice-cold distilled water
1% methylene blue solution
1 mL glass pipet
Plastic squeezer pipet
Transfer pipets (padl-pet)
Eppendorf tubes
Pipet bulbs
Eppendorf microfuge
Table top clinical centrifuge
Spectrophotometer
Microscope
Hemocytometer and cover slips
Vortexer mixer
10×75 mm test tubes
Test tube racks
Laboratory marking pens
Two pair of scissors and forceps
Dissecting pans and pins 2 mice (Swiss)
Three 15 mL centrifuge tubes
Six 10 mL pipet
Hank's balanced salt solution (HBSS)
Six Petri dishes with wire mesh screens
One 200 mL beaker
Coplin jars with absolute methanol and Giemsa stain
Twelve 10 mL syringes
Biohazard bags
Gloves
Roll of Bench Paper

Procedure

Part A

1. Using a 1 mL pipet, transfer 1 mL of the 5% mouse erythrocyte suspension from the provided stock cell suspension into two Eppendorf tubes. In a separate Eppendorf tube, add 100 μL of PBS, then pipet 10 μL of the cell suspension from the stock suspension and add it to 100 μL of PBS for erythrocyte counts. Read and follow instructions for counting erythrocytes. Use the formula: Total # cells in 5 (80 smaller squares) squares $\times$ 5 $\times$ 10^4 $\times$ dilution used = # red blood cells/mL.

2. Arrange two rows of empty Eppendorf tubes. Each row should have eight tubes. One set of tubes will be used for a serial 1:10 dilution (Fig. 26.2a). The second set of tubes will be used for serial 1:2 dilutions (Fig. 26.2b). Label the first row; 10^{-1}, 10^{-2}...etc. Pipet 0.9 mL of PBS into each tube. Pipet 0.5 mL of PBS into each tube of the second set and label the tubes, 1:2, 1:4, 1:8 ... etc. (See Fig. 26.2)

3. Transfer 0.1 mL of the 5% cell suspension into tube #1 of the 1:10 series. Gently resuspend the cells. Using a different pipet transfer 0.1 mL of the cell suspension from tube #1 to tube #2. Repeat the transfer of cells using a different pipet for each transfer till tube #8 for the 1:10 dilutions. For the second set of tubes for the 1:2 dilution series, transfer 0.5 mL of the 5% cell suspension into tube #1. Gently resuspend the cells. Using a different pipet transfer 0.5 mL of the cell suspension from tube #1 to tube #2. Repeat the transfer of cells using a different pipet for each transfer till tube #8 of the for the 1:2 dilution series. Check to make sure that your pipetting is accurate.

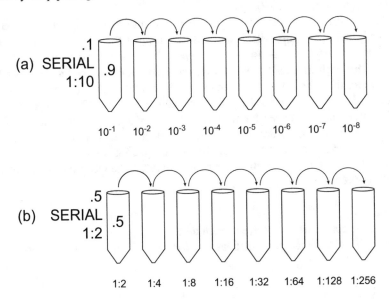

Fig. 26.2 Serial tenfold (**a**) and twofold (**b**) dilution scheme in 1 mL volumes. Tenfold dilutions are performed using red blood cells and twofold dilutions are performed using methylene blue to demonstrate the importance of dilutions in the immunology lab

4. Centrifuge all tubes in a microfuge for 5 min at 14,000 × g. Remove the supernatant with a plastic squeezer and discard it into the waste beaker provided.
5. Add 1 mL of ice-cold distilled water to the pellets in all the tubes. Cap the tubes tightly and invert them end-over-end, 2–3 times to lyse the erythrocytes. Place the tubes in a rack and incubate the tubes at room temperature for 15 min.
6. Switch on a spectrophotometer and set the wavelength to 690 nm. Place PBS in a cuvette, take an optical density (OD) reading in the spectrophotometer to calibrate the instrument. This is the blank reading. Using a different cuvet, add the contents of the dilution tubes, one at a time, place the tube in the spectrophotometer and record the OD at 690 nm to measure the amount of hemoglobin released from the lysed erythrocytes. Plot a graph of the absorbance versus dilution factor for both dilution schemes. The instructor will demonstrate the use of the spectrophotometer.

Part B

1. Using a 1 mL pipet, transfer 1 mL of the 0.5 % methylene blue suspension from the provided stock dye suspension into two Eppendorf tubes.
2. Arrange two rows of empty Eppendorf tubes. Each row should have eight tubes. One set of tubes will be used for a serial 1:10 dilution (Fig. 26.2a). The second set of tubes will be used for serial 1:2 dilutions (Fig. 26.2b). Label the first row; 1:10, 1:100 … etc. Pipet 0.9 mL of distilled water into each tube. Pipet 0.5 mL of distilled water into each tube of the second set and label the tubes, 1:2, 1:4, 1:8 … etc. (See Fig. 26.2)
3. Transfer 0.1 mL of the 0.5% dye suspension into tube #1 of the 1:10 series. Gently resuspend the cells. Using a different pipet transfer 0.1 mL of the dye suspension from tube #1 to tube #2. Repeat the transfer of dye using a different pipet for each transfer till tube #8 for the 1:10 dilutions. For the second set of tubes for the 1:2 dilution series, transfer 0.5 mL of the 0.5% dye suspension into tube #1. Gently resuspend the dye solution. Using a different pipet transfer 0.5 mL of the dye suspension from tube #1 to tube #2. Repeat the transfer of dye solution using a different pipet for each transfer till tube #8 of the for the 1:2 dilution series. Check to make sure that your pipetting is accurate.
   Mix the dye solutions by vortexing and observe the change in the color intensity of the dye in each tube.

Questions
What is the concentration of dye in each tube?
What is the dilution factor in the final tube for the 1:10 and 1:2 dilution series?

Part C

1. Sacrifice the mouse by placing it in a container with halothane soaked cotton (for halothane inhalation).

Fig. 26.3 Identification of mouse thymus and spleen, primary and secondary lymphoid organs, respectively

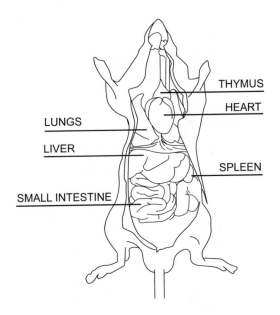

THYMUS

HEART

LUNGS

LIVER

SPLEEN

SMALL INTESTINE

2. Place the mouse on a dissecting board with the limbs extended. Secure the limbs to the dissecting board using dissecting pins. Use the illustration shown in Fig. 26.3 as a guide to locate and identify the lymphoid organs indicated.

3. Wet the mouse thoroughly with 70% ethanol, then make an incision in the ventral surface of the mouse to expose the peritoneal cavity. Locate the spleen on the left side underneath the liver. The spleen is the elongated reddish-brown organ. Carefully excise the spleen. To obtain the thymus extend the incision into the thoracic area. Expose the thoracic cage, cut through the bone structure to separate the chest and expose the thymic lobes directly above the heart and just beneath the sternum. For the mesenteric lymph nodes, extend the small intestines using a pair of forceps and carefully excise the lymph nodes from the network of mesenteric capillaries. The organ will appear elongated and cream colored. Remove the thymus, spleen and mesenteric lymph nodes and place each on the wire mesh screen placed within separate sterile petri dishes containing 10 mL of HBSS (the tissues should be placed in the center of the screen) (Fig. 26.4). Label all tubes correctly, with the lymphoid organ obtained. Using a plunger from a 10 mL syringe, gently press the tissue through the wire screens. Tilt the petri dishes to collect the cell suspension with a 10 mL pipet, and transfer it to 15 mL centrifuge tubes. Allow the large pieces of tissue to settle approximately I min, then transfer the cell suspension to fresh 15 mL centrifuge tubes.

4. Centrifuge the cells at 200 × g for 10 min. Remove the supernatant and discard it into the 200 mL waste beaker provided. Resupend the pellet in 200 μL of HBSS. Using a padl-pet, transfer a drop of the suspension to a clean glass slide, spread the drop with the flat end of the padl-pet, and allow the smear to air dry, then fix the smear in absolute methanol by placing the slide in a coplin jar containing absolute methanol. Fix the smears for 30 s, remove the slides from the jar

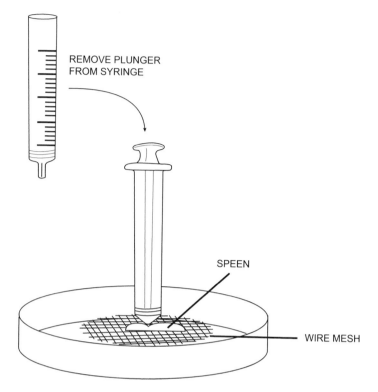

REMOVE PLUNGER
FROM SYRINGE

SPEEN

WIRE MESH

Fig. 26.4 Preparing a mouse spleen cell suspension using the plunger from a 10 mL syringe. Following splenectomy, the spleen is placed on a wire mesh contained in a petri dish with tissue culture medium. Using the plunger, spleen cells are gently teased into the medium

using a pair of forceps and let the smears air dry. When the smears are dry, place the slides in a coplin jar containing Giemsa stain and stain for 5 min.

5. Remove the slides from the coplin jar and wash the slides in distilled water for 30–40 s by squeezing distilled water over the smears until the water is clear. Let the smears air-dry, then observe the slides under oil immersion. Illustrate the cells and record your results in your notebooks. Note the differences in appearance of the cells obtained from the different lymphoid organs.

Question

Can you distinguish B and T lymphocytes based on morphology alone?

Selected References

Miller LE, Ludke HR, Peacock JE, Tomar RH (1991) Ch. 3, Introduction to serologic methods. In: Peacock JE, Tomar RH (eds) Manual of laboratory immunology, 2nd edn. Lea and Febiger, Philadelphia

Myers LR (1989) Immunology, a laboratory manual. Wm. C. Brown, Dubuque, IA. Exercise 2 The dilution concept

Chapter 27
Exercise 3: Blood Cell Preparation, Leukocyte Differentiation and ABO Blood Typing

Introduction

In this experiment, you will become familiar with the serologic technique of hemagglutination, and leukocyte differential analysis. We will use the method of ABO blood typing to demonstrate the technique of hemagglutination. The ABO group of antigens is important in blood transfusions in which the infusion of red cells carrying A or B antigens into a person with natural anti-A or anti-B antibodies (agglutinins) may result in a life-threatening transfusion reaction.

A second group of clinically important red blood cell antigens are the Rh (Rhesus) antigens for which there are more than 50. Unlike the ABO system, the antibodies against the Rh antigens are the products of authentic immunizations either through pregnancy or transfusions. The most clinically important of these antigens is the D antigen. In the newborn, this isoantigen accounts for over 90% of the cases of hemolytic disease due to maternal isoimmunization. Other Rh antigens are the C and E antigens. Although ABO-induced hemolytic disease occurs, the disease induced by the Rh system is usually more severe. The ABO system is useful in paternity determinations and forensic pathology, as these antigens are very stable. Both antigen systems will be studied in this experiment. Additional blood group antigens are the Kidd, Kell, Lewis and Duffy antigens. The Duffy antigens serve as receptors for *Plasmodium vivax*, a protozoan parasite that causes malaria in humans. Individuals lacking this receptor, such as most individuals in Western Africa, are refractory to this *Plasmodium* species (Table 27.1).

© Springer Nature Switzerland AG 2021
T. Y. Sam-Yellowe, *Immunology: Overview and Laboratory Manual*,
https://doi.org/10.1007/978-3-030-64686-8_27

Table 27.1 ABO blood antigens

Blood type	Antigen	Agglutinin	Acceptable donor	Acceptable recipient
A	A	Anti-B	Type A & O	Type A
B	B	Anti-A	Type B & O	Type B
AB	A + B	None	Type AB, A, B, O	Type AB
O	None	Anti-A	Type AB, O	Type O
		Anti-B		

Universal recipient (AB)
Universal donor (O)

Blood Components

Blood is connective tissue consisting of cellular elements and a number of molecules solubilized in the fluid portion or plasma. The fluid and cellular components can be separated by centrifugation. When blood is allowed to clot before centrifugation, clotting factors are removed from the plasma. The resulting fluid supernatant is referred to as serum. Serum contains immunoglobulin (antibodies), in addition to other macromolecules. Blood cells can be differentiated as erythrocytes (red cells) or leukocytes (white cells). Normal human blood contains $4-5 \times 10^6$ erythrocytes/mm^3 and $5-8 \times 10^3$ leukocytes/mm^3.

Cells of the Immune System

The cells of the immune system comprise three major categories: **Granulocytes, Monocytes,** and **Lymphocytes** (Fig. 27.1). Granulocytes contain distinctive granules in their cytoplasm. All three arise from the same stem cell originating primarily in the bone marrow. The stem cell is referred to as the hematopoietic stem cell. The process of cell differentiation from a pluripotent stem cell is referred to as hematopoiesis. Depending on the age of the animal, some of these cells may originate in the spleen or the liver.

The granulocyte series is distinguished by the structure of both nuclear and cytoplasmic components. The three distinct cell types comprising this group are **neutrophils, basophils,** and **eosinophils**.

Neutrophils (Polymorphonuclear Leukocytes, PMNs)

This is the most common of the granulocyte series (50–70% in human blood) and is characterized by a multi-lobed nucleus with densely packed chromatin. When stained with Giemsa stain, the cytoplasm is pale with pink or violet-pink granules. PMNs are generally the first cells to appear at the site of a foreign invasion and in the case of microbial infection will actively phagocytize the invading organism.

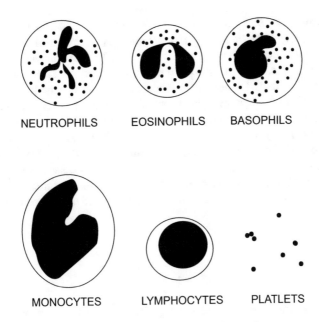

NEUTROPHILS   EOSINOPHILS   BASOPHILS

MONOCYTES   LYMPHOCYTES   PLATLETS

Fig. 27.1 Leukocytes (white blood cells) and platelets (thrombocytes)

Eosinophils

These cells are present in very low concentration in blood (1–5%). They are similar in appearance to neutrophils. However, the nucleus is typically bi-lobed. The cytoplasm contains orange-red granules and is more granular than the neutrophil. Eosinophils are found in the highest concentrations at sites of inflammatory reactions such as parasitic helminth infections or hypersensitivity reactions.

Basophils

These granulocytes have an irregular nucleus that is not lobulated. They are present in extremely low concentrations (0.5–1%). the most distinctive characteristic of basophils is the presence of large dense dark blue granules in the cytoplasm and overlying the nucleus. Tissue basophils (mast cells) are found in the deep tissues and are important in immediate hypersensitivity reactions.

The **Monocyte** series comprises 2–6% of white blood cells in human blood and is composed of functionally and morphologically distinct cell types. The blood monocytes enlarge and differentiate into macrophages and histiocytes. The term macrophage is generally applied to the form found free in peritoneal, pleural or alveolar spaces while the term histiocyte is most often used for those forms found fixed in tissue (lymph nodes, liver, spleen). Morphologically, monocytes have a large kidney shaped nucleus and light blue cytoplasm after Giemsa stain.

The **Lymphocyte** series comprises 20–30% of white blood cells in human blood. Approximately 70% of normal blood lymphocytes are thymus dependent (T cells) and the rest are B cells and natural killer cells. The lymphocytes are composed of highly specialized cells involved in the immune response. They possess most of the properties that make the immune mechanism in higher vertebrates unique among biological systems. Lymphocytes are capable of a wide variety of functions, including antibody production (humoral immunity), cell-mediated cytotoxicity (cell-mediated immunity), and cellular regulation. Morphologically, lymphocytes are divided into small, medium, and large lymphocytes and they contain a uniformly large round nucleus, with very small cytoplasmic area. As we shall see in later exercises, lymphocytes and their subsets can be separated using differential density centrifugation techniques. The cells can then be characterized using specific cell surface markers.

Platelets

These are small, anuclear, cell-like bodies found in the plasma portion of blood. They often appear in clusters. Platelets are important in blood clotting reactions and in allergic reactions.

The **first objective** of this exercise is to learn the technique of hemagglutination using human red blood cells. The **second objective** is to understand the clinical significance of the ABO and Rh antigens. The **third objective** is to learn to identify and morphologically differentiate the cells of the immune system.

Materials and Reagents (Per Pair)

Microscope
Warm slide box
Bunsen burner
Commercial anti-A, anti-B, and anti-Rh (D), C, E
Clean glass slides with frosted edges
Applicator sticks
Heparinized capillary tubes (sterile)
Grease pencils
70% ethanol
Cotton
Sterile lancets
Sterile gauze
Mouse blood (collected from tail snips)
Giemsa stain in coplin jar
Absolute methanol in coplin jar

Sterile alcohol pads
Cell counter/tally

Procedure

A. Blood typing

1. Warm 2 glass slides over the flame of a bunsen burner. On one slide draw three circles with a wax pencil. Label beneath each circle the letters A, B and RhD. On the second slide draw two circles. Label underneath each circle the letters RhC and RhE.
2. Clean the index finger with individually wrapped sterile alcohol pads. Wait for the alcohol to dry.
3. Carefully puncture the fingertip with a sterile lancet.
4. Wipe the first drop of blood with a sterile gauze and gently squeeze the finger to fill 3–4 heparinized capillary tubes with blood.
5. Add a drop of anti-A, anti-B, and anti-Rh antibodies to the appropriate circles on the glass slides.
6. Transfer drops of blood from the capillary tubes to sections labeled on the glass slide.
7. Mix well with applicator sticks (<u>use a different applicator stick for each circle on the slide</u>). Place the slides on a warm box and read the agglutination reaction after 2 min. Agglutinated cells should appear as clumps of cells on the slide (Fig. 27.2). Agglutination can also be performed in the round bottomed wells of a microtiter plate.

B. Blood smear for differential leukocyte count.

1. Add a drop of blood to the edge of a clean glass slide. Using a second clean glass slide, prepare a thin, evenly spread blood smear (your TA will demonstrate). Touch the drop of blood with the short edge of the second slide and quickly spread the blood in a thin film. Let the smear air dry. Prepare 2–3 slides and use the best one.
2. Immerse the slide in a coplin jar containing absolute methanol for 30 s to fix the cells.
3. Remove the slide from the coplin jar and let the smear air dry. Transfer the slide to a coplin jar containing Giemsa stain. Stain the smear for 5 min.
4. Remove the slide from the coplin jar and rinse the slide with distilled water by squeezing distilled water over the smear till the water is clear. Let the smear air dry.
5. When the smear is dry, observe the slide under oil immersion (100×). Note the morphology (appearance, shape and size) of the leukocytes. Distinguish the erythrocytes (red blood cells or normocytes) from leukocytes (Fig. 27.1). Cell morphology may be used to diagnose certain diseases such as leukemia.

Fig. 27.2 ABO and Rhesus (D) blood typing. Individuals with type A blood have the A antigen, lack anti-A antibodies but have anti-B antibodies. Individuals with type B blood have the B antigen, lack anti-B antibodies but have anti-A antibodies. Individuals with type AB blood have A and B antigens and lack anti-A and anti-B antibodies. Individuals with type O blood have anti-A and anti-B antibodies and lack A and B antigens. The presence of the D antigen on red cells will result in binding to anti-D antibodies which is a positive test

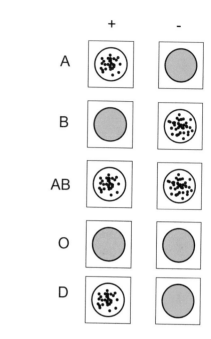

Table 27.2 Typical profile of a differential blood cell count from a peripheral human blood smear

Cell type	% Total Leukocytes	% Expected
Lymphocytes	28	20–30
Neutrophils (PMNS)	63	50–70
Eosinophils	4	1–5
Basophils	0	0.5–1
Monocytes	5	2–6
Total leukocytes	100	—

6. Count a total of 100 leukocytes and determine the percentage of the different cell types. A typical profile of leukocyte distribution is shown in Table 27.2. An increase or decrease in numbers of one or more types of leukocyte may be diagnostic in certain diseases or infections. Record the results in your notebook.

   Note: This exercise can also be performed using mouse blood. In this case, mouse blood will be collected from tail snips, thin smears will be prepared, air dried and fixed in absolute methanol and then stained with Giemsa stain. The slides will be visualized and the different blood cells counted and recorded. Simulated human blood can also be prepared and mixed with the antibodies to perform agglutination.

   Record agglutination results
   Positive result: (++) visible clumping of cells
   Negative result: (−) no clumping of cells

Sample tube #	Anti-A	Anti-B	Anti-RhD	Anti-RhC	Anti-Rh-E	Result significance
Tube 1						
Tube 2						
Tube 3						
Tube 4						

NOTES:

NOTES AND ILLUSTRATIONS:

Selected References

Avent ND, Reid ME (2000) The Rh blood group system: A review. Blood 95:375–387

Bellanti JA (1985) Immunology I 11. Saunders, New York. Ch. 3, Antigens and immunogenecity

Barrett JT (1988) Textbook of immunology. Mosby, St. Louis. Ch. 13, Agglutination and hemagglutination; Ch. 5, Macrophages and antigen-processing and presenting cells

Murphy K, Weaver C (2017) Janeway's immunobiology, 9th edn. Garland Press, New York

Punt J, Stranford SA, Jones PP, Owen JA (2019) Kuby immunology, 8th edn. W.H. Freeman and Company, New York. Ch. 2, Cells, organs, and microenvironments of the immune system

Chapter 28
Exercise 4: Single Suspension of Mouse Spleen Cells, Cell Viability Assays and Identification of Specific Cells Using Cell Surface Antigens

Introduction

Methods of lymphocyte quantitation and characterization are based on the determination of cell viability, quantitation, and detection of cell surface markers (Cluster of differentiation-CD antigens). Examples of CD antigens are summarized in Table 28.1. Cytoplasmic components, or nuclear material can also be used. Cell surface markers are the most commonly detected in the routine clinical laboratory. Lymphocytes and antigen presenting cells (APC) constitute important components of both the humoral and cell mediated branches of the immune system. B lymphocytes synthesize immunoglobulin (antibodies) along with some cytokines, and T lymphocytes produce and secrete a variety of cytokines that function in both branches of the immune system. The APCs, macrophages and dendritic cells also secrete a number of cytokines and reactive products following their binding to pathogen associated molecules (PAMPs) with their pathogen recognition receptors (PRRs). These immune cells and the components that they produce play a significant role in host defense against parasites, bacteria, fungi, viruses and some neoplastic disorders. Blood cells are prepared for analysis by the isolation of mononuclear cells using Ficoll-Hypaque or Histopaque density gradient centrifugation. Blood cells can also be prepared by the removal of red blood cells through lysis with a reagent such as ammonium chloride or acetic acid.

Particular cell types can be isolated using enrichment or depletion techniques followed by confirmation with immunofluorescence assays or flow cytometry.

Depletion techniques consist of the removal of a specific group of cells by cytotoxicity reactions in the presence of complement, leaving behind the desired population of cells e.g. removal of all T cells in a suspension by incubating the cells with anti-Thy-1 (CD90), Thy-1.2 (CD90.2) or anti-CD3 antibodies, to isolate B cells and other antigen presenting accessory cells or removal of all B cells and accessory cells by incubating the cells with anti-class II MHC or anti-CD19 antibodies to isolate T cells.

© Springer Nature Switzerland AG 2021
T. Y. Sam-Yellowe, *Immunology: Overview and Laboratory Manual*,
https://doi.org/10.1007/978-3-030-64686-8_28

Table 28.1 Summary of some frequently encountered types and sources of CD antigens

	B cell	TH cell	TC cell
CD2		+	+
CD3		+	+
CD4		+	− (also located on macrophages)
CD5	+	+	+
CD8			+
CD28		+	+
CD40	+		
CD45	+	+	+
CD54	+	+	+
CD19	+		

The antibodies used are of the IgM isotype. IgM antibodies are the most efficient for activating complement and thus are very efficient in cytotoxic elimination of cells. Particular cell populations can also be isolated using enrichment techniques such as panning for Thy-1+, Thy-1.2+ or Ig+ cells, for T and B lymphocytes, respectively, by incubating a cell suspension in a petri dish pre-coated with specific antibodies. CD4+ or CD8+ specific antibodies can also be used in the panning technique to isolate T cell subsets. The panning technique provides a precise method to isolate a given population of lymphocytes. T lymphocytes can also be isolated by passage through a nylon wool column or by rosetting. Human T cells bind to sheep red blood (SRBC) cells using the CD2 receptor, forming a rosette of 10–12 SRBC surrounding a single T lymphocyte. Sheep red blood cell rosetting also provides an easy method of counting T cells. Adherence techniques can also be used to enrich for a specific subset of cells. Macrophages and dendritic cells adhere to plastic. This property of adherence is used to recover them from a cell suspension. The adherent cells are then washed and recovered from the plastic surface for further analysis. In some cases, lymphocyte and macrophage continuous cell lines can be used to investigate cell function in vitro.

These laboratory analyses are an essential component of the clinical assessment of a variety of disorders, and are particularly useful in the diagnosis of lymphoproliferative malignancies, the diagnosis of primary immunodeficiency diseases and the diagnosis of acquired immunodeficiency disorders. Lymphocyte quantitation is most frequently performed on cells of the peripheral blood; (other specimens, e.g., lymph nodes, thymus, or bone marrow may be used when indicated).

In this exercise, students will prepare single cell suspensions from murine (Swiss Webster mice) lymphoid tissue (spleen). Lymphoid tissue can also be obtained from other sources such as the lymph nodes, Peyer's patches, thymus, or bone marrow.

Due to the nature of in vitro manipulations, it is especially important that care be taken to minimize trauma during the preparation of cell suspensions. Although some cells are killed or damaged during organ disruption, the techniques used generally yield cell suspensions that contain a high percentage of viable cells. We will also use the murine macrophage cell line, J774A.1 maintained by the American type culture collection (ATCC).

Cell viability may be determined for the spleen cell suspension and murine cell line by the following five methods: Various methods for determining cell viability are based on dye exclusion and can be evaluated by the light microscope. The dyes used are trypan blue, eosin Y, and nigrosin. Live cells will exclude the dyes, while dead cells take up and retain the dyes, appearing blue, red or brown-black, respectively. Fluorescein diacetate and acridine orange-ethidium bromide can be used to determine cell viability with the fluorescent microscope. Fluorescein diacetate is taken up by all cells, it is only hydrolyzed by live cells to reveal green fluorescence. Acridine orange is taken up by live cells whereas ethidium bromide is taken up by dead cells. Under ultraviolet (UV) light live cells appear green while dead cells appear orange-red. Cell viability is also determined using a **hemocytometer** counting chamber. Automatic cell counters are also used to count cells.

USING THE HEMOCYTOMETER: The standard hemocytometer chamber is for enumerating **erythrocytes** and **leukocytes**. There are two chambers, each consisting of ruled grids: four large squares subdivided into 16 smaller squares surrounding a central square divided into 25 small squares further subdivided into 16 smaller squares (see diagram below). Each chamber contains a V-shaped or beveled loading groove (Fig. 28.1). A coverslip is placed over the chambers before a cell suspension is loaded. With the cover-slip in place, each square of the hemocytometer represents a total volume of $0.1 \text{ mm}^3 = 10\text{--}4 \text{ cm}^2$ ($1 \text{ cm}^3 = 1 \text{ mL}$). The number

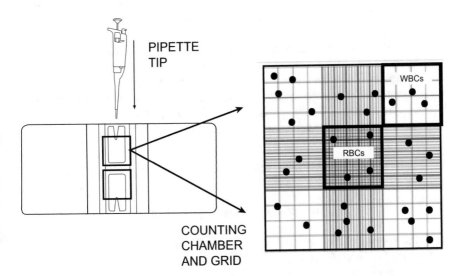

PIPETTE TIP

COUNTING CHAMBER AND GRID

Fig. 28.1 Hemocytometer showing the duplicate counting chambers with coverslips. Cells are added to the "V"-shaped groove. Capillary action moves the cells into the chamber. Enlarge counting chamber shows four large squares for counting white blood cells (WBCs). The center grid is used for counting red blood cells (RBCs)

of cells/mL can be calculated after cells have been counted using the hemocytometer.

Total leukocyte count (mononuclear cell count) and Trypan blue viability determination:

1. Prepare a lymphoid cell suspension as described, then prepare a dilution for counting. A suspension of J774A.1 cells obtained from cell culture can also be diluted for counting. Dilutions of 1:10 or 1:100 can be prepared depending on the concentration of the cell suspension. Mix the diluted cell suspension with 0.2–0.4% Trypan blue. Let the Trypan blue cell suspension stand for approximately 3–5 min (depending on the cell type the amount of time can be reduced). Prolonged incubation of cells in Trypan blue will result in viable cells also taking up dye.

    NOTE: Each group of students will receive cultured J774A.1 cells. After performing the cell count and determining the cell viability, students will perform subculture (passaging) of the cells to achieve the desired cell density, into 25 cm^2 flasks. If the tissue culture room is unavailable, subcultures will be performed by your TA under the laminar flow hood and incubated for use in the next lab meeting. The cells will be cultured at 37 °C, 5% CO_2, with humidity, till the next lab period.

2. Using a clean, dry hemocytometer with a clean coverslip in place, carefully load the chambers with the cell suspension using a yellow pipet tip (use Eppendorf or Gilson pipets), Pasteur pipet, padlpets or plastic squeezer (Fig. 28.1). The cell suspension will be drawn into the chamber by capillary action. **DO NOT EXCEED THE CAPACITY OF THE CHAMBERS AND DO NOT UNDERFILL THE CHAMBERS.** Both procedures will result in inaccurate counts.

3. Begin at the top left large square and count cells in all 16 squares. Use the 40× objective lens. To ensure accuracy, if cells on lines are counted, be consistent in counting cells only on left and top lines of the squares. Continue to second large square till all four large squares have been counted. Count the second chamber using same pattern. Count approximately 200 cells/chamber.

4. Determine the average cell count per square and multiply with the dilution factor and correction factor to obtain # cells/mL.

If 200 cells are counted in all four squares, the average count per square is 50 cells. If a 1:10 dilution was prepared, the # cell/mL is:

$$50 \times 10 \times 10^4 = 5,000,000 \, or \, 5 \times 10^6 \, cells \, / \, mL$$

If the volume of the total cell suspension is 6 mL, the total cell # is 6 (original volume) × 5,000,000 (cells/mL) = 3 × 10^7 cells.

Count both viable (unstained cells) and non-viable (blue stained) cells. This gives the total cell count. To calculate % viability:

$$\frac{\text{Total viable cells} \times 100}{\text{Total cell count}}$$

Total erythrocyte count:

1. Prepare an erythrocyte cell suspension then dilute the cells to be counted. Load a clean, dry hemocytometer with a coverslip in place as indicated above.
2. Move the hemocytometer to the central square and count the cells in five small squares (total of 80 smaller squares). The volume of the smallest squares = 2.5×10^4 mm^4. To calculate the number of cells in 1 mm multiply the volume by 4000. Since 80 squares were counted for cell #/mm, to get cells/mL multiply by a correction factor of 1000.

$$\# \text{RBCs} / \text{mL} = \# \text{cells in 80 squares} \times \text{dilution} \times 4000 / 80 \times 1000$$

$$\text{or} \# \text{RBCs} / \text{mL} = \# \text{cells in 80 squares} \times \text{dilution} \times 5 \times 10,000$$

E.g. If a total of 200 cells from a 1:2 dilution is counted in 80 squares from an original volume of 10 mL cell suspension, the number of red blood cells/mL would be:

$$200 \times 2 \times 5 \times 10^4 = 2 \times 10^7 \text{ cells} / \text{mL}$$

For the total cell count in 10 mL multiply cells/mL by 10 to obtain 2×10^8 cells.
The **first objective of** this exercise is to learn how to collect and prepare a single cell suspension of murine spleen cells and to determine the viability of the cells using Trypan blue. The **second objective** is to determine the viability of J774A.1 murine macrophages grown in Dulbecco's modifies eagle's medium (DMEM) containing 10 % fetal bovine serum. The **third objective** is to learn how to perform cell counts using the hemocytometer. The **fourth objective** is to isolate a mononuclear cell population and differentiate B and T lymphocytes by immunofluorescence assay (IFA).

Materials and Reagents (Per Pair)

Microscope
Clinical centrifuge
Balance
Bunsen burner
1 mouse
1 sterile glass petri dish with stainless steel wire mesh
10 mL plastic syringe
1 pair of scissors
2 pair of forceps

2 15 mL plastic sterile centrifuge tubes
3 1 mL glass pipets
6 sterile squeezers
Dissecting pans and pins
70% ethanol (squeeze bottle)
Gloves
1 Hemocytometer and Cover Slip
Glass slides with frosted edges
Methanol
0.2% Trypan Blue
Earl's Balanced Salt Solution (EBBS)
Disposable bag for mouse carcass
Kimwipes
Paper towel
Bench cover
One 200 mL beaker
Two 100 mL beakers
Ice bucket
Antibody conjugates
UV microscope
Histopaque
Clear nail polish
Glycerol mounting solution (or commercially available mounting solution with DAPI)

Procedure

Part A

Collection of Lymphoid Cells

1. Sacrifice the mouse by placing it in a container containing halothane soaked cotton (halothane inhalation).
2. Remove the mouse from the container and wet the entire mouse with 70% ethanol.
3. Make a V-shaped cut with a pair of sterile scissors through the loose skin in the midsection of the mouse and pull skin gently with forceps toward the head until the peritoneal cavity is exposed. Flood the peritoneal cavity with 70% ethanol to remove any loose hair.
4. Fold back the peritoneum, and lift the spleen with a pair of sterile forceps to separate it from the blood vessels and connecting tissue. Cut out the spleen, and place it on top of the wire mesh placed in a sterile plastic dish containing 10 mL of EBSS.

5. Gently press the spleen through the wire screen with the plastic plunger from a 10 mL syringe (**see** Fig. 26.4 in Exercise 2). Tilt the plate and collect the cell suspension using a sterile plastic squeezer. Transfer the cell suspension into a 15 ml centrifuge tube. Wait 1 min for large clumps of tissue to settle to the bottom of the tube, then transfer the suspension without disturbing the clumps, into a second 15 mL centrifuge tube.
6. Centrifuge the cells at $200 \times g$ for 10 min on the tabletop clinical centrifuge.
7. Remove and discard the supernatant into the 200 mL waste beaker provided. Record the volume of the cell pellet.
8. Resuspend the pellet in 10 mL of EBSS and repeat the centrifugation as in #7. Remove and discard the supernatant as in #7.
9. Resuspend the pellet in 0.5 mL of ammonium chloride-lysis buffer to lyse the red blood cells (this volume may be changed depending on the volume of the pellet or if commercially obtained lysis buffer is used).
Wait for 1 min, then add 10 mL of EBSS, centrifuge as above and discard the supernatant.

Proceed to **part B** for determination of cell viability or to **part D** for identification of B and T lymphocytes using antibodies specific for cell surface antigens.

Part B

Determination of Cell Viability by Trypan Blue Exclusion

10. Resuspend the pellet (from #9) in 1 ml of EBSS.
    NOTE: A suspension of J774A.1 cells will be centrifuged and resuspended in DMEM. Students will follow steps 11–15 for cell viability determination and counting.
11. From the suspension, prepare a 1:10 dilution of cells in EBSS, e.g. 50 µL of cells in 450 µL of EBSS or 500 µL in 4500 µL of EBSS, followed by a 1:2 dilution with the trypan blue solution.
    For example using 0.1 mL of cell suspension plus 0.1 mL of dye.
12. Wait for 30 s–1 min then load the cells into the hemocytometer by placing one small drop of the cell suspension using a plastic squeezer or pipet tip attached to a pipetman, into the v-shaped loading groove. Do not flood the counting chambers. Proceed to count the cells using the large squares on the hemocytometer (Your TA will demonstrate). Use a tally counter to keep track of cell counts. After counting in the first chamber, continue counting in the second, third and fourth chambers. Read and follow instructions for loading the counting chamber. Your instructor will demonstrate. Depending on the suspension and the number of cells present, each group of students will have to use a different dilution scheme to obtain a countable grid on the hemocytometer.
13. Count the number of unstained (viable) and stained (dead) cells separately in the four large squares. Divide the total number of cells by four to obtain the

Table 28.2 Average cell count and viability determination obtained from a typical experiment where the cell suspension was diluted 1:20 (Experiment 1) and 1:50 (Experiment 2)

Large squares	# Viable cells		# Non-viable cells		Total# cells	
	#1	#2	#1	#2	#1	#2
Square 1	152	32	32	11	184	43
Square 2	179	36	39	7	218	43
Square 3	109	23	39	13	148	46
Square 4	115	27	22	3	137	30
Average in 4 squares	139	118	33	34	172	152

average number of cells. For greater accuracy, count approximately 200 cells. Using the formula provided above, calculate the total number of cells/mL in the cell suspension, the percent viable and the percent non-viable (Table 28.2). Students will compare the cell counts obtained manually with counts obtained using the automatic cell counter.

14. The cells in culture will be evaluated for apoptosis using Annexin V labeling or DNA gel electrophoresis to identify DNA fragmentation. Evaluation of the culture for apoptosis using Annexin V will depend on the availability of the flow cytometer.

Part C

Giemsa Stain of Lymphoid Cells

15. Centrifuge the remaining cell suspension, discard the supernatant, and add an equal volume of EBBS to the cell pellet. This prepares a 50% cell suspension.
16. Prepare a thick smear on a clean glass slide, by placing a drop of the cell suspension in the middle of the slide using a padlpet and then spreading the drop gently with the flat end of the padlpet. Allow the smear to air dry, then fix the cells in absolute methanol for 30 s. Allow the smear to air dry.
17. Stain the smear in Giemsa stain for 5 min. Wash the slide with distilled water by squeezing water over the smear till the water is clear. Let the smear air dry.
18. Observe the smear under oil immersion. Record and illustrate your observations.

Part D

Differentiation of T and B lymphocytes using cell surface markers (cluster of differentiation-CD antigens) by immunofluorescence assays (IFA),

Continuing from #9 above. Resuspend each lymphoid cell suspension in 3 mL of HBSS.

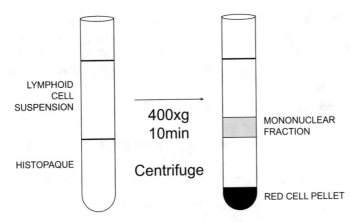

LYMPHOID
CELL
SUSPENSION

400xg
10min

Centrifuge

HISTOPAQUE

MONONUCLEAR
FRACTION

RED CELL PELLET

Fig. 28.2 Separation of blood cells on Histopaque. Following centrifugation, the mononuclear cell fraction is located at the interface Histopaque and the medium and the red blood cells are found in the pellet fraction

19. Layer the cell suspension on 3 mL of Histopaque (Fig. 28.2) and centrifuge for 10 min at 400 × *g*. Remove the mononuclear cell fraction into a clean 15 mL centrifuge tube and wash once by centrifugation in HBSS. After the last wash, resuspend the cells to 50% with HBSS.

20. Prepare three sets of smears from each cell suspension by pipetting a drop onto slides with a padlpet, followed by spreading the smear with the flat part of the pipet. Allow the smears to airdry, fix the slides in absolute methanol for 5 min.

21. Stain one set of slides with Giemsa stain. Use the second and third sets of slides for immunofluorescence by fixing the smears in absolute methanol, air drying the smears and then incubating the smears with rabbit anti-mouse IgM-FITC and anti-mouse Thy-1.2-TRITC for 1 h in a plastic container with tight fitting lid for direct IFA. Place moist kimwipes in the container (humid chamber) and then place the slides smear side facing up on the kimwipes. Incubate the chamber at room temperature. After the 1 h incubation, wash slides in 1× PBS, by placing the slides in a coplin jar containing 1× PBS. Shake the coplin jar gently, discard the PBS and repeat the wash step two more time for a total of three washes. Perform a fourth wash in distilled water.

22. Remove the slides from the coplin jar and place them on paper towel with the smear side facing up. Add a drop of mounting solution to the smear and cover the smear with a coverslip. Usin clear nail polish, seal the edges of the coverslip. Let the nail polish dry then observe the smear under a UV microscope. Sealed slides can be stored at −20 °C.

23. Mouse antibodies against CD4, CD8, or CD3 proteins conjugated to fluorochromes may also be used for T cell identification. Anti-mouse CD19 antibodies conjugated to fluorochromes may be used for B cell identification. Indirect IFA may also be performed using rabbit or goat anti-mouse IgG secondary antibodies conjugated to fluorochrome if the mouse antibodies to the markers are unconjugated to fluorochrome.

24. Determine the number of T and B lymphocytes by dividing the number of cells reacting with anti-Thy-1.2-TRITC or anti-mouse-IgM-FITC by the total number of lymphocytes and multiplying by 100. Anti-CD3 and anti-CD19 antibodies can also be used for identification of T and B cells, respectively.

Calculations:
Experiment #1

$$\% \text{viability} = \frac{139}{172} \times 100 = 80.8\%$$

Number of cells / mL : $172 / 4 \left(\text{average} \# \text{total cells}\right) \times 20 \left(\text{dilution factor}\right)$
$\times 10^4 \left(\text{correction factor}\right)$

$$= 3.44 \times 10^7 \text{ cells / mL in a total volume of 1 mL.}$$

Experiment #2:

$$\% \text{viability} = \frac{118}{152} \times 100 = 77.6\%$$

Number of cells / mL $152 / 4 \left(\text{average} \# \text{total cells}\right) \times 50 \left(\text{dilution factor}\right)$
$\times 10^4 \left(\text{correction factor}\right)$

$$= 1.9 \times 10^7 \text{ cell / mL}$$

Total volume of cell suspension for Experiment #2 $= 3.5 \, \text{mL.} \# \text{cells in } 3.5 \, \text{mL}$
$$= 1.9 \times 10^7 \times 3.5 = 6.65 \times 10^7 \text{ cells.}$$

Selected References

Mishell BB, Shiigi M (1980) Selected methods in cellular immunology. W. H. Freeman, San Francisco

Murphy K, Weaver C (2017) Janeway's immunobiology, 9th edn. Garland Press, New York

Punt J, Stranford SA, Jones PP, Owen JA (2019) Kuby immunology, 8th edn. W.H. Freeman and Company, New York. Ch. 2, Cells, organs, and microenvironments of the immune system

NOTES AND ILLUSTRATIONS:

.

Chapter 29
Exercise 5: Isolation of Mouse Peritoneal Macrophages: In Vitro

Phagocytosis of Bacterial Cells

Introduction

Macrophages are highly specialized phagocytic cells that are differentiated from monocytes. In their role as phagocytic cells, and major constituents of the reticulo-endothelial system (RES, also known as the mononuclear phagocyte system, MPS), they also serve as antigen presenting cells along with related phagocytic cells such as dendritic cells, and Langerhans cells. In this capacity, they function to process antigen for presentation to naïve T helper cells, and to secrete cytokines among other substances. Macrophages are located at strategic sites throughout the body and with their ability to circulate, are able to reach different locations throughout the body e.g. in the spleen, lymph nodes, skin, kidney, liver, brain, lungs, peritoneum, etc. Macrophages are named based on where they are found. In the RES system, macrophages also function in antibody-mediated cellular cytotoxicity reactions and in cell-mediated immune reactions along with cytotoxic T cells. Antibodies bound to antigen bind to Fc receptors on the surface of macrophages resulting in the uptake of the antigen into the cytoplasm. Macrophages function in the clearance of blood borne pathogens, insoluble particles, activated clotting factors and in the removal of aging erythrocytes, damaged cells, and other debris from the blood. Macrophages differentiate from monocytes into proinflammatory (M1) macrophages or anti-inflammatory (M2) macrophages in response to specific cytokines and transcription factors.

Phagocytosis is distinct from endocytosis, which is performed by many other cells and it occurs in the following sequence: Macrophages migrate towards the extracellular particle by chemotaxis, adhere to the particle, and then engulf the particle using pseudopodia. The vacuole formed, knowns as the phagosome fuses with a lysosome leading to the formation of a phagolysosome in which the engulfed material is digested by lysosomal enzymes. Elimination of digested material then occurs by exocytosis.

© Springer Nature Switzerland AG 2021
T. Y. Sam-Yellowe, *Immunology: Overview and Laboratory Manual*,
https://doi.org/10.1007/978-3-030-64686-8_29

In this exercise, students will observe the adherence of macrophages to plastic petri dishes and the engulfment of bacteria by the macrophages. Macrophages isolated from the peritoneal cavity of mice or a murine macrophage cell line (ATCC J774A.1) will be used to demonstrate phagocytosis. The **first objective** of this exercise is to learn how to enrich for macrophages in mouse peritoneal cavity. The **second objective** is to observe and evaluate the process of phagocytosis. The **third objective** is to detect proteins involved in phagocytosis and cell signaling following PRR binding to a pathogen with the use of fluorescent labels. The **fourth objective** is to determine the effect of cytokines on the process of phagocytosis.

Materials and Reagents (Per Group)

Two mice (Swiss) 8–10 weeks old
Halothane chamber
Six 25 cm^2 flasks of J774A.1 (ATCC) murine macrophage cell line in culture
   (DMEM, 10% Fetal bovine serum)
Trypan blue
Hemocytometer and cover slips
Automatic cell counter
Six Tally counters
Two 10 mL syringes with 25 gauge needles
Two 20 mL syringes with 20 gauge needles
Two sterile petri dishes containing microscope slides
Two empty petri dishes
Two 15 mL centrifuge tubes
One small test tube (15 × 100 mm) containing 5 mL of a 24 h culture of *Serratia marcescens* or *Bacillus subtilis* in nutrient broth
Three 50 mL tubes containing Eagle's Minimal Essential Medium (EMEM) at 37 °C
Four 10 mL serological pipets
Three 50 mL tubes containing Dulbecco's minimal essential medium (DMEM)
Two sleeves of 25 cm^2 tissue culture flasks
One sleeve of 75 cm^2 tissue culture flasks
Four 1 mL pipets
Centrifuge
Microscope
Vortexer
Six Coplin jars containing absolute methanol
Six Coplin jars containing Giemsa stain
One 500 mL beaker for waste collection
One disposable plastic bag for mouse carcass
Kimwipes, bench paper, and paper towels
One 15 mL centrifuge tube containing 5 mL EMEM

Procedure: (Fig. 29.1)

1. Kill mice by placing them in halothane chamber.
2. Inject 8 mL of pre-warmed EMEM intraperitoneally (i. p.) into each mouse abdomen. (Your laboratory instructor will demonstrate).
3. Massage the abdominal area for 1 min to resuspend peritoneal cells.
4. Using a 20 mL syringe and a 20 gauge needle, carefully withdraw the EMEM containing resuspended cells from both mice. The cell suspension contains mostly macrophages and lymphocytes and a few erythrocytes. See Fig. 29.1.
5. Transfer the cell suspension to a sterile 15 mL centrifuge tube and centrifuge at 1000 × *g* for 5 min. Use both tubes to balance each other.
   NOTE: If using J774A.1 cell line, scrape cells adhered to flask, collect and place cells into 15 ml tubes for centrifugation as in #5 and proceed with the rest of the steps. Instead of EMEM, DMEM will be used with the cell line.

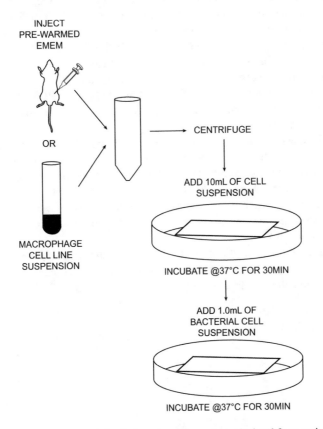

Fig. 29.1 Phagocytosis of bacterial cells by mouse macrophages isolated from peritoneal cavity and macrophage cell line suspension. Cells are centrifuged, resuspended in medium and incubated with bacteria

6. Discard the supernatant and add 10 mL of EMEM to the pellet in each tube. Resuspend the cells gently by vortexing at the low speed setting (3–4 setting) on the vortexer.

7. Prepare a 1:20 dilution of the cell suspension from each tube for counting and viability determination.

8. Pipet 10 mL of the cell suspension (1×10^5 cells per mL) into a petri dish containing clean glass slides. Place the cell suspension directly onto the slide. (Fig. 29.1)

9. Incubate the petri dish for 30 min at 37 ° C

10. Tilt the petri dish and pipet the EMEM cell suspension from the petri dish and discard into the waste container provided. Wash the glass slide with warm EMEM, by pipetting 10 mL EMEM into the petri dish, swirling the dish gently and then discarding the suspension by pipetting it into the waste container. Non adherent cells will be washed away, while adherent cells i.e. macrophages will be left on the slide. **DO NOT ALLOW THE SLIDE TO DRY.**

11. Pipet 1 mL of the bacterial suspension into the petri dish and incubate the petri dish for an additional 30 min. After incubation, carefully discard the EMEM as in #10. Remove the slides with a pair of forceps and wash once with EMEM by gently squeezing EMEM over the slide. Allow the slide to air dry, then place the slide in a coplin jar containing absolute methanol for 30 s to fix the cells. Remove the slides from the coplin jar and allow the slide to air dry. Place the slide in a coplin jar containing Giemsa stain. Stain the cell for 5 min, remove the slide and wash with distilled water. Let the slides air dry and then observe the cells under the microscope.

NOTE: macrophages can be processed for immunofluorescence staining using antibodies specific for markers on macrophage surface, e.g. anti-MHC class II, anti-Fc, or in the cytoplasm, anti-MyD88. In addition, macrophages can be formalin fixed or treated with chloroquine or IFNγ before the addition of bacterial cells. Live cell imaging using fluorescent tracking dyes for cytoskeletal proteins and lysosomes can be performed. Cells undergoing apoptosis can be detected using Annexin V.

12. Using oil immersion, observe the stained macrophages for the presence of small rod-shaped bacteria within (intracellular) the macrophages.

13. Record and illustrate your observations. Indicate if phagocytosis occurred or not.

Negative Control:

Positive Control:

Test Sample 1:

Test Sample 2:

For this exercise we will be using the murine macrophage cell line (ATCC) to demonstrate phagocytosis. However, students need to know how cells are collected from mice and how mice can be perturbed with various treatments in vivo before harvesting cells.

Cell culture supernatants from J774A.1 cultures will also be collected for ELISAs.

Cells will be formalin fixed and permeabilized for immunofluorescence using anti-MyD88 antibodies.

Cell pellets will be collected for SDS-PAGE and western blotting to detect MyD88.

Selected References

Miller LE, Ludke HR, Peacock JE, Tomar RH (1991) Manual of laboratory immunology, 2nd edn. Lea and Febiger, Philadelphia. Ch. 4, lymphocyte quantitation and function

Murphy K, Weaver C (2017) Janeway's immunobiology, 9th edn. Garland Press, New York

Punt J, Stranford SA, Jones PP, Owen JA (2019) Kuby immunology, 8th edn. W.H. Freeman and Company, New York. Ch. 2, Cells, organs, and microenvironments of the immune system

Valerio MS, Minderman H, Mace T, Awad AB (2013) β-Sitosterol modulates TLR4 receptor expression and intracellular MyD88-dependent pathway activation in J774A.1 murine macrophages. Cell Immunol 285:76–83

NOTES AND ILLUSTRATIONS:

Chapter 30
Exercise 6: Clearance of Bacteria from Mouse Blood by the Reticuloendothelial System (RES)

Introduction

The reticuloendothelial system (RES) also known as the mononuclear phagocyte system (MPS) is a functional network of phagocytic tissue macrophages. Mononuclear phagocytes include tissue phagocytes located primarily in the reticular connective tissue framework of the spleen, liver, and lymphoid tissues. The most easily obtainable form is the immature peripheral blood monocyte, found circulating in the blood system. The RES system is responsible for the removal of foreign particulate material or other debris from the blood system. These include old or injured erythrocytes, leukocytes and platelets, bacteria, antigen-antibody complexes and degenerated or damaged cell membranes. The most active phagocytic cells in the RES system are the Kupffer cells of the liver and the splenic macrophages. Others include the alveolar (pulmonary) macrophages, histiocytes, mesangial cells (kidney), microglial cells (brain) and macrophages of the lymph nodes and peritoneum.

Organs rich in tissue macrophages become involved when the RES system is actively engaged in clearing debris from the blood system, resulting in splenomegaly (enlarged spleen), hepatomegaly (enlarged liver) and lymphadenopathy (enlarged lymph nodes). The activity of macrophages can be observed following the injection of bacteria or carbon particles intravenously into a mouse. The bacteria or particles become localized within organs rich with the macrophages. In this experiment, we will examine the blood and RES organs from mice (Swiss Webster) that have been injected with viable bacteria, *Serratia marcescens*. The **first objective** of this experiment is to determine the rate of clearance of foreign material (bacteria) from mouse blood by the RES system. A **second objective** is to identify the organs participating in the RES network.

© Springer Nature Switzerland AG 2021
T. Y. Sam-Yellowe, *Immunology: Overview and Laboratory Manual*,
https://doi.org/10.1007/978-3-030-64686-8_30

Materials and Reagents (Per Group)

One mouse already injected with 0.1 mL of 1×10^9 cells/mL i.v.
20 heparinized capillary tubes
Four sterile small capped test tubes or Eppendorf tubes
Four sterile plastic petri dishes
30 sterile 1 mL glass pipet
One sterile large capped test tube with 10 mL sterile saline
2 sterile mortar and pestles
Two 27 G needles
1 mL syringes
Mouse holders
250 mL beakers
Plastic containers
Two pair of scissors and two pair of forceps in a beaker of 70% ethanol
24 capped tubes each containing 9.0 mL sterile saline
Six capped tubes each containing 9.9 mL sterile saline
30 nutrient agar plates
Bench paper
Bunsen burner 70% ethanol
Four test tube racks
Halothane
Cotton
Gloves
Four sterile glass spreaders
Kimwipes
Paper towel
Disposable plastic bags
Balance

Procedure

1. Place the mouse (already injected with bacterial cells) in the mouse holder so that the tail is accessible. Hold on to the tail and wipe the tip of the mouse (live mouse) tail with 70% ethanol immediately after receiving it from the instructor.
2. Snip the mouse tail with a pair of sterile scissors and collect blood into five heparinized capillary tubes. Massage the mouse tail to increase blood flow into the capillary tubes.
3. Empty the blood into the small, capped sterile test tube (or sterile eppendorf tubes), using a small rubber bulb to force the blood out of the capillary tubes. This has to be done very carefully otherwise the blood will not come out of the capillary tube easily. You need approximately 0.2 mL of blood.

4. With a sterile 1 mL glass pipet, quickly transfer 0.1 mL of blood into a tube containing 9.9 mL of sterile saline (this is a 1:100 dilution = 10^{-2} dilution) and mix thoroughly (Fig. 30.1). Using another sterile pipet and four 9.0 mL saline tubes prepare serial 1:10 dilutions (1 mL transfers) from 10^{-2} dilution of blood. Label these 10^{-3}, 10^{-4}, 10^{-5}, 10^{-6}. (Fig. 30.1)

5. Using another sterile pipet and starting with the 10^{-6} dilution, transfer 0.1 mL from each dilution tube to a separate nutrient agar plate. Spread the drop evenly using a sterile glass spreader. Incubate plates at 37 °C. Your dilutions in the plates are 10^{-3}, 10^{-4}, 10^{-5}, 10^{-6} and 10^{-7} to account for the 0.1 mL transferred from each tube.

6. After 10, 20, and 30 min repeat the bleeding, dilutions and plating as in step# 5. Label the plates and incubate as before.

7. After the 30 min collection (i.e., immediately after the last bleeding) place the mouse in the halothane chamber to kill the mouse (your TA will help with this step) and soak the ventral surface of the mouse with 70% ethanol. Open the abdominal and thoracic cavities of the mouse with a sterile pair of scissors and forceps (disinfected in 70% ethanol and passed over flame or use autoclaved forceps and scissors), and remove the spleen plus one other organ e.g. liver,

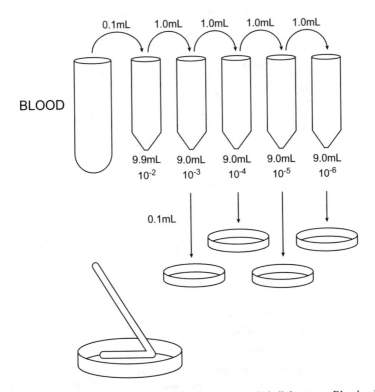

Fig. 30.1 Clearance of bacteria from blood by the reticuloendothelial system. Blood collected after injection of bacteria is diluted tenfold, then plated onto agar using the spread plate method

kidneys, thymus, heart, or lungs and place each in a sterile plastic dish. Cut small sections from each organ and transfer to separate tared sterile mortars containing 5 mL of sterile saline. Determine the weight of the mortar containing the piece of tissue.

8. Grind the tissue well with a pestle and allow the particulate material to settle. Then, using one 9.9 mL and four 9.0 mL saline tubes for each tissue, perform dilutions as with the blood samples (**see# 5 and** Fig. 30.2), plate out the cells and incubate the plates at 37 °C.

9. After 24 h, examine the plates for typical colonies of *Serratia marcescens*. Colonies will have a red-orange pigment. Determine the initial number of bacterial cells/ml of blood immediately after injection. Calculate the clearance rate as the number of viable cells/mL of blood/minute which were removed following injection. Compare the relative numbers of bacteria recovered from each organ and calculate the number of bacterial cells cleared by the RES/gram of each tissue. Plot a graph of your results (number of colonies vs. time), and record the data in your notebook. Use graph paper to plot the graph. Do not use plain notebook paper.

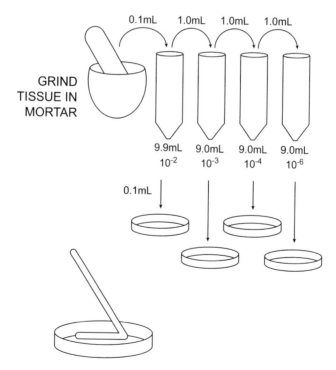

Fig. 30.2 Clearance of bacteria from blood by the reticuloendothelial system. Tissues (liver, spleen, lungs, thymus, and kidneys) collected from mouse after bacterial injection and blood collection are ground in a mortar containing saline. The saline suspension is diluted tenfold and plated onto agar plates using the spread plate method

Selected References

Miller LE, Ludke HR, Peacock JE, Tomar RH (1991) Manual of laboratory immunology, 2nd edn. Lea and Febiger, Philadelphia. Ch. 8, Phagocytosis

Murphy K, Weaver C (2017) Janeway's immunobiology, 9th edn. Garland press, New York

Punt J, Stranford SA, Jones PP, Owen JA (2019) Kuby immunology, 8th edn. W.H. Freeman and Company, New York. Ch. 2, Cells, organs, and microenvironments of the immune system

Roitt IM, Brostoff J, Male DK (1989) Immunology. J.B. Lippincott Company, Philadelphia, Ch. 2, Cells involved in the immune response

NOTES AND ILLUSTRATIONS:

Chapter 31
Exercise 7: Hemolytic Plaque Assay (The Jerne Plaque Assay)

Introduction

The hemolytic plaque assay (also known as localized hemolysis in gel or Jerne plaque assay) can be used to demonstrate that individual plasma cells are monospecific. The assay permits the visualization of the small amount of antibody released in the vicinity of a single plasma cell.

One principle of the modern theory of clonal selection is that each plasma cell is a member of a single clone of cells and secretes antibody molecules of a single kind (at one time). The technique has had a wide impact on several areas of immunology research.

The technique has the advantage of permitting the screening, counting and studying of individual antibody forming cells (AFC), even when they are a small minority of the lymphocyte population.

In this experiment, we will examine the antibody response in mice immunized with sheep red blood cells (SRBC). Two groups of mice will be immunized with 0.5 mL of SRBCS. One group will be immunized for 4 days and the second group for one week. A third group will receive a sham injection (control group). Four days after immunizing mice with SRBC, mice will be killed and their spleens will be removed to prepare a single cell suspension. The spleen cell suspension containing lymphocytes, plasma cells and macrophages will be mixed with SRBCs and solid media (agar) and then poured into a petri dish. The cells will then be overlaid with guinea pig complement. The interaction of complement with antibodies bound to the red cell antigens results in the lysis of the red cells and causes the areas around the antibody secreting cell to become clear. The clear areas in the red lawn of SRBC are called plaques.

Examination under the light microscope reveals a single antibody secreting cell at the center of each plaque. This is the antibody secreting cell.

The assay is very sensitive. As few as one in a million spleen cells secreting anti-SRBC antibodies can be detected. Also, one antibody-secreting cell may form a

© Springer Nature Switzerland AG 2021
T. Y. Sam-Yellowe, *Immunology: Overview and Laboratory Manual*,
https://doi.org/10.1007/978-3-030-64686-8_31

visible plaque after releasing as few as 10^1 antibody molecules (10^3–10^6 antibody molecules can be detected).

The assay described above is called the direct plaque assay. The direct assay measures only cells secreting IgM antibodies.

The assumption that the direct method measures only cells secreting IgM antibodies is based on the following facts:

1. IgM is extremely efficient at fixing complement. A single molecule of IgM bound to the surface of a red cell is sufficient to trigger the classical complement cascade.
2. The increase in the number of cells that form plaques directly and the rise in serum titer of specific IgM both peak 4 days after a primary immunization with a large dose of SRBCs in vitro

Plasma cells secreting other classes of specific antibodies attach to the antibody molecules, which have already been fixed to the red blood cells during an initial incubation period. The presence of these Ig-anti-Ig complexes facilitates hemolysis upon subsequent treatment with complement. The number of cells forming plaques indirectly can be estimated by the indirect method. Alternatively, the number of IgM plaques can be inhibited before performing the indirect assay, in order to obtain the precise number of indirect plaque forming cells.

The hemolytic plaque assay is not limited to the detection of plasma cells secreting antibodies to SRBCS. Cells secreting antibodies to haptens, polysaccharides, cell surface antigens or heterologous proteins can be detected by attaching these antigens to the surface of the red blood cells.

The **objective** of this experiment is to learn the hemolytic plaque assay technique.

Materials and Reagents (Per Group)

One Balb/cJ mice (1 immunized with 5 % sheep red blood cells-SRBC and 1 control/unimmunized mouse)
Microscopes (Light and dissecting)
2 hemocytometers with cover slips
2 tally counters
20 sterile 1 mL glass pipets
10 sterile 1 mL plastic squeezers and 4 small squeezers (50 μL/drop)
Four 15 mL centrifuge tubes
Two 50 mL tubes containing Hanks balanced salt solution without phenol red (HBSS)
6 plates of 1.5% purified agar in HBSS (underlay agar at 37 °C)
6 tubes of 4 mL top agar (0.7% purified agar) in HBSS at 45 °C containing 1 mg/mL final concentration, diethylaminoethyl (DEAE)—dextran
One 15 mL tube containing 20% washed SRBC in HBSS

1 tube containing pre-adsorbed diluted guinea pig complement 0.2% Trypan blue in water
Kimwipes, bench paper and paper towels
Sterile scissors and forceps (4 pair each), two 10 mL syringes
One empty 500 mL beaker
Two sterile petri dishes with wire mesh screens
1 ice bucket
37 and 45 °C and water baths
Moist chamber for incubation and 37 °C incubator
1 small plastic bag for mice
Centrifuge
Halothane chamber

Procedure

Part A

1. Kill mice by halothane inhalation (mark the mice with a laboratory marker to distinguish the SRBC immunized mouse from the control mouse). Wet the left dorsal side of each mouse with 70% ethanol.
2. Pipet 10 mL of HBSS into a sterile petri dish containing a wire mesh screen. Label the plates.
3. Remove spleens aseptically and transfer them to petri dishes containing screens. Place spleens in the center of the screens. (**Same procedure used in Exercise 3** (see Chap. 27), see Fig. 31.1)
4. Using the plunger from the 10 mL syringe, gently press spleens through the wire mesh to disperse spleen cells. Transfer the spleen cell suspension to 15 mL centrifuge tubes. Wait 1 min for large clumps to settle, then transfer cell suspension (without disturbing pellet) to a fresh 15 mL tube.
5. Centrifuge cells, 10 min at $200 \times g$. Discard the supernatant and resuspend cells in 3 mL of HBSS.
6. Prepare a 1:100 dilution of the spleen cell suspension in 5 mL of HBSS in a 15 mL centrifuge tube for counting and determination of cell viability.

Steps 7–9 must be performed rapidly to prevent solidification of soft agar in the tubes.

7. Using sterile graduated squeezers, add 0.25 mL of 20% SRBC suspension into each of seven tubes containing 4 mL of top agar from 45 °C water bath.
8. Using a 1 mL sterile glass pipet, add 0.1 0.2, 0.3, 0.4, 0.5, 0.6, and 0.8 mL of the spleen suspension to seven tubes and label properly (e.g. tube #1, 0.1 mL; tube #2, 0.2 mL; tube #3, 0.3 mL etc.). Cap tubes and invert 2–3 times to mix. **DO NOT PIPET TO MIX. AVOID FOAMING**

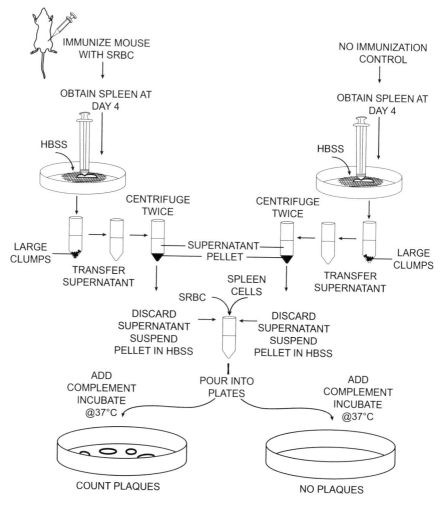

Fig. 31.1 Hemolytic plaque assay. Spleen cells obtained from a mouse immunized with sheep red blood cells (SRBCs) after 4 days are incubated with SRBCs and Guinea pig complement and poured on an agar plate. The formation of plaques indicates positive IgM antibody production. No plaques are formed in the negative control

9. Pour agar-SRBC-spleen cell mixture gently but rapidly into agar plates and rotate carefully to cover surface of agar evenly. **AVOID BUBBLES** as this may produce artifacts on the plates.

10. Allow agar to solidify then add 1.5 mL of diluted complement to plates. Rotate plates gently to spread complement over the surface of the agar overlay. All plates should be properly labeled. Place plates in humid chambers (plastic containers lined with moist paper towels) and incubate chambers in 37 °C incubator for 1 h.

NOTE: Spleen cells, SRBCs and complement can also be mixed together and poured directly onto the surface of the agar plates. Plates will be incubated upright at 37 °C (Fig. 31.1).

11. After 1 h, check plates for the presence of plaques. If plaques are not clear, let the plates stand for 15–30 min at room temperature, then observe plaques.

12. Plates may be stored overnight at 4 °C and the plaques counted the next day. Arrangements should be made by each group to have the plaques counted the next day.

Part B

Plaques are clear areas against a lawn of SRBC, resulting from lysis of SRBC by complement. The clearing will appear small and circular. For better visualization, a dissecting microscope or the low power objective (4×) of a light microscope can be used to view and count the plaques.

At a higher magnification, a plasma cell can be seen at the center of the plaque. A countable plate contains between 100 and 200 plaques. Express your results as plaque forming cells (PFC) per spleen (per# of spleen cells added). Calculate dilution of cells used for each of the six tubes. Tabulate your results.

Selected References

Baig MA, Ansari AA, Malling HV (1982) A hemolytic plaque assa for the detection of red blood cells carrying abnormal or mutant hemoglobin. J Immunol Methods 55:43–50

Barrett JT (1988) Textbook of immunology. Mosby, St. Louis. Ch.9, Biological aspects of the immune response

DeToma FJ, Macdonald AB (1987) Experimental immunology: a guidebook. Macmillan Publishing Company, New York, Chapter 11, Hemolytic plaque assay

Hudson L, Hay FC Practical immunology, 3rd edn. Blackwell Scientific Publications, Oxford, London. Chapter 4

Kimball JW (1990) Introduction to immunology. Macmillan, New York. Ch. 7, B lymphocytes

Miller LE, Ludke HR, Peacock JE, Tomar RH (1991) Manual of laboratory immunology, 2nd edn. Lea and Febiger, Philadelphia. Ch. 6, Complement

Mishell, B.B. and Shiigi, M. 1980. Selected methods in cellular immunology. W.H.Freeman, San Francisco.

Myers RL (1989) Immunology: a laboratory manual. Wm. C. Brown Publishers, Dubuque, IA. Exercises 18, Hemolytic plaque assay

Punt J, Stranford SA, Jones PP, Owen JA (2019) Kuby immunology, 8th edn. W.H. Freeman and Company, New York. Ch. 2, Cells, organs, and microenvironments of the immune system

NOTES AND ILLUSTRATIONS:

Chapter 32
Exercise 8: Rabbit and Mouse Immunizations: Preparation of Polyclonal Antibodies and Screening Assays

Introduction

Polyclonal antibodies in general are specific to multiple epitopes on a single antigen and may also be specific to several epitopes on different antigens. **Monospecific polyclonal antibodies** can also be prepared. These antibodies are usually prepared against a single purified protein and the specificity is usually against different epitopes on the protein. These antibodies are different from **monoclonal antibodies** which are the products of single B cell clones and are much more specific usually for a single epitope on an antigen. The production of monoclonal antibodies has become a routine part of many immunology laboratories. However, it is a complex, labor-intensive process requiring tissue culture methods and often expensive reagents and equipment (we will discuss monoclonal antibodies in the tissue culture section).

For this exercise polyclonal antibodies will be prepared using parasite antigens from *Plasmodium chabaudi adami* or *P. falciparum* schizonts, causative agents of rodent and human malaria, respectively. We will be using two different **adjuvants** for immunization. Adjuvants enhance the immunogenicity of immunogens and can act as immunopotentiators or immunomodulators. Other antigens and adjuvants can be substituted for this exercise depending on the goals of the immunization project for class or research purposes. Several types of adjuvants are in use. In general adjuvants act by promoting a slow release of the antigen in the body. A "depot" or focus of antigen is formed at the site of injection. A macrophage-enriched granuloma forms at the site of injection, usually enhancing antigen processing. A common type of adjuvant is a **water-in-oil emulsion** that can be combined with the immunogen. **Oil emulsions** are also used and **liposomes** coated with the immunogen or encapsulated with the immunogen are also used. Many bacterial products e.g. lipopolysaccharide (LPS), muramyl dipeptide, complex carbohydrates, surfactants and aluminum salts are used as adjuvants. Not all adjuvants are acceptable for human use. We will be using Freund's complete and incomplete adjuvant, a water-in-oil

© Springer Nature Switzerland AG 2021
T. Y. Sam-Yellowe, *Immunology: Overview and Laboratory Manual*,
https://doi.org/10.1007/978-3-030-64686-8_32

emulsion. The complete adjuvant is a water-in-oil emulsion that contains whole *Mycobacterium* and the incomplete adjuvant is the oil-in-water emulsion alone. We will also be using TiterMax Gold adjuvant (Sigma-Aldrich) also a water-in-oil formulation containing copolymers. Both of these adjuvants enhance the production of IgG which is the antibody of choice for most research procedures.

Rabbits are widely used for the production of high titer, highly specific polyclonal antibodies. An added advantage of using rabbits for antibody production is that assays can be developed using protein-A which binds specifically to the Fc region of rabbit IgG. The IgG produced can be affinity purified, easily and efficiently using protein-A conjugated to a solid matrix such as CNBr-activated sepharose or magnetic beads.

Handling of Experimental Animals

The correct procedures for handling, injecting and bleeding animals (mice and rabbits) will be demonstrated by your instructor. Animals are to be handled carefully, firmly and safely. Laboratory animals are not pets and should not be treated as such (avoid getting attached to them). However, the animals should be handled gently and treated humanely at all times, in accordance with the strict rules, IUACUC approved protocols and regulations that govern the use of experimental animals which will be elaborated in classes. When in doubt about a particular procedure concerning the animals, be sure to find out before performing the procedure.

Blood Collection and Immunization

We will be collecting blood from the marginal ear vein or artery of the rabbit using a 20 G needle. Before blood collection the rabbit ear will be carefully shaved with a single edge razor blade and the area wiped with sterile 70% alcohol pads. The ear will be manipulated by brisk rubbing, thumping or heating to dilate blood vessels and increase the flow of blood. Xylene (optional, may not be needed) may also be used to dilate vessels, but must be removed thoroughly after bleeding the rabbit. Blood will be collected by drip method through the needle into sterile 50 mL centrifuge tubes and allowed to clot for serum collection. After the desired volume of blood has been collected, withdraw the needle carefully and apply a steady pressure with sterile cotton or gauze until the bleeding ceases. The clotted blood will be separated by "ringing" the clot using applicator sticks followed by centrifugation for 10 min at 1500 rpms. The serum (supernatant) will be collected into a fresh 15 mL centrifuge tube, properly labeled and stored at −20 °C until required. The blood clot which is the pellet, may be discarded.

Rabbits can be immunized using several different routes. These can be intramuscular (i. m.), intraperitoneal (i. p.), subcutaneous (s. c.), intradermal (i. d.) and intravenous (i. v.). For all injections the needle is placed bevel up, and slightly angled for s. c. injections. For i. m. injections, the needle is inserted into the upper thigh in the gluteal muscles. To prevent tissue damage, nicking veins or arteries, apply moderate pressure to the syringe and inject the antigen gently but rapidly. Withdraw the syringe and apply even pressure to the injection site to disperse the antigen. For s. c. injections, the needle is inserted in the area between the ears (interscapular), in the back of the neck or in the inguinal and axillary regions. For i. d. injections, the needle is inserted underneath the superficial layer of the epidermis and the antigen is injected. If multiple sites are to be injected, proper spacing of the sites will be necessary to avoid coalescing of lesions. This is very important when adjuvants are used. All injections will be performed with sterile needles of the correct size (gauge). Initial injections can be performed s. c. at the inguinal and axillary regions of the body or i. m. in the upper thigh.

These areas are very close to the regional lymph nodes and therefore enhance antigen uptake and processing. Alternatively, the initial injection can be administered s. c. on the dorsal/neck region of the rabbit in combination with i. m. injections.

The sera collected throughout the quarter will be analyzed using various primary (western blotting, immunofluorescence and ELISA), and secondary (precipitation and agglutination) assays. The antibody titer from each collection will be monitored using ELISA and western blotting. IgM and IgG can be purified from the serum and the antibody titers determined also by agglutination and enzyme-linked immunosorbent assays respectively.

Mice may also be used for the preparation of polyclonal antibodies. Similar injection routes, as described-for rabbits are used. Since the blood vessels are smaller in a mouse, needles of a smaller gauge are used. For i. v. injections into the lateral tail vein, 25–30 G needles are used. With the bevel up, the needle is inserted in the lumen, parallel to the vein. Mice will be immunized by a combination of i. p., s. c. and i. v. injections at 1 week intervals for three weeks, and the serum collected analyzed. Blood collection 1st by tail snips to monitor antibody production and then by cardiac puncture to collect blood for immune serum.

In both mice and rabbits, surgical implantation of antigen can also be performed, where the antigen is deposited intrasplenically. Nitrocellulose paper or sepharose beads coated with the antigen is placed in the exposed caudal end of the spleen in an anesthetized animal, followed by booster injections i. v. at 1–2 week intervals.

Recombinant proteins or peptides (alone or combined with large protein carriers/backbones) can also be used as antigen following the same directions discussed above. In addition, plasmid constructs containing DNA encoding a recombinant protein of interest and under the influence of an active promoter, can be injected as a DNA antigen i.e. DNA vaccine. In some cases DNA encoding proteins that possess adjuvant properties e.g. certain cytokines, can also be engineered onto the plasmid construct before use in injections. Follow the instructions provided for the particular host animal that will be used.

Materials (Per Group)

1 New Zealand white rabbit
Immunogen (parasite extract in CFA, IFA or TiterMax Gold)
Complete Freund's adjuvant
TiterMax Gold
2 sterile double hub needles
50 mL centrifuge tubes
20 and 18 G needles
Single-edge razor blades
Sterile alcohol pads
Cotton balls
Applicator sticks
1, 3 and 10 mL syringes
Marking pens and Notebooks

For mouse immunizations:
Same items above and including those listed below

Swiss mice or BALB/c mice
Mouse holders
Vortex
26 and 27 G needles
1 mL syringes

NOTE: Carefully record the rabbit identification number from the ear tags, cage number and other information on the cage card provided. Write down the room number where the rabbit is housed. Depending on the record keeping of your particular animal facility, record all pertinent identifiers for the rabbit as appropriate. For mice record the information provided on the cage card any required identifiers. Also record the type of adjuvant used for immunization. In some exercises, the class will conduct an experiment to compare the efficiency of two adjuvants administered with *P. chabaudi adami* or *P. falciparum* schizonts, Freund's adjuvant and TiterMax Gold. Other adjuvants can be substituted. In other exercises, the class will compare the immunogenicity of antigens treated in different ways. For example denatured, native or peptide antigens may be compared. The class may analyze the effectiveness of soluble versus particulate antigen, routes of antigen administration, the course of the immune responses and the quality of the response generated.

Procedure

Collection of pre-immune serum

The rabbit needs to be restrained in an approved rabbit restraint or two individuals need to work together to obtain the blood. One individual will hold the rabbit while the other collects the blood.

1. Collect blood for pre-immune serum from marginal ear vein, with the needle pointed towards the base of the ear or from the central auricular artery on the ear of rabbit.

   Using a clean new single edge razor blade, carefully shave the rabbit's ear and wipe the shaved area with a sterile alcohol pad.

2. Rub or thump the rabbit ear briskly to dilate blood vessels and increase blood flow to the ear. Your instructor will demonstrate. When the blood vessels appear distended and the rabbit ear appears slightly red, hold the ear firmly and carefully insert a 20 G needle approximately 5 mm into the vein (or artery) with the bevel facing upwards. Do not touch the tip of the needle. Hold on to the ear firmly, and hold a 50 mL tube below the needle. The blood will drip through the needle into the tube. Collect approximately 20 mL of blood.

3. Place a cotton ball against the needle and carefully withdraw the needle. Apply pressure to the cotton ball to initiate hemostasis and to stop the flow of blood. After approximately 1 min., remove the cotton ball and examine the ear to make sure bleeding has stopped. **DO NOT PUT THE RABBIT BACK INTO ITS CAGE IF BLEEDING HAS NOT STOPPED.**

4. Moisten a fresh cotton ball with water and wipe the rabbit's ear to remove all traces of blood.

5. Administer vaccine (immunogen) mixed in complete Freund's or Titermax Gold adjuvant using a 1 mL syringe attached to an 18 G needle. For vaccine in CFA, inject 0.25 mL of immunogen at four sites s. c. in the neck region of the rabbit (total of 1 mL). For vaccine in TiterMax Gold, inject 40 µL of immunogen at two sites also s. c. in the neck region (total 80 µL). For s. c. injections, pick up a fold skin in the neck region and inject vaccine under the skin, not in between skin. Massage the area lightly. To ensure that the needle has been properly inserted, you should feel the resistance of the skin give way as the needle penetrates the skin. You may also hear a slight "popping" sound. Slowly inject the vaccine at this point. Carefully withdraw the needle and observe for bleeding. If capillaries are nicked, slight bleeding will occur, but this usually clots rapidly. If bleeding is observed, clean the area with cotton before placing the rabbit back in its cage.

Blood Processing for Serum Collection

6. After 10–15 min, the blood in the centrifuge tube should be clotted. Using a wooden applicator stick, "ring" the clot to retract it from the sides of the centrifuge tube. Make sure the applicator stick is inserted all the way to the bottom of the tube. Incubate the tube at 4 °C for 12–24 h. We will place tubes in the cold room.

7. After 24 h remove the tubes from the cold room, "ring" the clot again and centrifuge the tubes for 10 min. at 2000 rpm. Collect serum into clean 15 mL centrifuge tube. Serum should be straw colored. If serum appears red, this may be due to hemolysis of erythrocytes or incomplete sedimentation of erythrocytes. Divide the serum into Eppendorf tubes and centrifuge for 2 min at 14,000 rpm. Collect serum and transfer 0.5–1 mL aliquots to Eppendorf tubes. Aliquot 100 µL of the serum into 2–3 tubes. Store serum at −20 °C.

8. For obtaining serum on the same day, "ring" the blood clot and incubate the centrifuge tube at 37 °C for 30–60 min. Centrifuge the tube as above and collect serum. The overnight procedure yields more serum.

9. The rabbits will be boosted with the same vaccine four times at 7–14 day intervals to increase antibody yield and antibody specificity. After the fourth boost, the anti-serum will be collected for IgG purification and further characterization. We will then compare the antibody titers, specificity and how rapidly IgG was produced using the two adjuvants. Follow the vaccination and blood collection schedule outlined in the laboratory schedule that you receive at the beginning of the term.

Selected References

Myers RL (1989) Immunology a laboratory manual. Exercise 1, Vaccination-a semester project. Wm. C. Brown Publishers, Dubuque, IA, p 3

Nilsson BO et al Immunization of mice and rabbits by intrasplenic deposition of nanogram quantities of protein attached to sepharose beads or nitrocellulose paper strips. J Immunol Methods 99:67–75

Sam-Yellowe TY, Fujioka H, Aikawa M, Hall T, Drazbar JA (2001) *Plasmodium falciparum* protein located in Maurer's clefts underneath knobs and protein localization in association with Rhop-3 and SERA in the intracellular network of infected erythrocytes. Parasitol Res 87:173–185

Ternynck T, Avrameas S (1990) Techniques in immunology. Vol. Immunoenzymatic techniques. Elsevier, New York

Walker JM (1984) Chapter 32, Production of antisera. In: Bailey GS (ed) Methods in molecular biology, Vol. I Proteins. Humana Press, Clifton, NJ, pp 295–300

NOTES AND ILLUSTRATIONS:

Chapter 33
Exercise 9: Determination of Antibody Titer and Screening Techniques

Introduction

The amount of antibody present in an antiserum can be determined by a variety of serologic reactions that are based on the detection of antigen-antibody complexes (immune complexes). When antigens are mixed with specific antisera in the right ratio, insoluble immune complexes are formed. These antigen-antibody reactions vary in their sensitivity, specificity and simplicity, and can be performed in liquid or gel media.

In the experiments described below, we will perform precipitation and agglutination reactions using soluble (for precipitations) and particulate (for agglutinations) antigens with their respective antisera. These tests form the basis for many antigen-antibody reactions that are performed in the clinical and research laboratory.

Maximum precipitation occurs when the antigen and antibody concentrations are in the **zone of equivalence**. When the antigen concentration is greater than the concentration of antibody, precipitation may be reduced or absent. This is known as a **postzone** reaction. When the antibody concentration is greater than the concentration of antigen, this is known as a **prozone** (also known as prezone) reaction, and like the postzone reaction, there may be reduced precipitation or no precipitation (Fig. 33.1).

The development of a precipitate depends on the formation of cross-links between antigen and antibody resulting in a lattice. In order for there to be a precipitation or agglutination reaction, the antigen must have at least two antigenic determinants. Examples of precipitation reactions include: double diffusion, capillary tube precipitation, double diffusion Ouchterlony, radial immunodiffusion (RID) (Mancini immunodiffusion test), rocket immunoelectrophoresis and immunoelectrophoresis (IEP).

In general, precipitation techniques are less sensitive in detecting the presence of specific antibodies than agglutination reactions.

© Springer Nature Switzerland AG 2021
T. Y. Sam-Yellowe, *Immunology: Overview and Laboratory Manual*,
https://doi.org/10.1007/978-3-030-64686-8_33

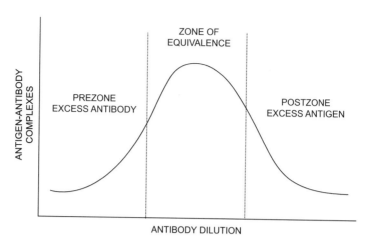

Fig. 33.1 Precipitation curve. Immune complexes form leading to precipitation at the zone of equivalence. In the presence of excess antibody (prezone) or excess antigen (postzone) precipitate will not form

The **first objective** is to determine the titer of an antiserum using the precipitation technique. The **second objective** is to determine the titer of an antiserum by direct hemagglutination and passive hemagglutination techniques.

Part A

Ring precipitin test: This is a quick and simple qualitative technique used to screen undiluted samples of antisera for the presence of specific antibody. More quantitative methods can then be used to determine the titer of the antisera.

Materials and Reagents (Per Pair)

12 small test tubes
Kimwipes
Eppendorf pipet (0–200 μL)
Pipet tips (yellow tips)
12 Pasteur pipets
2 small test tube racks
2 tubes of antisera: anti-bovine serum albumin (BSA) and anti-goat serum (GS)
2 tubes of soluble antigen: BSA and goat serum
I tube of normal control serum
Paper towel

Bench cover
Eppendorf tubes
Small test tube rack
Spectrophotometer
100 mL 0.1 M NaOH
100 mL lx PBS
37 °C water bath

Procedure

1. Using a micropipette (Eppendorf pipet), transfer 100 μL of anti-BSA, anti-goat serum and normal rabbit serum (NRS) into three separate 1.5 mL Eppendorf tubes. Label the tubes. Transfer the antisera and NRS to each of three small glass test tubes (Durham tubes) using a Pasteur pipet attached to a rubber bulb. Use a different Pasteur pipet for each transfer. As you add antisera and NRS to the Durham tubes, touch the bottom of the tube with the Pasteur pipet. Take care not to wet the sides of the tubes.

2. Using a micropipette, transfer 100 μL of BSA and goat serum into two 1.5 mL Eppendorf tubes. Add 0.1 mL of goat serum into a third 1.5 mL tube. Using a Pasteur pipet, carefully overlay the anti-serum samples with an equal volume of the specific soluble antigen, taking care not to mix the two samples at the interface. For example, in the Durham tube containing anti-BSA, overlay it with BSA antigen solution. In the Durham tube containing anti-goat serum, overlay it with goat serum. In the Durham tube containing normal rabbit serum, overlay it with goat serum.

3. Incubate the tubes at room temperature and observe frequently. A white precipitation (precipitin) ring at the antiserum-antigen interface will form. This indicates a positive test.

4. The tubes may be stored overnight at 4 °C and checked for the formation of the precipitin ring. The precipitate may form very fast and become so thick that it falls to the bottom of the tube rather than remain at the interface.

5. Record your observations.

Part B

Quantitation of precipitin reaction (see materials in Part A)
   In this section students will quantitate the antigen-antibody reaction obtained by precipitation. Increasing amounts of antigen will be added to a constant concentration of antibody. The resulting precipitate that forms will be measured.

Procedure

1. Obtain six precipitin tubes and label them 1–6.
2. To each tube add 0, 5, 10, 20, 50, 100 μL of the antigen (BSA) (note concentration of stock BSA concentration provided in class).
3. To each tube add 1× PBS to make a total volume of 400 μL.
4. Add 100 μL of anti-BSA to each tube (note the dilution/concentration of antibody provided in class).
5. Incubate the tubes at 37 °C for 1h followed by incubation on ice for 1 h.
6. Centrifuge the tubes for 10 min at 3000 rpm using the bench top centrifuge. Collect the supernatant and place in fresh tubes. Save them on ice. Save the precipitin pellets.
7. Add 1× PBS to the pellets, resuspend gently and centrifuge as in step 6. Discard the wash supernatant.
8. Vortex the tubes and add 2 mL of 0.1 M NaOH to the pellets. Resuspend to dissolve the pellets.
9. Transfer the tube contents to cuvettes to read the O.D. at 280 nm using a spectrophotometer. The blank will be NaOH without protein.
10. Plot a graph of BSA concentration (μg BSA) on the x-axis against the O.D. (or protein precipitate in μg) on the y-axis. Determine the zone of equivalence, antigen excess/postzone and antibody excess/prozone (Fig. 33.1).

Part C

Capillary precipitin test: This technique can be used to determine the titer of an antisera specific for a given soluble antigen. The antiserum is serially diluted in saline solution, and a constant amount of soluble antigen is added to the dilutions. The titer of the antiserum is obtained by determining the end point dilution that gives a precipitation reaction.

Materials and Reagents (Per Pair)

26 small test tubes
2 test tube racks
26 capillary tubes
100 mL of saline
2 tubes of antisera: anti-BSA and anti-GS
2 tubes of soluble antigen (BSA and GS)
1 tube of normal rabbit serum (NRS)
2 clay blocks

Four 1 mL pipets
Kimwipes
Paper towel
Bench cover

Procedure

1. Place 24 small test tubes in a rack. Number the tubes and label with the specific antigen (BSA or GS) and antibody (anti-BSA or anti-GS). Add 0.2 mL of saline to each tube with an l mL glass pipet.
2. Using a l mL glass pipet, add 0.2 mL of antiserum to tube #1, and add 0.2 mL of normal control serum to tube #12.
3. Make a serial twofold dilution of the antiserum from tube #2 through tube# 11.
4. Starting with the most dilute antiserum, fill a capillary tube about 1/3 full by touching the end of the tube to the surface of the liquid. Wipe off the excess antiserum with a kimwipe.
5. Carefully layer the specific soluble antigen on top of the antiserum by touching the end of the tube to the antigen solution. Carefully tilt the capillary tube so that an air pocket forms in both ends of the capillary tube, and seal one end with a plug of clay. Seal the side nearest the antiserum.
6. Wipe the tube with a kimwipe and stand it upright in the clay block. Repeat the process with all the dilutions. Prepare an additional control tube from tube #1. Fill a second capillary tube with the 1:2 diluted antiserum and overlay it with saline.
7. Incubate the tubes at 37 °C for 1 h and observe for the presence or absence of precipitation. Incubate the tubes overnight at 4 °C and read the results again. Record your results. What are the titers of both antisera?

Agglutination

Agglutination may be defined as the cross-linking of a particulate or insoluble antigen and the corresponding antibody. In agglutination reactions, a suspension of cells (erythrocytes, bacteria, protozoa, etc.), when mixed with specific antisera under suitable conditions, leads to the clumping or agglutination of the cells. Specific agglutination reactions have been extensively used in the identification and classification of microorganisms.

As with precipitation reactions, excess antibody or antigen in agglutination reactions results in prozone and postzone reactions, respectively.

IgM antibodies agglutinate particles very readily since their large size of five basic immunoglobulin units allows the attachment of up to five antigens. IgG antibodies are poor agglutinins. However, the assay conditions can be modified to produce good agglutinations with IgG.

Agglutination reactions are classified into four major types: **direct agglutination (bacterial agglutination), viral hemagglutination, passive (indirect) hemagglutination** and **reverse passive agglutination.** Patient serum can be screened for the presence of antibodies specific to bacterial, parasite or viral antigens using agglutination reactions lending clinical relevance to agglutination reactions. Antibody titers obtained can provide significant data regarding exposure to a pathogen or a deficiency in antibody response indicating poor B cell activation.

Part D

Slide agglutination test: This is a rapid test that requires very little reagents. It is used as a basis for preliminary reports. However, results are confirmed by a titrated agglutination test that is more precise.

Materials and Reagents (Per Pair)

2 clean glass slides (microscope slides) with frosted edges
1 grease pencil
4 Pasteur pipets
4 applicator sticks
Warm slide box
1 tube of particulate antigen (sheep red blood cells, SRBCs)
1 tube of antisera (anti-SRBCs, Hemolysin)
1 tube of control serum (Normal Rabbit Serum)
Plastic squeezers (Padl-pets) or Pasteur pipets with rubber bulbs
Kimwipes
Paper towel
Bench cover

Procedure

1. Using a grease pencil, divide a clean microscope slide into 2 sections, and draw a small (15 mm) diameter circle in each section. In one circle, place 1 drop of antiserum, and in the other, place 1 drop of normal rabbit serum using a Pasteur pipet.
2. Add 1 drop of SRBC suspension to each of the serum samples. Mix the contents in each circle with an applicator stick (use a different stick for each circle) and gently rotate the slide for 2–3 min. Observe for visible clumping of cells.
3. Slides may be placed on warm slide boxes to speed up the reaction. Record your observations. Agglutinated cells appear as large clumps while unagglutinated

cells remain in a cloudy suspension. Observe the test circle and compare it to the control circle.

Tanning and Coating Sheep Red Blood Cells

Tanning cells with tannic acid

1. Prepare a 1% tannic acid stock solution in 1× PBS. Tannic acid can be used at a final concentration of 0.003–0.007%.
2. Wash SRBCs suspended in Alsevar's solution three times by centrifugation using PBS, 5 min at 1500 rpm in an IEC table top centrifuge at room temperature. After the last wash, resuspend cells to 5% in PBS.
3. Add tannic acid to SRBCs for a final concentration of 0.007% and incubate cells in a 37 °C water bath for 10 min.
4. Centrifuge cells as in step 2, and discard supernatant. Wash the cells twice by centrifugation with PBS. After the last wash, resuspend cells in 10 mL of PBS and store at 4 °C.

Coating Tanned Cells with Bovine Serum Albumin (BSA)

1. Prepare a 10 mL 5% SRBC suspension in PBS. Add 27.5 mg BSA (or ovalbumin) to the cell suspension.
2. Incubate the cell mixture in a 37 °C water bath for 15 min. Centrifuge the cells at 750 rpm for 5 min. Discard supernatant. Wash the cells twice with PBS and after the last wash, resuspend cell pellet to a 5% final concentration in PBS. The cells may be stored at 4 °C or used immediately for passive hemagglutination assays.

Part E

Direct hemagglutination and passive hemagglutination tests: The direct assay uses antigens found naturally on the surface of cells, such as red blood cells and bacteria. An example of this is the ABO, Rh blood typing that was performed in Exercise 4 (see Chap. 28). In passive hemagglutination, soluble antigen is attached to a red cell carrier or beads and then incubated with the specific antiserum. This increases the sensitivity of the assay. Some antigens attach to the cell surface spontaneously, while others attach to the red cell after the cells have been treated with specific reagents such as tannic acid (see procedure described above). An important clinical test used to identify antibodies against the bacterial toxin, streptolysin O (SLO) produced by β-hemolytic streptococci relies on the use of beads bound with

SLO. Upon incubation of the SLO-beads with human serum containing antibodies against SLO (ASO), agglutination occurs, indicating the presence of specific antibodies in the patient's serum. Similarly, the indirect agglutination technique can be used to detect the presence of C-reactive protein (CRP). Antibodies against CRP are bound to beads and then incubated with human serum. The occurrence of agglutination indicates the presence of CRP in the serum; a major indicator of inflammation. We will perform both types of agglutination reactions in this exercise.

Materials and Reagents (Per Pair)

3 U-bottomed microliter plates
3 0.05 mL microdiluters (50 μL)
1 micropipette (Eppendorf)
(0–200 μL) pipet tips
50 mL sterile saline or 1× PBS
1 tube of untreated SRBC—10% suspension ("A") in 5 mL
1 tube of BSA adsorbed to tanned SRBC—10% suspension ("B") in 5 mL
1 tube of anti-SRBC antibody—200 μL (hemolysin)
1 tube of anti-BSA antibody—200 μL
One tube of normal control serum—200 μL
Gloves

Procedure

1. Label 3—96 well U-bottomed microliter plates for direct hemagglutination and passive hemagglutination (Fig. 33.2).
2. Using the Eppendorf pipet, add 50 μL of saline (or 1× PBS) to wells numbered 2–22 in rows 1 and 2 of the two 96 well microtiter plates.
     NOTE: Plates may already contain saline or PBS in the wells. If that is the case, label the plates and begin the procedure at step 3.
3. Using the pipet, add 50 μL of normal serum to well #24 in each second row in all plates. Add 50 μL of anti-SRBC antibody to wells #1 and #2 of row 1 in the first plate.
4. Using the 50 μL microdiluter, make a serial twofold dilution of each antiserum starting with well #2 and ending at well #22. (Instructor will demonstrate the use of microdiluters) Fig. 33.2.
     NOTE: if microdiluters are unavailable, serial 1:2 dilutions can be performed using the Eppendorf pipet pre-set at 50 μL. Use a yellow tip with the pipet. (Instructor will demonstrate the use of pipets for dilution)

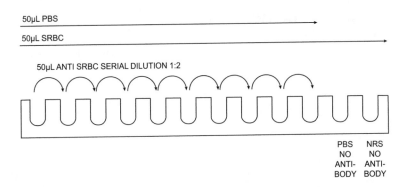

Fig. 33.2 Dilution scheme for SRBC agglutination in round bottomed 96-well microtiter plates. Anti-SRBC (hemolysin) serially diluted in a two-fold dilution scheme are incubated with SRBC. Control wells contain PBS or saline and normal rabbit serum (NRS)

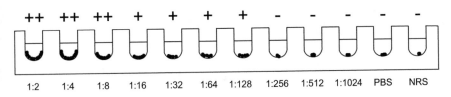

Fig. 33.3 Determination of hemolysin titer in SRBC agglutination. Positive agglutination is shown in wells 1-7 for a titer of 1:128

5. Using the pipet set at 50 μL, add 50 μL of normal SRBC to all 24 wells in rows 1 and 2. To the second plate add 50 μL of BSA-absorbed SRBC to all 24 wells in rows 1 and 2. Mix well by gently rotating the plate.

6. The dilution in well #1 is now 1:2, well #2 is 1:4, etc. Well #23 is a saline control and well #24 is a normal serum control.

7. Cover the plate and incubate at 37 °C for 1 h. Check for agglutination. Incubate plates at 4 °C overnight and examine on the next day for agglutination. Agglutinated cells will form a matted network at the bottom of the wells. Figure 33.3 shows an illustration of a completed agglutination reaction in microtiter wells. In positive wells agglutinated cells form a "mat" at the bottom of the wells unlike cells in negative wells.

Questions

1. What is the agglutination titer of the different antisera?
2. How does it compare to the precipitation titer of the same antiserum? Which procedure is more sensitive?
3. What is the advantage of performing a passive agglutination assay?

NOTES AND ILLUSTRATIONS:

NOTES AND ILLUSTRATIONS:

Selected References

Barret JT Textbook of immunology. Mosey, St. Louis. Ch. 12, Precipitation; Ch. 13, Agglutination and hemagglutination

MacLeod I (1965) Specific agglutination of tanned red cells coated with globulin fraction of an antithyroid serum by saline extracts of thyroid glands. J. Clin Path 18:813–816

Murphy K, Weaver C (2017) Janeway's immunobiology, 9th edn. Garland Press, New York

Punt J, Stranford SA, Jones PP, Owen JA (2019) Kuby immunology, 8th edn. W.H. Freeman and Company, New York. Ch. 20, Antigen-antibody interactions

Sheehan C (1990) Principles and laboratory diagnosis: clinical immunology. J.B. Lippincott Company, Philadelphia. Ch. 11, Precipitation; Ch. 12, Agglutination and agglutination inhibition

NOTES AND QUIZZES:

Chapter 34
Exercise 10: Immunodiffusion and Immun oelectrophoresis

Introduction

The Ouchterlony gel immunodiffusion technique (double immunodiffusion) and immunoelectrophoresis assays both use a semi-solid medium such as agar or agarose for the diffusion of antibody and antigen. Soluble antigens and antibodies diffuse through the semisolid medium until they reach the optimum concentration to form a visible precipitation line.

The precipitation line (precipitate) is the result of lattice formation, between antigen and antibody. A single antibody reacting with its cognate antigen will give rise to single precipitin line. If several precipitin lines are observed, this indicates that several antigen-antibody complexes are present. The molecular size of the antibody-antigen components determines the rate of diffusion through the gel matrix. Smaller molecules diffuse faster than larger molecules. In addition, the rate of diffusion of antigen and antibody increases in direct proportion to their concentrations in the gels.

Other factors affect the rate of diffusion on antigen-antibody through the gel mix; temperature, gel viscosity, and hydration and interactions between the gel matrix and the reactants. The distance between antigen-antibody wells may also affect the rate of diffusion. Immunodiffusion techniques can be divided into two groups based on the number of components diffusing at any given time. Simple diffusion systems in which only one of the reactants-either antigen or antibody-is diffusing and double-diffusion systems in which both of the reactants are diffusing. In both systems, diffusion can occur in one dimension or in two dimensions.

In the Ouchterlony technique developed by Orjan Ouchterlony both antigen and antibody diffuse. Antigen is placed in one well and antibody in another well. Diffusion occurs, and where both molecules meet in the equivalence zone, a precipitin line develops. Where there are multiple wells of antigen present opposite an antibody (e.g., 2 antigens, 1 Ab), three main patterns of precipitation are possible (Fig. 34.1):

© Springer Nature Switzerland AG 2021
T. Y. Sam-Yellowe, *Immunology: Overview and Laboratory Manual*,
https://doi.org/10.1007/978-3-030-64686-8_34

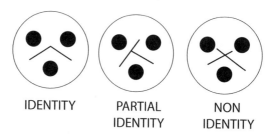

IDENTITY   PARTIAL   NON
                  IDENTITY   IDENTITY

Fig. 34.1 Illustration of double diffusion immunoprecipitation (Ouchterlony) of antibody and antigens. Antibody in the lower well and antigens in the top two wells. Patterns of identity, partial identity and non-identity are shown

(a) **Identity,** where a solid continuous smooth line between antigen wells indicates that both antigens are the same

(b) If the antigens in both wells are different, then both lines cross, forming a double spur. This is referred to as **non-identity**

(c) If both antigens share some cross reactivity, a single spur is formed. This is known as **partial identity.**

The double diffusion technique has many applications. In general, they can be grouped as follows:

(a) Determining the homogeneity of antibody-antigen systems
(b) Determining the minimum number of antibody-antigen complexes present
(c) Following the purification of an antigen from a mixture of substance
(d) Determining whether a given antigen shares structural characteristics (i.e., cross-reacts) with other molecules of interest.

Immunoelectrophoresis (IEP)

Immunoelectrophoresis is a modification of the double gel diffusion technique developed by Graber and Williams. A mixture of antigens is placed in a well cut in agar (or agarose) and then separated electrophoretically. A solution containing the homologous antibodies is placed in a trough cut parallel to the path of electrophoretic migration (also cut in the gel) and allowed to diffuse through the gel toward the electrophoresed antigen (**double immunodiffusion**). Precipitin arcs form wherever homologous antigens and antibodies meet and form insoluble immune complexes. IEP may be used to test for the presence of myelomas, a condition where excess of one or more immunoglobulin is produced, urine proteins can also be identified using IEPs.

Examples of single immunodiffusion assays include **single radial immunodiffusion** and electroimmunoassay (rocket immunoelectrophoresis). In this exercise, we will perform two double immunodiffusion assays using the Ouchterlony and immunoelectrophoretic techniques and one single immunodiffusion assay, rocket immunoelectrophoresis. We will also perform double immunodiffusion assays using commercially available pre-poured plates. The objective of this exercise is to learn gel immunodiffusion techniques.

Ouchterlony Double Diffusion

Materials and reagents (Per Pair)

One Petri dish containing 2% agarose
Two tubes containing 5 mL 1% agarose kept in a 60 °C water bath
Three tubes each containing soluble antigen: Bovine serum albumin (BSA), goat
   serum, horse serum
One tube of antisera: rabbit anti-BSA
Water aspirator and trap
Pasteur pipets
Pipetman 0–200 μL
Pipetman 0–20 μL
0.85% NaCl
Two pre-poured agarose plates with four wells

Procedure

1. Pour a tube of 1% agar into a petri dish containing 2% solid agar. Gently swirl
   the petri dish to spread the agar and cover the entire surface of the petri dish. Be
   sure to avoid bubbles or uneven spreading of agar. Repeat the process for a
   second plate. Set both plates aside for 5 min to let the agar cool and harden.
      Using a pasteur pipet (large end), punch wells out of the agar in the pattern
   shown. Using the smaller end of the pipet, punch another hole above the pattern
   to indicate the top and bottom orientation. Be careful not to punch wells clear to
   the bottom of the plates. Instructor will illustrate patterns on the board.
2. Using a pasteur pipet attached to a water aspirator, remove the agar plugs from
   inside the wells, taking care to remove all gel pieces.
3. Use a pipetman to add 100 μL of antiserum into the center well. Add antigens as
   indicated in the outer wells. Incubate plates in a humidity chamber (provided by
   instructor) for 1 h at 37 °C. Place the gels at 4 °C overnight and check for
   precipitin lines. Record your results. Prepare an illustration of the wells and
   precipitin lines on each plate. If necessary, refill antibody or antigen wells and
   read the plates again after 24 h.
4. Plates with wells arranged in the pattern shown in Fig. 34.2 will also be used.
   Add antibody and antigens as shown on the template. Incubate plates in a
   humidity chamber (provided by instructor) for 1 hour at 37 °C. Place the gels at
   4 °C overnight and check for precipitin lines. Record your results. Prepare an
   illustration of the wells and precipitin lines on each plate. If necessary, refill
   antibody or antigen wells and read the plates again after 24 h.

Fig. 34.2 Well template for Ouchterlony immunoprecipitation. In a petri dish containing agarose, punch holes as shown in the template and using a Pasteur pipet with a rubber bulb or an aspirator, remove the agarose plugs. Fill the wells with the antibodies and antigens shown. Antigens: *BSA* Bovine serum albumin, *FBS* Fetal bovine serum, *OVA* Ovalbumin, *HS* Human serum, *DS* Donkey serum, *CHS* Chicken serum, *GS* Goat serum, *RPL* Rabbit plasma, *NRS* Normal rabbit serum. Antibodies: Anti-bovine serum albumin and anti-goat serum

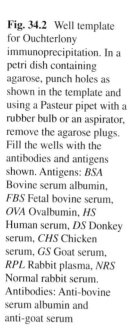
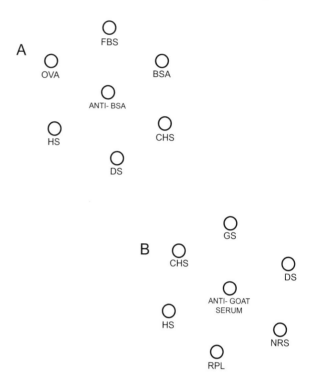

Immunoelectrophoresis

Materials and Reagents (Per Pair)

Two thin agarose coated glass slides in humid chamber
Template
Power supply
IEP chamber
100 mL 2% agarose in Tris-Tricine buffer pH 8.6 kept in 60 °C water bath
4 L Tris-Tricine buffer
Three 1 mL sterile glass pipet
100 mL Coomassie Blue G 2.5%
IL destaining solution
IL wash solution
Two tubes of soluble antigen
1 tube of antisera
Kimwipes
Paper towel

Procedure

1. Pipet 4 mL of 2% agarose onto glass slides pre-coated with 1% agarose. Using the tip of a 1 ml pipet, carefully and quickly spread agar to cover the glass slide. Allow the agarose to solidify.
2. Using a template with a center trough and one or more wells on either side of the trough, cut patterns in agarose. Antiserum will be placed in the center trough and antigens will be placed in the wells. Remove the agarose plug from antigen wells only (as indicated), using a pipet attached to a water aspirator. **Do not aspirate the trough at this time.**
3. Fill the wells with soluble antigen samples (approximately 3 μL). Place the slides in an IEP chamber and electrophorese (instructor will perform electrophoresis) for 1 h.
4. After electrophoresis, disconnect current, aspirate antiserum troughs and fill with antiserum (approximately 100 μL).
5. Place the slides in a humid chamber and examine within 24 h for precipitin lines. Record your results. Illustrate the pattern of precipitin lines. On your drawings indicate the contents of each well and trough. (Fig. 34.3a)

   Note: Ouchterlony gels and IEP slides will be washed with wash solution, pressed, stained with Coomassie dye, destained, and dried as indicated.

Rocket Immunoelectrophoresis

Materials and Reagents (Per Pair)

Two 10 mL tubes of 2% agarose in Tris-Tricine buffer pH 8.6 kept in 60 °C water bath
4L Tris-Tricine buffer
Power supply
IEP chamber
Two thin coated glass plates
Two 10 mL pipet
One tube of anti-goat serum
One tube of goat serum
One tube of unknown antigen
Parafilm
Scissors

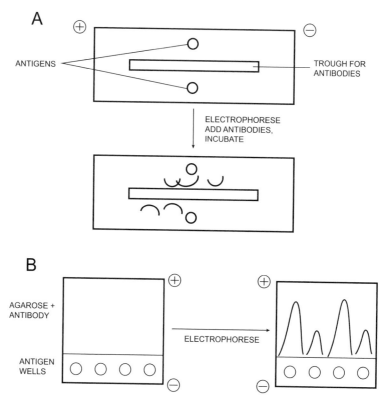

Fig. 34.3 Illustration of electrophoresis of antigens and precipitation by antibodies. (**a**) Immunoelectrophoresis of antigens placed in wells alongside a trough that is filled with antibody after antigens are electrophoresed. Precipitin arcs form after antibody diffuses and combines with antigen. (**b**) Rocket immunoelectrophresis of antigens placed in wells and electrophoresed in agar mixed with antibody. Incubation of agar results in "rockets" showing antigen reactivity with the antibody

Procedure

1. Remove a tube containing 10 mL of 2% agarose from a 60 °C water bath. Allow the tube to cool slightly. Quickly add 300 μL of antiserum to the tube. Cover the tube with parafilm and gently invert 2–3 times to mix. Quickly pour the solution onto a glass plate pre-coated with 1% agarose. Spread the agarose-antiserum mixture on the slide up to the edges of the glass plate.

2. Allow the agarose to solidify, and then use the tip of a Pasteur pipet to punch 4 wells as indicated (Fig. 34.3b). Just before electrophoresis, aspirate the gel plugs. Fill three of the wells with 2 μL of the appropriate soluble antigens. Fill the 4th well with an unknown soluble antigen provided by the instructor.

3. Electrophorese the proteins for 30 min at 15mA per plate.

4. Immediately following electrophoresis, measure and record the heights of the precipitin arcs ("rockets") and make an illustration of them. On your illustrations, indicate the contents of the wells. The gels may be washed and stained as with Ouchterlony and IEP gels (Fig. 34.3b).

Selected References

Barrett JT (1988) Textbook of Immunology. Mosby, St. Louis. Ch. 12, Precipitation.

De Toma FJ, MacDonald AB (1987) Experimental immunology. A guidebook. Macmillan, New York. Ch. 4, Analysis of antigens by immunodiffusion and immunoelectrophoresis.

Murphy K, Weaver C (2017) Janeway's immunobiology, 9th edn. Garland Press, New York

Myers RL (1989) Immunology. A laboratory manual. WM. C. Brown Publishers, Dubuque, Iowa. Exercise 16, Column chromatography.

Punt J, Stranford SA, Jones PP, Owen JA (2019) Kuby immunology, 8th edn. W. H. Freeman and Company, New York, Antigen-antibody interactions, Ch. 20.

Sheehan C (1990) Principles and laboratory diagnosis: clinical immunology. J.B. Lippincott, Philadelphia. Ch. 11, Precipitation.

NOTES AND ILLUSTRATIONS:

Chapter 35
Exercise 11: Protein-A Affinity Purification of Rabbit IgG

Introduction

In experiments where other serum proteins may interfere with antibody reactivity, having purified immunoglobulins is important. Immunoglobulin G (IgG) is the most commonly used isotype in the laboratory. In this exercise, rabbit IgG will be purified from rabbit antiserum using affinity binding. The Fc region of IgG binds to a number of molecules most notably protein A which is found in certain strains of *Staphylococcus aureus*. We will use affinity methods to remove IgG from whole antiserum. Incubation of antiserum with sepharose beads previously complexed with protein A will allow IgG to bind the beads. IgG will then be eluted from the beads using low pH. Glycine (0.1 M) at pH of 2 or 0.58% acetic acid is used for elution of IgG. Once IgG is purified, the antibody molecule can be fractionated with papain or pepsin to obtain the antibody binding regions. The specificity of the antibodies can then be evaluated using different immunoassays. Magnetic beads conjugated to protein A or secondary antibodies may also be used to isolate IgG from antiserum. After incubating magnetic beads conjugated to protein A with antiserum, a magnetic separator is used to remove IgG-bound beads. Unbound proteins are washed off and the bound IgG is eluted from the beads. Affinity purification of IgG can be performed using columns packed with protein A-sepharose or a batch method can be used where the protein A beads are contained in centrifuge tubes. Large volumes of beads such as 1 mL of beads in 15 mL centrifuge tubes can be used or volumes as little as 100 µL can be used. The **first objective** of this exercise is to isolate IgG from rabbit antiserum using affinity purification. The **second objective** is to fractionate IgG using pepsin to obtain the F(ab')$_2$ region of the antibody.

© Springer Nature Switzerland AG 2021
T. Y. Sam-Yellowe, *Immunology: Overview and Laboratory Manual*,
https://doi.org/10.1007/978-3-030-64686-8_35

Materials and Reagents (Per Pair)

200 μL protein-A sepharose beads in 1× PBS, in a 1.5 mL Eppendorf (microfuge) tube
1 mL of rabbit antisera
Quartz cuvettes (3)
Spectrophotometers (3)
Bench top microfuge
500 mL 1× PBS
50 mL 0.58% glacial acetic acid
Sleeve of 50 mL centrifuge tubes
Sleeve of 15 mL centrifuge tubes
Shaker/Nutator (end-over-end shaker)
10 mL glass pipets
Plastic squeezer pipets (1 box)
Waste beaker (empty 500 mL beaker)
15 mL tube containing 5 mL 1 M NaHCO₃
15 mL tube containing 1 mL Sodium azide in 1× PBS

Procedure

Part A

1. Pipet 1 mL of antiserum into a clean dry quartz cuvette and then measure and record the absorbance or optical density (OD) of the rabbit antiserum (at 280 nm). **DO NOT DISCARD THE ANTISERA.** Pipet 100 μL of the antiserum into a clean Eppendorf tube and save. This is your starting material to include in your protein analysis. Figure 35.1 illustrates the protocol for IgG isolation using protein A beads.
2. Place the tube containing 200 μL of protein-A beads (provided in a 1.5 mL microfuge tube) in a microfuge. Balance the tube with tubes from other groups in the lab. Centrifuge the protein-A beads for 5 min at 13,000 rpm. Using a plastic 1 mL squeezer, discard the PBS supernatant into the waste beaker provided.
3. Using a plastic 1 mL squeezer, add 1 mL of rabbit antiserum to the protein-A beads, cap the tube tightly and invert end-over-end 3–4 times to mix and resuspend the beads. **DO NOT VORTEX OR PIPET TO RESUSPEND.**
4. Incubate the tube containing the protein-A beads plus antiserum on an end-over-end shaker for 30 min at room temperature.
5. Centrifuge the tube for 5 min as in step #2, collect the flow-through i.e. supernatant containing unbound proteins and save it in a clean 1.5 mL Eppendorf tube.

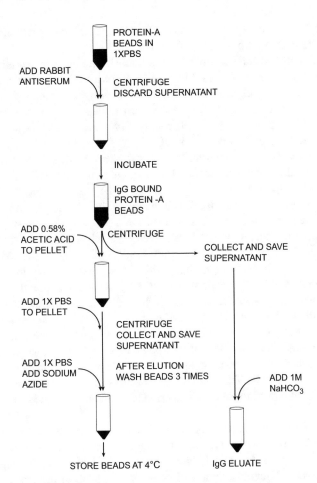

Fig. 35.1 Protein-A affinity purification of rabbit IgG. Rabbit antiserum is incubated with protein A beads, followed by washes and elution of bound IgG with 0.58% acetic acid or 0.2 M glycine, pH 2

6. Add 1 ml of 1× PBS to the bead pellet form #5, resuspend the beads as in step #3 and centrifuge for 5 min at 13,000 rpm. This is the first wash step. Repeat the washes three more times using 1 mL of I× PBS for each wash. Save the supernatants from each wash in a clean 1.5 mL microfuge tube. The OD (optical density) will be measured for each wash. The OD of the 4th wash should be at background level approximately 0.1 OD. When collecting the supernatant from the 4th wash, collect to about 1 mm of the bead surface but do not let the beads run dry.

7. Add 400 μL of 0.58% acetic acid to the bead pellet from #6, to elute the bound IgG. Cap the tube, invert end-over-end 3–4 times, then incubate on the end-to-end shaker for 5 min. After the incubation, centrifuge the microfuge tube

containing the beads as in #2, then collect the supernatant containing the IgG eluate into a clean 1.5 mL microfuge tube.

8. Add 35 μL of 1 M NaHCO$_3$ into the IgG eluate from step #7 to neutralize the pH.

9. Repeat the elution step i.e. #7 by adding 400 μL of 0.58% acetic acid to the bead pellet, mix the tube as in step 7, centrifuge the tube and collect the supernatant containing the IgG eluate into a clean 1.5 mL microfuge tube. **NOTE**: The second elution will remove any remaining IgG on the beads. Neutralize the eluate by adding 35 μL of 1 M NaHCO$_3$ in to the eluate.

10. Pool both eluates by pipetting the second eluate from step 9, into the tube containing the first elute in step 7. There should be a total of 870 μL of total IgG eluate. Place the tube containing the eluate in the ice bucket provided.

11. Wash the protein-A beads by centrifugation, twice by adding 1 mL of 1× PBS to the beads using a 1 mL plastic squeezer and centrifuging as in step 2. Collect the wash supernatants into 1.5 mL microfuge tubes and save. After the last wash, add 1 mL of 1× PBS to the beads. Cap the microfuge tube and invert end-over-end 3–4 times. Add sodium azide to the bead suspension, to a final concentration of 0.02%. The tubes will be collected and stored at 4 °C. The beads may be reused after washing off the sodium azide preservative.

12. There should be nine tubes for analysis: tube 1 = 100 μL antiserum (starting material, SM); tube 2 = flow through (FT) supernatant containing unbound proteins; tubes 3–6 = washes; tube 7 = pooled IgG eluate and tubes 8–9 = washes. Measure the OD of each sample using the spectrophotometer at 280 nm wavelength. **NOTE**: The OD 280 nm readings may not be performed on the first day, but moved to the next lab period. Collect all tubes and store at 4 °C for analysis.

13. The pooled eluate may be dialyzed before analysis. Add the pooled eluate to the dialysis tubing provided making sure that the ends of the tubing are properly secured. Leave approximately half volume of the tubing free for expansion of the dialysate. Your instructor will demonstrate. Dialyze the eluate overnight against distilled water with two changes.

14. After 24 h collect the eluate from the dialysis bag by cutting one end of the dialysis bag with a pair of scissors and pipetting the eluate into a clean 50 mL tube. Freeze the eluate at −70° C overnight.

15. After 24 h lyophilize the eluate overnight to dryness and reconstitute the protein in 300 μL of 1× PBS. Vortex briskly i.e. 2–3 short pulses to resuspend. Store at −20 °C until required.

Part B

Digestion of rabbit IgG with pepsin for generation of F(ab′)$_2$ fragments

16. Resuspend lyophilized IgG in 1 mL of 20 mM sodium acetate pH 4.

17. Add 125 μL of immobilized pepsin and incubate at 37 °C for 4 h.

18. Centrifuge the beads for 5 min at 14,000 rpm in an eppendorf microfuge. Collect the supernatant and add to 1 mL of hydrated protein A beads. Fc fragments generated in # 17 will bind to the protein A beads.

19. Centrifuge the protein beads, collect the supernatant and transfer to a fresh 15 mL centrifuge tube. Prepare a dialysis bag as indicated in #11 and dialyze the F(ab')$_2$ fragments against distilled water.

20. Collect the dialysate and freeze on dry-ice, lyophilize and reconstitute in 1 mL PBS.

21. Determine the protein concentration using the Coomassie blue dye binding assay. Analyze the fractionated IgG on SDS-PAGE gels stained with Coomassie blue.

22. The collected samples will be analyzed by sodium dodecyl sulfate–polyacrylamide gel electrophoresis (SDS-PAGE), western blotting and determination of protein concentration using the Bradford protein assay.

NOTES AND ILLUSTRATIONS:

Selected References

Murphy K, Weaver C (2017) Janeway's immunobiology, 9th edn. Garland Press, New York
Punt J, Stranford SA, Jones PP, Owen JA (2019) Kuby immunology, 8th edn. W.H. Freeman and
  Company, New York. Ch. 20, Antigen-antibody interactions

Chapter 36
Exercise 12: Sodium Dodecyl Sulfate Polyacrylamide Gel Electrophoresis (SDS-PAGE)

Introduction

Complex mixtures of proteins (heterogeneous population of proteins) can be separated and analyzed by a variety of methods. Individual proteins can then be purified or identified by specific antibodies. Electrophoresis is a routine procedure used for separating and analyzing complex mixtures of proteins in the laboratory. A semi-solid gel matrix consisting of either starch, agarose (polysaccharide) or polyacrylamide is used for separation. One of the most commonly used electrophoretic techniques is sodium dodecyl sulfate polyacrylamide gel electrophoresis (SDS-PAGE). Acrylamide is a water soluble polymer that is used to prepare gels by polymerization with bis-acrylamide (N^1,N′-methylene-bis-acrylamide) in the presence of catalysts, TEMED (tetramethylethylenediamine) and ammonium persulfate. The resulting crosslinked gel polymer consists of a porous meshwork through which proteins of different molecular weights can migrate according to their size. The porosity i.e. the size of the meshwork in the matrix, depends on the concentration of acrylamide in the mixture. Polyacrylamide gels are electrophoresed vertically and are routinely poured or cast in between two glass plates and placed in gel chambers containing the appropriate buffers for electrophoresis. Depression wells are created at the top of the gel for sample loading. SDS-PAGE gels can be prepared from scratch or purchased as pre-made or pre-cast gels.

Proteins can be separated under denaturing (non-native) conditions or non-denaturing (native) conditions. In this exercise, we will perform denaturing SDS-PAGE. Sodium dodecyl sulfate is an anionic detergent that binds to proteins and imparts a net negative charge to the protein, in effect nullifying the overall intrinsic charge of the protein (Fig. 36.1). In the presence of an electric charge the proteins therefore migrate from the negatively charged cathode (−) usually colored black, to the positively charged anode (+), usually colored red. The binding of the detergent to the proteins also denatures the proteins exposing the primary structure of the proteins. Protein samples to be electrophoresed are mixed with electrophoresis

© Springer Nature Switzerland AG 2021
T. Y. Sam-Yellowe, *Immunology: Overview and Laboratory Manual*,
https://doi.org/10.1007/978-3-030-64686-8_36

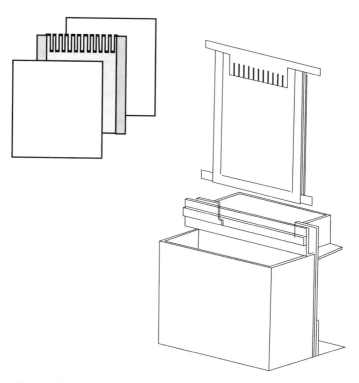

Fig. 36.1 SDS-PAGE gel preparation. A mixture of acrylamide and bis-acrylamide prepared in Tris-glycine-SDS buffer is poured into front and back plates assembled with spacers, first the separating or running gel followed by the stacking gel. A comb used to form the wells is inserted into the stacking gel before the gel polymerizes (top left). The comb and bottom spacer are removed before the gel is placed in a gel chamber with buffer. Proteins loaded in the gel are electrophoresed

buffer containing a dense substance such as glycerol or sucrose, to facilitate gel loading. To further separate individual polypeptides, proteins are also treated with a reducing agent such as 2-mercptoethanol (2-ME) or dithiothreitol (DTT) to reduce disulfide bonds, followed by alkylation with iodoacetamide to keep bonds separated. A tracking dye is also added to monitor progress of protein migration. The samples are boiled to further denature the proteins. The mobility of the protein is influenced by the length of the protein, with longer/larger proteins migrating slower (will form bands at the top of the gel), and shorter/smaller proteins migrating faster (will form bands at the bottom of the gel). Protein standards are also loaded in lanes of the gel for estimation of the molecular weight of the separated protein samples. With a ruler measure the distance migrated by the individual proteins in the molecular weight mixture, and the distance migrated by the dye front. Using the formula shown below calculate the Rm. Plot a standard curve using the values. Measure the distance migrated by the individual protein (s) in your sample and determine their molecular weights from the standard curve. The relative migration, Rm (Rf value) of the proteins can be calculated using the following formula:

$$Rm = \frac{\text{distance migrated by protein}}{\text{distance migrated by the dye front}}$$

Separated proteins are visualized by a variety of staining techniques such as the quantitative dye Coomassie blue dye, and other non-quantitative stains such as silver staining which is an enhancement stain and exquisitely sensitive and very useful for staining low abundance proteins and for confirming the purity of isolated proteins. Stains-all (Sigma Aldrich) is another dye that can be used. Individual proteins can be separated from the gel matrix for further analysis or the separated proteins can be transferred to nitrocellulose paper or nylon matrices for western blotting using specific antibodies. Specific protein bands can be excised (cut out) and the proteins electroeluted (the proteins are removed from the acrylamide matrix). Contents of a specific lane can also be electroeluted and analyzed.

Define or Explain the Following Terms

Homogeneous gels
Gradient gels
One-dimensional gel electrophoresis
Two-dimensional gel electrophoresis
Resolving gel

The **first objective** of this exercise is to learn how to prepare and perform SDS-PAGE electrophoresis using a 1% Nonidet P-40 (NP-40) or 1% Triton X-100 detergent extract of *P. yoelii* or *P. chabaudi* proteins. Extracts can be prepared from other organisms for analysis on SDS-PAGE gels. Also, recombinant proteins and purified native proteins can be separated and analyzed by SDS-PAGE gels. Purified rabbit IgG or IgG fragments can also be analyzed on SDS-PAGE gels. Protein samples for electrophoresis will be solubilized with or without reduction with DTT or mercaptoethanol. A **second objective** is to learn how to perform Coomassie blue and silver staining of separated proteins.

Materials and Reagents (Per Pair)

One pair of front and back plates
Three spacers
One squeeze bottle containing absolute ethanol
Erhlenmyer flask containing 30 mL
30%:0.8% bis-acrylamide mixture
1 M Tris pH 8.8
1 M Tris pH 6.8

10% SDS

Combs

TEMED

10% Ammonium persulfate prepared fresh on the day of the experiment

Two 10% SDS-PAGE gels with stacking gels/10 well combs (sometimes the gels are prepared out of the lab by the TA)

Plastic dish to collect glass plates and spacers

10 mL syringe with bent 18 G needle

Hot plate, tube holder and 500 mL beaker (1 set for the whole class)

100 mL of 2% agarose in 70 °C water bath

10× SDS running buffer

Distilled water

One tube of molecular weight standards (prestained and unstained)

Two tubes of sample buffer (one with DTT and one without)

50 mL of Coomassie Blue

500 mL destain solution

Samples from IgG purification: SM, FT, all washes, eluted IgG.

Micropipettes 20, 200, 1000 μL

Pipet tips 20, 200, 1000 μL

Power supply, cables/electrodes

Electrophoresis chambers (double chambers)

Waste beaker

Single edge razor blade

One large spatula

Four large weigh boats

Three large bull-clamps

All materials for protein assay (see Exercise 15, Chap. 39)

NOTE: If **pre-cast gels** are available, students will proceed to assemble the gels in the gel chambers and use the buffer recommended by the manufacturer for electrophoresis. Students will also use the sample buffer recommended by the manufacturer for denaturing the protein sample before loading the gels.

Assembling SDS-PAGE Gels

Procedure

1. Clean both front and back plates and spacers with absolute ethanol using lint-free paper e.g. kimwipes.
2. To assemble the plates, place the plates and spacers on the surface of clean bench paper, taking care not to touch the surface of the plates after cleaning. Handle the plates by the edges.

3. Place the three spacers at the sides and bottom of the front plate, then place the back plate which is notched, on top of the front plate forming a sandwich with the spacers in between. See Fig. 36.1.

4. Clamp both plates together, at both sides and at the bottom of the plate. Open the clamps using the bottom clamp as a stand.

5. Seal the sides of the plate sandwich with 2% agarose using a pipetman.

6. Prepare a homogeneous 10% acrylamide mixture in a 50 mL Ehrlenmeyer flask using the volumes shown in Table 36.1. Add the catalysts immediately before casting the gel.

7. Pipet 6 mL of the acrylamide mixture into the plates, and carefully add a layer of distilled water onto the surface of the acrylamide.

8. Carefully place the comb in between the plates and allow the gel to polymerize in approximately 30 min. While the gel is polymerizing prepare the stacking gel in a 50 mL Ehrlenmeyer flask without the catalysts. Once a line of retraction forms at the interface of the water and the gel indicating that the gel is polymerized, pour out the water and blot the sides of the plate dry with kimwipes. Add the TEMED and Ammonium persulfate to the stacking gel mixture and pour the mixture on top of the separating (=running) gel. Allow the stacking gel to polymerize for approximately 10–20 min.

9. Carefully remove the bottom spacers and combs from SDS-PAGE gels and attach gels to electrophoresis chamber with back plate facing gel chamber. Add running buffer to the top chamber and observe for a few minutes for leaks into the bottom chamber. If you observe any leaks, seal the sides of the glass plates with 2% agarose. Add running buffer to the bottom chamber such that the lower part of the gel is completely immersed in the buffer. Remove air bubbles that form in between the plates using a 10 mL syringe with a bent 18 G needle.

10. If precast gels are available, the gel protector strips will be removed from the bottom of the gels, the combs will be removed to expose the loading wells and the gels will be assembled in the electrophoresis chambers using the clamps provided.

11. Connect the electrodes to the gel chamber and to the power supply. **DO NOT TURN THE POWER SUPPLY ON.** Connect the red electrode (+), cathode to

Table 36.1 Components required for preparing separating and stacking acrylamide gel mixtures

Components	Gel concentration		
	10%	**15%**	Stacking gel
Distilled water	4.5 mL	2 mL	11.1 mL
Acrylamide	5 mL	7.5 mL	1.95 mL
1 M Tris pH 8.8	5.5 mL	5.5 mL	
1 M Tris pH 6.8			1.8 mL
10% SDS	0. 15 mL	0. 15 mL	0.075 mL
TEMED	0.01 mL	0.01 mL	0.018 mL
Ammonium persulfate (0.1 g in 1 mL distilled water)	0.05 mL	0.05 mL	0.075 ml

the bottom of the chamber and the black electrode (−) anode, to the top of the chamber. Your proteins will be covered with a net negative charge from the SDS in the sample buffer and will migrate downwards towards the cathode.

12. Pipet 20 μL of your samples and molecular weight standards into two sets of microfuge tubes. Add 20 μL of sample buffer to each tube. Use sample buffer containing DTT for one set and sample buffer without DTT for the second set.

13. Place the tubes in a floating tube holder. Place the tube holder in a 1 L beaker containing boiling water and boil the samples for 2 min (set a timer). Allow the samples to cool for approximately 1 min, then load 20 μL of each sample in each well of the gel using the loading pattern indicated by your instructor (Fig. 36.2). Record this pattern on the gel form provided. The SM, FT, washes, IgG eluate and washes after elution, will be analyzed by SDS-PAGE.

14. Turn the power supply on and electrophorese the gel for 45 min at 25 mA per gel.

15. Turn the power supply off, detach the gel from the chamber and carefully pry the front plate apart using a spatula. Using a razor blade, remove the stacking gel and then mark the orientation of the sample loading pattern by cutting a small piece from the lower left corner of the gel.

16. Place the gels in large weigh boats containing 0.75% Coomassie Blue. Stain for 30 min, pour the dye out and add destain. Continue to destain gels in the next few days till the gel background is clean. For silver staining fix the gel in 50% methanol for 2 h or overnight and follow the silver staining procedure. If the gel is to be transferred to nitrocellulose paper, follow the procedure for western blotting.

17. Record the pattern of the stained proteins on the gels.

Determine the approximate molecular weight of the IgG from both gels. **Is there a difference in the bands seen in the gel with DTT and the one without? What is the reason for the difference?**

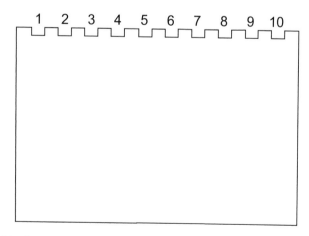

Fig. 36.2 Gel loading template for SDS-PAGE gel

18. Using the samples from the IgG purification determine the protein concentration in duplicate using 10 μL of the samples. BSA standards will be provided to generate a standard curve from which the concentration of IgG will be determined. Determine the protein concentration from the standard curve by extrapolating the values from the curve. Compare the OD readings with those obtained on the first day of the IgG experiment, measured at 280 nm.

19. **NOTE:** In rabbit immunization experiments, the titer of the IgG will be determined using parasite antigen coated plates by ELISA and the specificity of the antibodies will be determined by immunoblotting schizont antigens on nitrocellulose paper. In addition, the antibody will be used to detect parasite epitopes on acetone fixed smears of schizont- infected blood smears by immunofluorescence assay. The sera from the different bleedings will also be used to perform Ouchterlony double diffusion assays to determine the time of IgG appearance in the rabbit serum.

Silver Staining

1. Place the gel in a clean plastic container and fix the gel in 50% methanol for at least 2 h or overnight at RT.
2. Wash the gel five times for 5 min each wash.
3. Stain the gel for 15 min on a shaker using the following staining solution prepared fresh:
   Solution A-0.8 g silver nitrate in 4 mL distilled water
   Solution B-21 mL of 0.36% sodium hydroxide, 1.4 mL ammonium hydroxide
   Add solution A into–solution B dropwise by titration into an Ehrlenmyer flask, while mixing on a stir plate. Do not allow the solution to precipitate. Look for a brown flashpoint and continue to stir until the solution clears up.
   Bring the volume up to 100 mL with distilled water.
4. Wash the gel five times, each wash at 5 min.
5. Develop the gel for 10 min using the following solution:
   2.5 mL 1.0% citric acid
   0.25 mL 37% formaldehyde
   Bring the volume to 500 mL with distilled water.
   Mix the solution thoroughly
6. Wrap the plastic container with foil during development.
   Check for developed bands within the first 2–3 min as the bands may become overdeveloped if the protein concentration is high.
7. Wash the gel three times for 10 min each wash in distilled water.
8. Store the gel in 50% methanol, wrapped in foil at room temperature.

Chapter 37
Exercise 13: Immunoblotting (Western Blotting)

Introduction

Western blotting (also known as immunoblotting), is a highly sensitive, solid-phase assay that is performed routinely in research and clinical laboratories. It is routinely performed to detect the presence of specific antibodies to an antigen or to identify a specific antigen in a complex mixture of proteins. For example, a specific viral, bacterial or parasite antigen can be identified by its reactivity with specific antibodies from an individual patient's serum. In general, a specific antibody is used to identify a specific cognate antigen from a heterogeneous mixture of proteins. The protein identified is in a denatured, linear conformation on transfer to nitrocellulose paper or nylon membrane from a replica SDS-PAGE gel. Polyclonal, monospecific polyclonal or monoclonal antibodies (primary antibodies) are employed in western blotting assays, and incubated with the transferred proteins on nitrocellulose paper following blocking of non-reactive sites on the paper by albumin, gelatin or milk proteins in the presence of Tween to reduce nonspecific binding. The primary antibodies are detected by species-specific secondary antibody conjugated to an enzyme such as **alkaline phosphatase, horseradish peroxidase or biotin-labeled** antibodies can be detected by the specific interaction of enzyme conjugated streptavidin. Cleavage of an enzyme substrate, results in the development of an insoluble colored product that precipitates on the protein bands, making the specific reactive protein bands visible against the white background of the nitrocellulose paper. The secondary antibodies may also be labeled with a radioactive substrate such as ^{125}I iodine and the antigen–antibody complexes detected on X-ray film by autoradiography. For safety reasons, detection is now commonly detected by colorimetry, by chemiluminescence or by fluorescence. Levels of antibody reactivity and the intensity of protein bands detected can be quantitated when chemiluminescenc or fluorescence is used for detection.

Pre-stained protein standards separated on the same gel serves as good indicators of efficient transfer. However, due to the size, concentration and other properties of

© Springer Nature Switzerland AG 2021
T. Y. Sam-Yellowe, *Immunology: Overview and Laboratory Manual*,
https://doi.org/10.1007/978-3-030-64686-8_37

the proteins to be analyzed, transfer may be inefficient. In addition, if the antibody reactivity is dependent on tertiary conformation of the protein epitopes, there may be no reaction or antibody reactivity may be reduced. Blocking the un-reacted sites on the nitrocellulose paper is also necessary to reduce background and to increase the sensitivity of the assay. Control reactions on western blots treated with positive and negative control antibodies are also necessary to allow for correct interpretations of results obtained. An advantage of this highly sensitive assay is that very small concentrations of antibodies are required to detect the protein of interest, and in cases where antibody detection is desired small concentrations of labeled antigen can be used to detect separated antibody on NCP.

The western blot technique is similar to other blotting techniques such as Southern blotting which is a hybridization technique used to detect DNA (gDNA or cDNA) fragments and Northern blotting which is used to detect RNA.

The **objective** of this exercise is to learn how to perform a western blot and identify proteins reactive with a specific antibody.

Materials and Reagents (Per Pair)

All materials for SDS-PAGE gel electrophoresis
SDS-PAGE gel with separated proteins
Transblot chamber
Power supply
Nitrocellulose paper (NCP)
4 pieces of 3 MM Whatman filter paper
2 Scotch brite sponges
Cassette holders
Absolute methanol (1.2 L)
Distilled water (4 L)
10× transfer buffer (1 L)
10× tris buffered saline (Blot buffer) (1 L)
Plastic tupperware trays with lids
Primary antibodies
Secondary antibodies
Carnation milk powder
Tween-20
Fetal bovine serum
Large plastic container or tray (for assembling transfer "sandwich")
Bench paper
Scissors
Gloves
Pencils
Kimwipes
Plastic "ziploc" storage bags

Large weigh boats
Plastic bag sealer

For some experiments each pair of students will begin the blotting procedure from step #9.
Nitrocellulose paper containing already transferred proteins will be provided stored in Tris buffered saline (TBS). Proceed to the blocking step and continue with the rest of the assay. One piece of NCP will be incubated in test antiserum and the other piece in control preimmune rabbit serum. Both papers will have the same protein loading pattern in all lanes.

For some experiments each pair of students will begin the procedure from step # 1 and continue to the antibody detection of proteins on NCP. Follow the instructions contained in the laboratory schedule or announced in class.

The primary antibody is rabbit antiserum prepared against *Plasmodium* sp. proteins or commercially obtained rabbit antibodies specific for the serum samples listed below for the evaluation of immunophylogenetic relationships of proteins.

The following antigens may be separated in different combinations by SDS-PAGE to determine the relationship of serum proteins among different species:

Fetal bovine serum (FBS), chicken serum (CHS), human serum (HS), human albumin (HA), ovalabumin (OVA), bovine serum albumin (BSA), horse serum (HRS), donkey serum (DKYS), goat serum (GS), sheep serum (SHPS), mouse serum (MS), rat serum, (RA), hamster serum (HMS), rabbit serum (RS), cat serum (CTS), catfish serum (CFS), dog serum (DS), monkey serum (MKYS), pig serum (PS), and Kangaroo serum (KS).

Depending on the source of the primary antibody, the Secondary antibody will be a goat anti-rabbit IgG conjugated to horseradish peroxidase (GAR-HRP), or alkaline phosphatase (AP) or rabbit anti-mouse IgG conjugated to horseradish peroxidase (RAM-HRP), or alkaline phosphatase (AP). Protein A-conjugated to either enzyme may also be used. Protein A binds specifically and with high affinity to the Fc region of rabbit IgG and with varying levels of affinity for IgG from other species. If the antisera obtained has been produced in different species such as a goat or horse, then the appropriate secondary antibody, in this case sheep anti-goat IgG or sheep anti-horse IgG antibodies will be used. The western blot procedure may be performed as a direct assay, in which case the primary antibody is conjugated to the enzyme. An indirect western blot may also be performed. In an indirect assay, the primary antibody is unconjugated. However, the secondary antibody specific to the primary antibody is conjugated with the enzyme. The substrate for peroxidase is 4-chloro-1-naphthol provided as a lyophilized powder or as tablets. The substrate ophenylenediamine dihydrochloride (OPD) is used for AP-conjugated antibodies. (Other substrates may be substituted depending on commercial availability).

NOTE: This exercise may be performed simultaneously with a genotyping exercise using genomic DNA isolated from cells of specific organisms whose serum is being analyzed. The rabbit IgG isolated by affinity binding to protein-A sepharose beads will be analyzed by western blotting using goat anti-rabbit IgG-HRP in a direct western blotting procedure. Isolated IgG will also be tested to identify stage specific antigens using extracts from the ring, young trophozoite, mature schizont and segmented schizont stages of *P. falciparum* and *P. chabaudi*.

Procedure

1. Separate protein samples on a 10% SDS-PAGE gel, using the SDS-PAGE protocol outlined above. If commercial pre-cast gels are available, they can be assembled directly in to the gel chambers and the wells loaded with the protein samples to be separated.

2. Cut the NCP and 3 MM Whatman filter paper to the size of the gel to be transferred and equilibrate in 1× transfer buffer. Transfers can be performed as wet transfers or semi-dry transfers. For wet transfers of large gels, up to 6 L of buffer is required. Small wet transfer chambers require 3 L of buffer. Semi-dry chambers need approximately 300–500 mL of buffer for soaking and saturating NCP and filter papers. Buffer is not needed during the transfer process for semi-dry protocols. The 1× transfer buffer is prepared by adding the following reagents to distilled water (volumes can be adjusted to make more or less volumes as needed):

   (a) 10% of 10× transfer buffer 20% absolute methanol
   (b) 70% distilled water Total volume 6000 mL

3. Once the electrophoresis is complete, separate the glass plates by gently prying the plates apart using a spatula. Remove the front plate carefully, and with the gel positioned in the same orientation as when it was loaded, cut a piece of the gel at the bottom left corner of the gel to mark the orientation. Carefully pick up the gel by holding the bottom part of the gel, taking care not to tear the gel. Place the gel on top of the NCP. See orientation of western components in step 4 (Figs. 37.1 and 37.2)

4. Proceed to prepare a transfer sandwich for wet transfer in the orientation shown below.

5. Place filter papers, Scotch brite sponges and nitrocellulose paper in a large plastic container (provided) containing 1× transfer buffer to equilibrate (Fig. 37.1)

   (a) Place the plastic cassette on the bench (A tray may be provided for this). **The bench should have bench paper covering your work space.**
   (b) Place one Scotch brite sponge equilibrated in 1× transfer buffer on top of the cassette.
   (c) Place two pieces of 3 MM Whatman paper equilibrated in 1× transfer buffer on top of the sponge. Depending on the thickness of the filter paper, only one piece will be used.
   (d) Place the NCP equilibrated in 1× transfer buffer on top of the 3 MM filter paper.
   (e) Place the SDS-PAGE gel on the NCP paper. Avoid the formation of air bubbles. If bubbles form, these can be removed by *gently* pressing down on

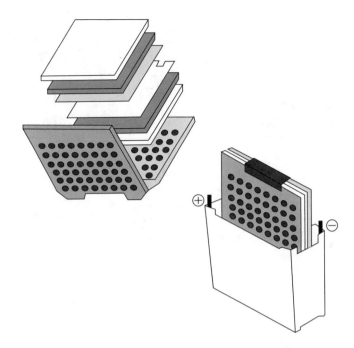

Fig. 37.1 Western blot sandwich assembly showing SDS-PAGE gel "sandwiched" between filter papers and cassettes. Locked cassette is placed vertically in a wet transfer buffer system contained in an electrophoresis chamber

the gel, smoothing them out toward the edges of the gel with your fingers. Moisten your gloved fingers with transfer buffer before pushing the bubbles to the edge.

(f) Place two pieces of 3 MM filter paper equilibrated in 1× transfer buffer on top of gel (depending on the thickness of the filter paper, only one may be used).

(g) Place one Scotch brite sponge equilibrated in 1× transfer buffer on top of the 3 MM filter paper.

(h) Place the second cassette on top of the sandwich and lock in place into the bottom cassette (some cassettes have a sliding lock, snap lock or other interlocking fastners; some require rubberbands to secure the sandwich).

6. Add 1× transfer buffer into the transblot chamber to approximately ¾ full, and place a stir bar in the chamber.

7. Check to make sure that the entire sandwich is secured with a rubber band or other interlocking fasteners on the cassettes. Gently pick up the sandwich and **with the NCP positioned closest to the positive electrode**, slide the cassette into the transblot chamber. It is important not to dislodge the components of the sandwich at this point.

8. Place the transblot chamber on a stir plate, turn it on to medium speed and connect the electrodes to a power supply set at constant current and transfer at

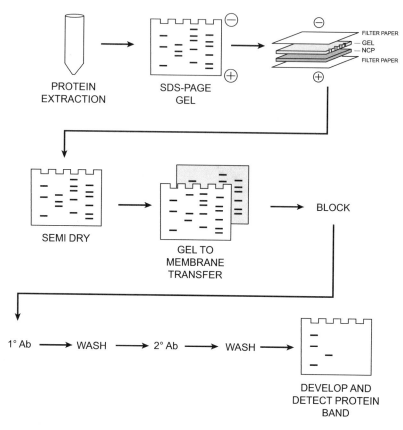

Fig. 37.2 Schematic illustration of SDS-PAGE and western plot procedure showing antibody identification of a single protein band from a heterogeneous mixture of proteins

300–400 mA for 4 h. For semi-dry chambers, electrophoresis will be performed for 2 h at 100 mA.

9. At the completion of the transfer, remove the cassette and carefully dismantle the sandwich. Place the transferred SDS-PAGE gel in a plastic container, add Coomassie blue to cover the gel and stain for 30 min on an orbital shaker. **NOTE:** <u>Proceed to step 9 while the gel is staining</u>. After 30 min, pour out the stain into flask (labeled used stain). Gently press down the gel with a gloved hand as you pour out the stain, to prevent the gel from sliding out of the container. Add destain solution to the gel, cover the container and place the container on the orbital shaker. After 30 min, check the gel. The background of the gel should begin to clear so that the blue stained protein bans are visible against the clear background. Pour out the destain solution and replace with fresh destain.

10. Place the transferred NCP in a plastic container containing blocking solution. Incubate the NCP for 30 min on an orbital shaker, at room temperature (RT), to block unreacted sites on the NCP. A large plastic weigh boat can be used in

place of the plastic container. We will use 2% milk/0.1% Tween 20 in Tris buffered saline (TBS, blocking buffer). Other blocking solutions that can be used are 1% bovine serum albumin (BSA), 1% gelatin, or 1% hemoglobin.

11. After blocking, incubate the NCP in primary antibody diluted at 1:200 in 5 mL of 5% fetal bovine serum/TBS, for 1 h, in a plastic bag, at RT or overnight at 4 °C. If performing a direct western blot procedure, incubate the blocked NCP in antibody conjugated with enzyme. In order to detect the purified IgG, the NCP containing separated proteins will be incubated in 1:1000 goat anti-rabbit HRP for 1 h or overnight at 4 °C.

12. After antibody incubation, pipet the antibody solution from the NCP using a plastic 1 mL squeezer and place the used antibody in a 15 mL centrifuge tube. Add 1× blot buffer to the NCP, enough to cover the paper and place the container containing the NCP on the orbital shaker. Incubate for 5 min, pour out the wash buffer into the waste container provided and repeat the wash step 3 more times using the procedure shown below.

   (a) First wash in 1× TBS
   (b) Second wash in 1× TBS
   (c) Third wash in 0.5% Triton X-100 in 1× TBS
   (d) Fourth wash in 1× TBS

13. If you are performing a direct assay, proceed to step 14 to develop the NCP (For the detection of the purified IgG, we will be performing a direct assay). If performing an indirect assay, incubate the NCP in GAR-HRP diluted at 1:1000 in 5 mL of 5% fetal bovine serum/TBS for 30 min at RT or overnight at 4 °C, then proceed to step 14.

14. Wash the NCP as in step 11, but leave the NCP in the last wash until the substrate solution has been prepared. The substrate solution should be prepared fresh.

15. Preparing the substrate solution:

(a) **Solution A:** Add a 30 mg tablet (substrate is also available in powder form and can be weighed also 30 mg) of 4-chloro-1-naphthol to 10 mL of ice-cold methanol in a 200 mL Erlenmeyer flask and mix to dissolve.

(b) **Solution B:** Add 30 μL of 30% Hydrogen peroxide to 50 mL of ice-cold TBS in a 100 mL Erlenmeyer flask.

(c) **Add solution B to solution A.** Mix properly by gently swirling the solution around in the flask, and use it immediately.

Pour out the last wash from your NCP then add the substrate solution to the NCP. Incubate the NCP in the dark for 10 min on a shaker e.g. cover the plastic container with aluminum foil while it is on the shaker (the plastic tray can also be incubated in a bench drawer). Observe the color development of the bands and prolong or shorten development appropriately. Stop the color development by pouring off the substrate solution and adding distilled water to the NCP. Record your results. Compare the NCP that was treated with test antiserum to the one that was treated with control serum. Do you observe any differences in the number or the intensity of the bands seen on the NCP? Also compare the number of antibody reactive bands on the NCP with the bands remaining on the destained gel.

Chapter 38
Exercise 14: Protein Assay

Introduction

The Coomassie Blue dye binding assay is a sensitive assay for determining protein concentration in samples and is based on the method originally developed by Bradford. The assay is reproducible, straightforward and easy to perform. Furthermore, the dye is compatible with various biochemical reagents, e.g. detergent solutions, buffers, chaotropic salts, preservatives such as sodium azide, some acids such as HCl etc. The proteins dissolved or mixed in any of these reagents can be measured. The assay is based on the principle of an absorbance shift resulting from an acidic Coomassie Brilliant Blue G-250 solution. When the dye solution is added to a protein sample interaction of the dye's sulfonic groups with the protein results in a color change from brown to blue. This change can be measured at 595, 650 and 470 nm corresponding to anionic, neutral and cationic equilibrium states respectively for the Coomassie Blue dye.

The color response is non-linear over wide ranges of protein concentration and the color produced by a given amount of protein is influenced by temperature changes. So a standard curve is prepared with each assay. Other than the standard assay, the procedure can be modified and performed as a micro assay or performed in microliter plates. Protein concentrations of less than 1 μg/mL can be measured. The **first objective** of this exercise is to learn how to prepare a standard curve for protein determination and the **second objective** is to learn how to use the spectrophotometer.

Materials and Reagents (Per Group)

20 glass test tubes, 16 × 100 mm
10 mL glass pipets

© Springer Nature Switzerland AG 2021
T. Y. Sam-Yellowe, *Immunology: Overview and Laboratory Manual*,
https://doi.org/10.1007/978-3-030-64686-8_38

Micropipette 200 µL, 20 µL
Pipet tips
Dye solution-100 mL (this is a commercial reagent from Biorad or Pierce)
BSA or Ig protein standard-1.5 mg/mL or 2.0 mg/mL
Unknown samples
500 mL beakers
Erlenmeyer flasks with 100 mL distilled water
Vortex
Spectrophotometer
Cuvettes

Procedure

1. Pipet protein standards into duplicate labeled test tubes using the following volumes: 0, 5, 6.6, 16.6, 26.6, 33.3, 66.6 and 100 µL (depending on the standard protein provided, the volumes will be changed). Pipet 10 and 20 µL of your unknown sample also into duplicate test tubes. The tube without a protein standard solution will be used as your blank.
2. Add distilled water to the protein standards for a final volume of 100 µL.
3. Add 5 mL of protein dye to each tube and vortex briskly. Cover the tubes with parafilm and incubate for 10–20 min at room temperature.
4. Using the cuvettes provided, measure the optical density (O.D.) (Absorbance) of the samples at 595 nm and record the values in your notebook or in a chart provided by your TA.
5. Calculate the average for the blank tubes, each pair of standards and the unknowns. Subtract the average O.D. of the blanks from the standards and unknowns and plot the values on linear graph paper to prepare a standard curve. Extrapolate the values of your unknowns from the standard curve and determine the protein concentration of your unknowns.

PROTEIN DETERMINATION ASSAY TABLE:

DATE:						
NATURE OF SAMPLES:						
NAME:						
Tube#	sample vol.	vol.dH$_2$O 595nm	O.D.	X O.D.	X-Blank O.D.	µg protein

NOTES:

Selected References

Bradford M (1976) A rapid and sensitive method for the quantitation of microgram quantities of protein utilizing the principle of protein-dye binding. Anal Biochem 72:248

Spector T (1978) Refinement of the Coomassie blue method of protein quantitation. A simple and linear spectrophotometric assay for less than or equal to 0.5 to 50 microgram of protein. Anal Biochem 86:142

Chapter 39
Exercise 15: Enzyme-Linked Immunosorbent Assay (ELISA)

Introduction

The **enzyme-linked immunosorbent** assay (ELISA) is a highly sensitive, rapid, relatively cheap solid-phase immunoassay that is used to screen for the presence of, and specificity of a given antibody to an antigen, or to quantitatively determine the concentrations of antibodies and soluble antigens from sources such as patient sera, immunized hosts or antibody secretion by hybridomas. The ELISA can also measure the affinity of an antibody to an antigen. When known amounts of specific antibodies are available, unknown antigens can be detected and their concentrations determined. Protein antigens between 100 pg/mL and 1 ng/mL can be detected. The ELISA is also used to determine the titer of antibodies, most routinely used for antibodies such as monoclonal antibodies.

The assay is based on the **radioimmunoassay (RIA)** developed by Berson and Yalow. In RIA the competitive binding of a saturable concentration of ^{125}I-labeled antigen to a high affinity specific antibody is evaluated in the presence of increasing amounts of unlabeled antigen. The concentration of the unlabeled antigen is unknown and since both antibodies are the same, the unlabeled antigens will displace the labeled antigen from the binding site. The concentration of labeled antigen free in solution is used to determine the concentration of unlabeled antigen. The basic principle of the ELISA although similar to RIA, involves the use of an enzyme-conjugated antibody, rather than a radioactively labeled antibody to detect the interaction of the antibody to its cognate antigen. The antigen is usually attached to a solid phase support such as a polystyrene tube or microtiter plate, or microtiter pins. Addition of a chromogenic enzyme substrate e.g. pnitrophenyl phosphate (NPP), the secondary reagent (not to be confused with secondary antibody) results in hydrolysis of the substrate and the formation of a colored product which can be visualized and also measured spectrophotometrically (schematic illustration of the assay—Fig. 39.1). Fluorogenic enzyme substrates are also used, and are 10–100 times faster than chromogenic assay. A commonly used fluorochrome is

© Springer Nature Switzerland AG 2021
T. Y. Sam-Yellowe, *Immunology: Overview and Laboratory Manual*,
https://doi.org/10.1007/978-3-030-64686-8_39

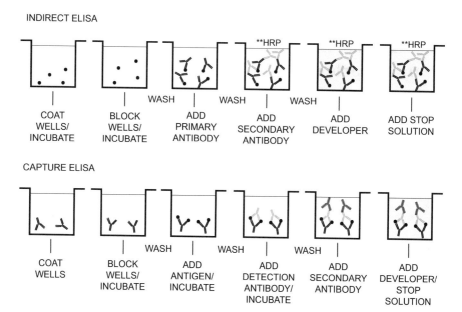

Fig. 39.1 Indirect and capture ELISA. In indirect ELISA, antigen is coated to wells of a microtiter plate, wells are blocked and primary antibody is added to wells. Secondary antibody conjugated to HRP is added and following the addition of substrate, reactive wells are identified. In capture ELISA, capture antibody is coated to wells of a 96 well plate, wells are blocked, antigen is added followed by detection antibody. Biotinylated secondary antibody is added followed by streptavidin-HRP. After substrate addition, wells are developed to detect antigen

4-methylurnbelliferyl phosphate (MUP). Enzyme-labeled antigens may also be used in a capture assay. Several types of ELISA washers and readers are available to provide reproducible wash steps and to quantitate the degree of enzyme hydrolysis following substrate addition. Following coating of the wells with antibody or antigen, the nonreactive sites on the plates are blocked with bovine serum albumin (BSA), and in between incubations with each reagent, the wells are washed several times to remove unbound reagents. Positive and negative controls are included in the assay to aid in proper interpretation of results. In antibody sandwich assays or indirect assays, an enzyme-conjugated secondary antibody (tertiary reagent), is also added and this binds to antigen-primary antibody complex.

Several enzymes are used for the ELISA, however some of the most commonly used are horseradish peroxidase (HRP), alkaline phosphatase (AP), urease, beta-galatosidase and glucoamylase. Both HRP and AP are two of the most widely used.

Due to the sensitivity of the assay, several precautions are undertaken to ensure the reproducibility of the assay and facilitate interpretation of the assay. The concentration of antigen and antibody is optimized by performing crisscross serial 1:2 dilutions also referred to as checker board titrations. A constant concentration of antigen or antibody is reacted with serially diluted antigen or antibody, respectively, and the degree of enzyme hydrolysis is measured or visualized. The criss-cross assay is particularly valuable when strictly polyclonal antibodies, monospecific polyclonal antibodies or heterogeneous mixtures of antigen solutions are used. The concentrations of antibody and antigen resulting in an OD of 0.5 when NPP is used is considered as optimal. For most assays the antigen does not have to be pure, however, the desired epitope(s) should represent at least 1–3% of the protein in the antigen mixture.

Several variations of the assay are performed, and depend on the nature of the question or experiment. The assay can be performed as a direct antibody-antigen interaction where the primary antibody is enzyme-labeled, or the sensitive indirect antibody-sandwich assay, where an enzyme-labeled species specific secondary antibody is used to detect the interaction between the antigen and the primary antibody. In both assays the antigen is coated on the surface of a 96-well microtiter plate. The antibody sandwich method can also be performed to detect specific antigen. In this form, the antibody is coated to the wells of a microtiter plate (capture antibody), followed by the addition of the soluble antigen solution, and an antibody-enzyme conjugate.

Competitive ELISAs are also performed, and are used to determine the close similarity or differences between antigen epitopes or between antibodies. Epitopes can be mapped using this method. Immunoglobulin G fragments obtained by pepsin or papain digestion, F(ab')2 or Fab fragments, respectively, can also be used directly in ELISAs or conjugated to HRP or AP as labeled secondary antibodies, providing a highly specific reaction.

Some of the more practical concerns for ensuring reproducible results include maintaining constant experimental conditions from start to finish, and using the same batch of reagents for a given experiment. Reagents should be prepared as stock solutions filtered or autoclaved, and stored to be diluted to working concentrations as needed. The concentrations should be kept constant, incubation times and temperature, as well as wash times and temperature should also be kept constant. Samples should be run in triplicates or at least in duplicates to facilitate statistical analysis of the data. It is also desirable to include a standard curve in all plates to control for microenvironmental variations among different plates. The **objective** of this exercise is to learn how to perform the ELISA assay.

Materials and Reagents (Per Pair)

Spectrophotometer
ELISA plate washer
ELISA plate reader
Vortex
Distilled water
13 × 100 mm glass tubes
1 microfuge tube containing 150 µL of rabbit anti-Lipopolysaccharide (LPS)
1 microfuge tube containing 150 µL of rabbit anti-Goat serum (GS)

1 microfuge tube containing 150 µL of rabbit anti-Bovine serum albumin (BSA)
1 microfuge tube containing 150 µL of rabbit anti-Chicken ovalbumin (OVA)

   NOTE: In some experiments rabbit antisera specific for human albumin, human serum or malaria parasite proteins will be used. Monoclonal antibodies (mouse antibodies) specific for a given protein may also be used. In some exercises, we will screen "human sera" for the presence of antibodies against an infectious pathogen and also determine the antibody isotype reacting with the antigens from the pathogen. Any change, usually due to availability or titer, of a particular reagent, will be announced in class.

Materials and Reagents (Per Pair)

One Erhlemeyer flask containing 500 mL of washing buffer
1 tube of secondary antibody—10 mL
One tube of antigen-lipopolysaccharide (LPS, endotoxin), goat serum (GS), ovalbumin (OVA), bovine serum albumin (BSA) and *E. coli* lysate diluted in coating buffer, 10 mL/plate
In some experiments as indicated above other antigens can be used for coating wells. This will be announced in class.
One tube of diluting buffer—10 mL/plate
One tube of substrate solution—10 mL/plate
One tube of stopping solution—10 mL/plate
Four 96-well microtiter plates plus lids
10 mL disposable pipets, microdiluters
Eppendorf
Plastic 1 mL squeezer pipets
Gloves
Bench paper
Scissors
Kimwipes
Ice bucket

   In some experiments, each pair will receive microtiter plates previously coated with antigen. In that case continue with the ELISA procedure from step 5. For experiments where antigen application will be performed in class the ELISA procedure will be started from step 1 (see Fig. 39.1)

Starting with Pre-Coated Plates

Each pair will receive four 96-well microtiter plates. One plate will contain coated antigens i.e. rows A–C coated with LPS and rows E–G coated with GS. A second plate will contain BSA in rows A–C and OVA in rows E–G. The second uncoated plate in each set will be used to perform serial 1:2 dilutions of the antibodies. To set up the serial dilutions, add 50 μL of PBS to all wells in the plate except well #1 in row A and well #1 in row E (these wells will contain your undiluted antibody). Add 50 μL of anti-LPS to well #1 and #2 in row A. Add 50 μL of anti-GS to well #1 and #2 in row E. in the second coated plate, add 50 μL of anti-BSA to well #1 and #2 in row A and 50 μL of anti-OVA to wells #1 and #2 in row E. In each case #1 contains undiluted antibody and #2 contains a 1:2 dilution of the antibody.

Beginning from well #2 start making serial 1:2 dilutions using a microdiluter and continue to well #10 in row C (for anti-LPS) and to well #10 in row G for anti-GS. To dilute the antibody twirl the microdiluter gently but briskly in the well and then transfer the microdiluter to the next well in the series. Fifty μL of antibody is transferred each time. When you get to the last well, burn off the excess antibody with the flame from a bunsen burner.

Add 50 μL of normal rabbit serum (NRS) (negative control) to well #11 in rows C and G. Well #12 will not receive any antibody.

To proceed, complete the serial dilutions and transfer the diluted antibodies to the same numbered wells in the antigen coated plates using the transfer pipets with the pointed tips. Use the same pipet to transfer the antibodies starting from the least dilute well backwards to the most concentrated well. Use a different pipet for each type of antibody i.e. one for anti-LPS, one for anti-GS, one for anti-OVA, one for anti-BSA and one for NRS. Also transfer the PBS in well #12. This is your second negative control.

For adding the secondary antibodies, substrate and stopping solution, use the small transfer pipets. Each drop is 50 μL, so for 100 μL add two drops. For washing the wells, use the graduated squeezer pipets to add the washing solution to each well.

Detection of LPS in Extracts of *E. coli* Lysates

Procedure

1. Prepare antigen solution in coating buffer (0.2 M sodium bicarbonate, pH 9.4) at a concentration of approximately 1 μg/mL. We will use *E. coli* LPS, BSA, GS, OVA and *E. coli* lysate as antigens.
2. Coat wells of 96-well microtiter plates by adding 100 μL of antigen with an Eppendorf micropipet to each well and incubating the plates for 2 h at RT (or overnight at 4 °C).
3. Remove unbound antigen by inverting the plates and tapping out antigen into a waste beaker, pan or in the sink. Remove the residual antigen by placing the plate upside down on blotting plate or on a stack of paper towels. Wash the wells three times by adding approximately 100 μL of wash buffer into each well, using a plastic squeezer, and shaking the plates gently from side to side to ensure the sides of the well are also washed. Discard the wash buffer as indicated above for the antigen. The residual wash buffer should be blotted as indicated after each wash.

4. Add 100 μL of blocking buffer (1% BSA in PBS/0.1% Tween) to each well and incubate the plates for 1 h at RT, then discard the blocking buffer as described above. This step in the procedure is critical. Insufficient blocking will lead to high backgrounds.

5. Add 50 μL of the diluted primary antibodies to each well, and incubate the plates for 45 min at 37 °C. For *E. coli* lysate, use anti-LPS antibodies. Antibodies will be diluted in buffer containing a carrier protein such as gelatin, BSA, fetal bovine serum (FBS) or horse serum at 0.1–0.5%. In addition, Tween 20 at 0.05–0.1% is added. Both components improve the sensitivity of the assay.

6. Discard the unbound antibody and wash the wells three times with wash buffer as described in #3. Make sure the residual wash buffer is blotted out. For antibodies, we will be using rabbit anti-LPS, rabbit anti-GS, rabbit anti-BSA and rabbit anti-OVA. Any changes to the antibodies will be announced.

7. Add 100 μL of the diluted secondary antibody, goat anti-rabbit IgG-horseradish peroxidase (HRP) 1:10,000 dilution to each well, and incubate the plates for 45 min at 37 °C. Secondary antibodies will also be diluted in a buffer containing a carrier protein plus Tween 20.

8. Discard the unbound antibodies, and wash the wells three times as in #3.

9. Add 100 μL of 1-step turbo TMB substrate solution (3,3′, 5,5′ tetramethylbenzidine)
   (Pierce) to each well and incubate the plates at RT in the dark for 10–20 min. The plates can be covered with foil. A graded blue color reaction will develop in the positive wells. Wells with more antibodies will be proportionately darker than wells with less antibodies. **DO NOT DISCARD THE SUBSTRATE SOLUTION.**
   A second substrate which can also be used in o-phenylenediamine dihydrochloride (OPD).

10. **Add 100 μL of I M H2SO4 to each well still containing the substrate solution**, to stop the enzyme reaction. The color in the wells will now change to yellow. The plates can now be placed in an ELISA reader to measure the OD at 450 nm in each well. A computer read out will be obtained showing the OD values in each well. For our purposes, we will read the plates visually and also measure the OD, then determine the titer (sensitivity) of the antibodies. This will be compared to the reaction in the control wells. If OPD is used the reaction will be stopped with I N HCI.

We will also measure the OD at 450 nm for one plate by transferring the contents of each well to 13 × 100 mm glass tubes, followed by the addition of 2 mL of distilled water. Vortex briefly, then measure the OD at 450 nm using disposable cuvets or by an aspirator attached to the spectrophotometer. Record the values for each tube. Compare the titers obtained by visual examination of the plates with that obtained by spectrophotometry. For the LPS ELISA, a serial twofold dilution of LPS can be prepared and coated in 96-well microtiter plates. *E. coli* lysate will also be added to the wells of the microtiter plate. After blocking the wells, the antibody titer obtained for anti-LPS in the ELISA procedure above can be added to the wells coated with LPS and *E. coli* lysates. Following incubation with the primary antibody, washing and incubation with the secondary anti-rabbit antibody conjugated to HRP, the wells will be developed. A standard curve of the OD readings obtained for LPS can be generated and used to determine the concentration of LPS present in the *E. coli* lysate. In experiments where recombinant proteins are expressed in *E. coli* host cells for immunization, the levels of endotoxin associated with the recombinant protein may be unsuitable for immunizations. The use of ELISA to determine levels of endotoxin remaining in the recombinant protein after passing the recombinant protein through commercial resins conjugated to polymyxin B, confirm the removal of endotoxin from the recombinant. This will ensure the safe use of the recombinant protein for immunization in rabbits or mice.

Direct ELISA Procedure

1. Prepare coating buffer by diluting 10× buffer 1:10 in distilled water. Prepare 10 mL.
2. Dilute antigen 1:5000 in 1× coating buffer.
3. Add 100 μL of diluted antigen into the wells of a 96 well microtiter plate (antigen may be titrated in this step).
4. Incubate the plate at room temperature (RT) for 45 min.
5. Prepare BSA blocking solution by diluting 10% BSA solution 1:10 in distilled water.
6. Discard unbound antigen from microtiter plate (by turning plate upside down and discarding antigen into a plastic container or directly into the sink).
7. Add 100 μL of blocking solution to microtiter wells.
8. Incubate plate for 10 min at 37 °C.
9. Prepare diluent for antibody conjugate dilution using blocking buffer. Prepare a 1:15 dilution of 10% BSA blocking solution to be used for diluting the antibody.
10. Dilute antibody conjugate 1:5000 (or prepare serial dilution of antibody in microtiter wells) in diluent (antibody may be titrated in this step)
11. Discard blocking buffer from microtiter wells.
12. Add 100 μL of antibody conjugate to microtiter wells and incubate for 45–60 min at RT
    Note: If performing an indirect ELISA, primary antibody without conjugate would be added at this step.
13. Prepare wash solution by diluting 20× wash solution 1:20 in distilled water. Discard antibody conjugate
14. Discard antibody conjugate
15. Wash wells 3× (for more stringency, wash 5×) with wash buffer.
    NOTE: If performing an indirect ELISA, secondary antibody conjugated to enzyme would be added at this step, followed by wash steps as above. The procedure would then continue as indicated in step 16.

16. Prepare the developing substrate by mixing equal volumes of peroxidase substrate solution 1 and peroxidase substrate solution 2 (obtained commercially).
17. Add 100 μL substrate solution to microtiter wells.
18. Incubate for plates 5–10 min and note that well contents will turn blue (record results visually) **DO NOT DISCARD SUBSTRATE SOLUTION IN WELLS.**
19. Add 100 μL of stop solution to wells and note that well contents will turn yellow.
20. Measure OD of wells within 30 min of reaction using an ELISA reader.
21. Read OD of wells in ELISA reader at wavelength of 450 run

    Note: For cytokine capture ELISAs (Fig. 39.1), capture antibodies specific for cytokines will be coated in microtiter wells followed by blocking of nonspecific sites and the application of cytokine standards or samples (such as tissue culture supernatants from cells secreting cytokines). Cytokine detection antibodies (enzyme or biotin conjugated antibodies) can then be used to bind to the cytokines, followed by the addition of developing reagent (substrate) to demonstrate antibody binding to cytokines.

Capture (Sandwich) ELISA

Materials (Per Pair)

High binding 96 well plates with lids
ELISA diluent buffer (1× PBS, 0.1% BSA) and block buffer
ELISA wash buffer (1× PBS, 0.05% Tween-20)
50 mL tubes
1 mL squeezers
1× PBS
Coating buffer
Capture antibodies (mouse anti-IFNγ and anti-IL-4)
Detection antibodies (mouse anti-IFNγ-biotin and anti-IL-4-biotin)
Streptavidin-HRP
Paper towels
Distilled water
Serological pipets (1 and 10 mL)
Timer
100 mL Ehrlenmeyer flasks
Pipetmen (200 μL)
Pipet tips (yellow)
TMB substrate solution (Tetramethylbenzidine)
2N H_2SO_4 (stop solution)
ELISA plate reader
2 L empty waste beaker
4 °C cold room or refrigerator
TH1/TH2 ELISA kits may be purchased from different vendors

Procedure

1. Coat 96 well plates with capture antibody diluted (1–10 μg/mL) in coating buffer.
2. Add 100 μL diluted capture antibody to each well of the microtiter plate.
3. Cover the plate with the plate lid and incubate the plate overnight at 4 °C (plates may also be incubated at RT for 2 or 1 h at 37 °C.
4. Remove lid from the plate, turn the plate upside down in to discard unbound antibody in the waste beaker.
5. Wash the wells three times with ELISA wash buffer by adding wash buffer to the wells, soaking for 1 min, shaking the plates from side to side then turning the plates upside down to discard the wash buffer. After the last wash, place the plate upside down on paper towels to absorb remaining wash buffer.
6. Add 100 μL of blocking solution to each well and incubate as in step 3.
7. Remove blocking solution by turning plate upside down to discard blocking solution. Wash once with wash buffer and block excess on paper towel as in step 5.
8. Add recombinant cytokine standard to wells of the 96 well plate in duplicate and perform a serial twofold dilution of the cytokine in duplicate (see dilution scheme below). Add test T cell culture supernatants to test wells and also perform a serial twofold dilution in duplicate. In negative control wells, add 1× PBS, normal mouse or rabbit serum and irrelevant non-specific antibody. Cover plate and incubate as in step 3.
9. Discard unbound proteins and wash plates as in step 5.
10. Add diluted detection antibody conjugated to biotin. Cover the plates and incubate as in step 5.
11. Discard unbound detection antibody and wash wells with wash buffer five times (form more stringency) as in step 5.
12. Add 100 μL of streptavidin conjugated to horseradish peroxidase (streptavidin-HRP) diluted in ELISA diluent buffer. Cover the plates and incubate at RT for 30 min.
13. Remove lid from plates, discard unbound streptavidin-HRP and wash plates five times as in step 5.
14. Add 100 μL of substrate solution (1× TMB) to wells. Cover plates and incubate at RT in the dark for 15 min. Contents of the wells will turn blue.
15. **DO NOT DISCARD SUBSTRATE SOLUTION**
16. Add 100 μL of the stop solution to the wells. Contents of the wells will turn yellow.
17. Place the plates in an ELISA reader and measure the OD in wells at a wavelength of 450 nm.

Serial Dilution of Cytokines for Step 8 Above

1. Using the plates coated with the capture antibodies and blocked, add 100 μL ELISA diluent buffer to two rows for each cytokine standard. For example, add 100 μL diluent buffer to wells E2 to E7, F2 to F7, G2 to G7 and H2 to H7. Rows E and F are duplicate wells for IFNγ and rows G and H are duplicate wells for IL-4.
2. Add 100 μL of IFNγ cytokine standards to wells E1 and E2 and F1 and F2. Add 100 μL of IL-4 cytokine standard to wells G1 and G2 and H1 and H2.
3. Using a pipettor and yellow pipet tip, perform serial 1:2 dilution from wells E2 to E7 by gently pipetting up and down the contents of well E2 and transferring 100 μL of the well contents to well E3. Repeat pipetting up and down and transfer 100 μL to well E4. Repeat and continue the transfers till well E7. Perform the same dilutions for wells F2 to F7, G2 to G7 and H2 to H7. Take care not to scratch the bottoms of the wells.
4. Add the test culture supernatants from T cell cultures or mouse serum to rows A and B. In rows C and D add PBS controls and blank control wells.
5. Continue the procedure by covering the plates and incubating them overnight at 4 °C (or 1h at 37 °C or 2 h at RT) and proceeding to step 9 as indicated above.

Questions

1. How does the ELISA assay differ from radioimmunoassays (RIA)?
2. How sensitive an assay is the ELISA compared to precipitation and agglutination reactions?
3. What is the advantage of using capture ELISA to quantitate the concentration of cytokine in culture supernatant obtained from activated T cell culture?

ELISA ASSAYS:

DATE:

PURPOSE OF EXPERIMENT:

Selected References

Kemeny DM (1992) Titration of antibodies. J Immunol Methods 150:57–76

Punt S, Jones O (2019) Kuby immunology, 8th edn. W. H. Freeman and Company, New York. Antigen-antibody interactions; Ch. 20

Venkatesan P, Wakelin D (1993) ELISAs for parasitologists: or lies damned lies and ELISAs. Parasitol Today 9:228–232

Chapter 40
Exercise 16: Enzyme-Linked Immunospot Assay (ELISPOT)

Introduction

The ELISPOT assay was developed for the detection of single antibody secreting cells (B lymphocytes) and in many ways it has replaced the hemolytic plaque assay. The ELISPOT assay is also used for the detection of single cytokine secreting cells (T lymphocytes). The ELISPOT assay can be used together with the ELISA assay (Enzyme linked immunosorbent assay) to estimate the production of antibody molecules and cytokines produced by a single cell and to obtain the titer. In the ELISPOT assay, antibody or cytokine secreting cells are added to each well of a 96 well microtiter plate coated with antigen or antibody. Instead of the usual polystyrene wells used for ELISA, the plates for ELISPOT have nitrocellulose membranes at the bottom of the wells. The cells are cultured for 3 h (up to 5 days if mitogen stimulated), removed and the wells washed in buffer. A second antibody conjugated to an enzyme is then added and in the final step, a substrate is added that results in an insoluble product visualized on the membrane as spots or plaques. These spots can be counted microscopically under low magnification to determine the number of antibody or cytokine secreting cells in the sample (Fig. 40.1). In the ELISA assay a soluble antigen is used to coat the wells and antibody is added in solution. The added substrate results in a soluble product that can be measured using a spectrophotometer i.e. an ELISA plate reader.

With the ELISPOT, two different cytokines or antibodies with different specificities can be detected simultaneously using substrates that result in different colored spots.

You will receive plates already coated with rabbit anti- mouse IL-2 (Plate #1) and chicken ovalbumin (Plate #2), and cultured with different dilutions of a mouse spleen cell suspension. Cells used for the detection of IL-2 will also be incubated in the presence of phorbol-12-myristate-13-acetate (PMA) 20 ng/mL and Concanavalin A (10 ug/mL). Control wells will be incubated without mitogen. You will begin the

© Springer Nature Switzerland AG 2021
T. Y. Sam-Yellowe, *Immunology: Overview and Laboratory Manual*,
https://doi.org/10.1007/978-3-030-64686-8_40

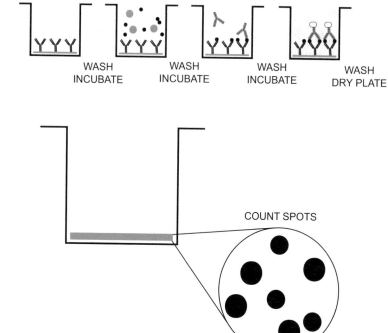

Fig. 40.1 ELISPOT Assay. Antibody or cytokine secreting cells will be identified as dark spots on the nitrocellulose membrane

procedure from step #3 below. The **objective** of the exercise is to learn how to perform ELISPOT assays.

Materials and Reagents (Per Pair)

Mouse spleen cell suspension
37 °C incubator
Phorbol-12-myristate-13-acetate (PMA)
Concanavalin A
1× PBS
Wash buffer (1× PBS with 0.5% Tween)
Blocking solution
10 and 1 mL serological pipets
Gilson pipettors (200 μL)
HRP-conjugated secondary antibody
Microtiter plates with PVDF membranes
Anti-IL-2 antibody

4-chloro-l-napthol solution (mixed in methanol and hydrogen peroxide solution in PBS)
Paper towels
Kimwipes
Waste beaker (empty 500 mL beaker)

Procedure

1. Wash plates three times with 1× PBS, 1× PBS plus 0.5% Tween and again with 1× PBS. Add 100 μL of the wash buffer to each well for each of the washes.
2. Add 200 μL of blocking buffer, 2% milk in 1× PBS, in each well and incubate for 30 min at 37 °C.
3. Discard blocking buffer and wash once in 1× PBS. Drain wells thoroughly by inverting plates and tapping dry on paper towel.
4. Add 50 μL of 1:3000 dilution of goat anti-rabbit lgG-HRP and 1:250 dilution of goat anti-mouse IgG-HRP to plate #1 and plate #2 respectively. Incubate for 90 min at 37 °C.
5. Wash three times as in step #1. Add 50 μl of 4-chloro-l-napthol. Incubate for 15–30 min, discard substrate and wash wells once with distilled water. Count spots or plaques under 4× magnification. Spots will be dark purple or blue.

Questions
How does the ELISPOT differ from ELISA?
What is an advantage of performing ELISPOT over ELISA?
Which of the two protocols is quantitative?

NOTES:

NOTES:

Selected References

Czerkinsky C et al (1988) Reverse ELISPOT assay for clonal analysis of cytokine production. I. Enumeration of gamma-interferon-secreting cells. J lmmunol Methods 110:29–36

Punt S, Jones O (2019) Kuby immunology, 8th edn. W. H. Freeman and Company, New York, Antigen-antibody interactions, Ch. 20

Slota M, Lim J, Dang Y, Disis MJ (2011) ELISpot for measuring human immune responses to vaccines. Expert Rev Vaccines 10:299–306

Streeck H, Frahm N, Walker BD (2009) The role of IFN-γ Elispot assay in HIV vaccine research. Nat Protocols 4:461–469

Chapter 41
Exercise 17: Immunofluorescence Assay (IFA)

Introduction

Antigens in cells or in tissue sections can be identified by incubating cell smear preparations on glass slides or fixed tissue section with specific antibodies. The site of antibody interaction can be visualized directly using primary antibody conjugated with a fluorochrome i.e. fluorescent dye or indirectly by using a species specific antibody conjugated to the fluorochrome. The stained sample is washed, mounted under a coverslip with mounting fluid and sealed with clear nail polish. An anti-fluorescent quenching agent may be included in the mounting fluid to prevent fluorescent bleaching when the sample is visualized by ultraviolet microscopy. Antibodies used can be derived from a variety of species. As with western blotting and ELISA assays, the appropriate species specific secondary antibody is required for detection in indirect assays. Protein A-conjugated to fluorochromes can also be used, and binds specifically to the Fc region of IgG. In some cases biotin-conjugated secondary antibodies are used to bind the primary antibody-antigen complex, followed by detection with streptavidin conjugated to a fluorochrome (**triple sandwich indirect method**). Streptavidin binds to biotin with very high affinity. The IFA is a rapid, sensitive and practical assay that can be used to confirm the location and specificity of an antigen. The titer of specific antibodies can also be obtained using IFA. Since an ultraviolet (UV) microscope is required for visualization of stained samples, it is not a very cheap procedure. However, in most settings such as a clinical laboratory, or research laboratory UV microscopes and the more sophisticated confocal microscope, is usually available. A modified IFA is also used in the detection of antigen by cell sorting techniques using a fluorescent activated cell sorter (FACs) or by flow cytometry. The cell sorting techniques allow for the separation of fluorescent cell subpopulation, based on the intensity of stain and also by size (FACS). Two or three different antibody stained cell subpopulations can be analyzed simultaneously. Each cell population is separated and grouped based on the fluorescence emitted. The groups are displayed on an oscilloscope.

© Springer Nature Switzerland AG 2021
T. Y. Sam-Yellowe, *Immunology: Overview and Laboratory Manual*,
https://doi.org/10.1007/978-3-030-64686-8_41

Fig. 41.1 Indirect
immunofluorescent
staining of *Plasmodium
falciparum* merozoite
rhoptries

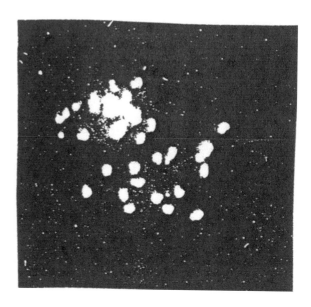

Membrane antigens, cytosolic antigens or other structural antigens can be detected using IFA on bacteria, parasites (protozoan or helminth), fungi, or virus-infected cells (Fig. 41.1). Developmental expression and localization or loss of proteins can be monitored using IFA. With specific antibodies to cell surface markers, e.g. cluster of differentiation (CD) antigens or to immunoglobulins (Ig), this technique can be used to identify B and T cell subpopulations from a mixture of lymphocytes contained in a lymphoid cell suspension.

Polyclonal or monoclonal antibodies against CD3, CD4 or CD8 can be used to detect T cells while anti-IgM or anti-IgD can be used to detect B cells. Some membrane proteins are mobile. This is an energy dependent process, therefore temperature dependent. At 4 °C only **patching** is observed, while at 37 °C both processes can be observed. When such proteins are cross linked as occurs when anti-IgM is incubated with B cells, the immune complexes formed are visualized as patches. The patches migrate to one pole of the cell and are either internalized or endocytosed or sloughed off, i. e. shed. **Capping** of immune complexes on B cells leads to cell proliferaction which ultimately results in immunoglobulin synthesis. Visualization of the patching and capping process is possible when IFA is performed in solution, followed by transfer of the cells to a glass slide.

The fluorochromes used, in IFA absorb light at a given wavelength and emit light at a different and longer wavelength. Fluorescein dyes such as **fluorescein isothiocyanate (FITC)**, a commonly used fluorochrome, absorbs blue light at 490 nm and emit a yellow-green fluorescent light at 519 nm. **Rhodamine dyes such as Tetramethyl rhodamine isothiocyanate (TRITC)** absorbs yellow-green light at 515 nm and emits a deep red fluorescence at 546 run. Other fluorochromes that are also used for IFA include **Texas red, phycoerythrin and Alexa Fluor dyes (available from various vendors).** Due to the differences in fluorescence of fluorchromes, antigens present in the same cell or tissue, or located in close proximity to one another on the cell surface can be identified by colocalization using the respective specific antibodies incubated simultaneously or together, and detected by secondary antibodies conjugated to different fluorochromes. With the appropriate exclusion filters on the UV microscope, images from either fluorochrome can be detected and recorded by photography using camera attachments on the microscope. Images can also be captured by digital scanning of the fluorescent image, visualized on a monitor screen, followed by storage of the image on a computer disc for further analysis. The samples can be couterstained with dyes that stain the nucleus i.e. DNA specifically, such as ethidium bromide or DAPI. These counterstains are useful, in providing a cellular orientation, staining nuclei and in confirming the cellular localization of the antigen.

Although easier to perform, cheaper and less time-consuming the **direct assay** is less sensitive than the **indirect methods** of IFA. For diagnostic work, the direct IFA is routinely used. The procedure can be completed in 30 min. However, background levels may be high in direct assays. The indirect method is more sensitive and relatively more expensive because the antibody signal is amplified by the presence of the secondary antibody which binds to more primary antibody sites. Furthermore the added step with the secondary antibody increases the assay time. The entire procedure may take up to 2 h. Since the dilution of the primary antibody required in the indirect assay is small, background levels are reduced and this makes up for the added cost of the secondary antibody. As with the other immunoassays described, both positive and negative controls are included in the assay to aid interpretation of results.

To ensure reproducibility, times and length of incubation, temperatures, pH of buffers used should remain constant between experiments. Inadequate washing, improper or inadequate fixation of samples e.g. with methanol, acetone, formaldehyde, gluteraldehyde also contribute to difficulties in interpretation of results. Insufficient antibodies, antigens, or conformational constraints to the specificity of the antibodies may also interfere with antibody reactivity. In some experiments, a blocking step may be included to reduce nonspecific or auto fluorescence of the sample. As with the other immunoassays fractionated immunoglobulin e.g. Fab or F(ab′)2 fragments can also be used for IFA.

In most studies, localization of antigen by IFA is followed by ultrastructural localization of the antigen by **immunoelectron microscopy** (IEM) (Fig. 41.2), using tissue prepared and processed for IEM. The basic principle of the immunoassay remains the same. Primary antibodies are incubated with fixed samples embedded in a substance such as lowicryl. The embedded samples are sectioned using a diamond knife attached to a microtome. The sections are captured on metal grids, incubated with a primary antibody followed by a secondary antibody conjugated to an electron dense material such as **colloidal gold** particles (520 nm) or **ferritin.** Under an electron microscope, the gold particles or ferritin absorb electrons under high vacuum. Electrons emitted are visualized as black dots. Due to the high cost of housing, and maintaining an electron microscope-an entire room is dedicated to the use of one microscope-IEM is not routinely performed in teaching laboratories.

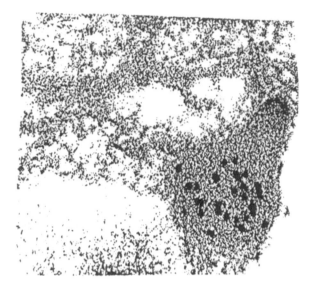

Fig. 41.2 Immunoelectron microscopy of *Plasmodium chabaudi* rhoptries

Unlike the assays described above, IEM requires many more steps than those described above to prepare cell samples. However, the same precautions and requirements for proper controls also apply.

The **first objective** of this exercise is to learn the procedure for IFA. The **second objective** is to learn to distinguish lymphocytes based on their cell surface markers.

Materials and Reagents (Per Pair)

Ultraviolet fluorescence microscope
1 mouse
Materials and reagents used in Exercise #3 (see Chap. 27)
Histopaque-1077 (Sigma)
Microscope glass slides
Glass cover slips
CD4 and CD8 specific polyclonal or monoclonal antibodies
FITC-conjugated anti-mouse antibodies (or Alexa Fluor 488 conjugated antibodies)
TRITC- conjugated anti rabbit antibodies (or Alexa Fluor 647conjugated antibodies)
FITC-conjugated anti-mouse IgM (μ chain specific) FITC-conjugated rabbit anti-mouse IgM
Unlabeled anti-mouse IgM (μ chain specific)
10× PBS
Distilled water
One 1 L graduated cylinder

One 100 mL graduated cylinder
One 1 L Erhlenmeyer flask
One 250 mL Erhlenmeyer flask
One 500 mL beaker
Coplin jar containing absolute methanol
Empty coplin for PBS washes
Solution of 50% glycerol in 1× PBS
Giemsa stain
15 mL centrifuge tubes

Procedure

1. Prepare a mouse spleen suspension as described in Exercise #4 (See Chap. 28).
2. Wash and resuspend the cells in 3 mL of RPMl/5% FBS. Remove 0.1 mL each into three eppendorf tubes for (1) Giemsa staining, (2) viability determination, and (3) IFA. Bring the volume in tube #2 to 1 mL for a 1:2 dilution and proceed with counting and viability determination procedures.
3. Centrifuge tubes #1 and #3 in a microfuge for 2 min. at 8000 rpm, remove and discard the supernatants, and resuspend the pellet to a 50% suspension in RPMI in preparation for making smears. E.g. if the pellet is 50 µL, add 50 µL of RPMl/5% FBS for a 50% suspension.
4. Resuspend the cells gently, then prepare thin smears on glass slides using a padlpet. Your instructor will demonstrate.
5. Prepare at least two slides from tube #1. Stain the slides using Giemsa stain.
6. Prepare six slides from tube #3. Let the slides air dry, then fix the smears in absolute methanol.
7. Place the two slides from tube #1 in Giemsa stain for 10 min. For the six slides from tube #3 for IFA proceed as follows:

   (a) Two slides will be incubated with 50 µL of a 1:50 dilution of goat anti-mouse IgM conjugated to fluorescein isothiocyanate (FITC) for 30 min in a humid chamber at 37 °C.(All incubations will be at this temperature).
   (b) One slide will be incubated with 50 µL of a 1:50 dilution of goat serum for 30 min as in #1.
   (c) One slide will be incubated with 50 µL of a 1:200 dilution of rabbit anti-mouse IgM for 30 min in a humid chamber. 1 slide will be incubated with 50 µL of rabbit anti-mouse CD3 for 30 min in a humid chamber.
   (d) One slide will be incubated with 50 µL of a 1:200 dilution of normal rabbit serum for 30 min in a humid chamber.

8. After incubation, wash slides from 7(a) and 7(b), three times with 1× PBS, and once with distilled water. Use a coplin jar for the washes.
9. Wash the slides from 7(c) and 7(d) three times with 1× PBS, then add 50 µL of anti-rabbit IgG-Alexa Fluor 488 diluted 1:000 to the smear incubated with

rabbit anti-mouse IgM and add 50 μL of anti-rabbit IgG-Alexa Fluor 647 diluted 1:1000 to the smear incubated with anti-mouse CD3. Incubate the smears for an additional 30 min in a humid chamber. Wash the slides three times in a coplin jar with IX PBS, and once with distilled water.

NOTE: Cells may also be fixed in 5% formalin for 10 min at room temperature, washed in 1× PBS by centrifugation and the pellets resuspended in 100 μL of 1× PBS for preparation of smears. Once the smears are air-dried, they can be place in a coplin jar containing 0.1% Triton X-100 to permeabilize the cells for 5 min. After permeabilization, the smear is blocked by placing the slide in 3% BSA for 30 min followed by two PBS washes. The smears can then be processed for IFA as described above.

10. Add 20 μL (a small drop) of 50% glycerol in 1× PBS (or commercial mounting solution containing DAPI) to the smears and cover with a coverslip, taking care to avoid bubbles. Seal the slides with clear nail polish.

11. After the nail polish is dry, store the slides at −20 °C in a plastic container wrapped in aluminum foil to protect from light. The slides will be observed using a UV and confocal microscope. This will be done in groups.

Questions

1. What is the difference between the two IFA procedures? What class of lymphocytes will be identified using anti-IgM and anti-CD3 antibodies? Are there any advantages or disadvantages to performing either procedure?
2. What is the difference between using methanol and formalin as fixatives for IFA?
3. How does permeabilization affect antibody binding to antigen on the cells?
4. Define or explain the following terms: Capping, Patching

NOTES:

NOTES:

NOTES AND ILLUSTRATIONS:

Chapter 42
Exercise 18: Flow Cytometry

Introduction

Flow cytometry is an important and essential laboratory technique used to sort and analyze cell populations bound to antibodies reacting with cell surface and intracellular antigens. The cell surface proteins, commonly referred to as cell surface markers are recognized by specific antibodies against the markers known as cluster of differentiation (CD) antigens. Antibodies used for detection are fluorescently labeled, and different antibodies conjugated to different colored fluorochromes can be used to identify different subpopulations of cells. Monoclonal antibodies are typically used for antigen detection. In the process of identifying fluorescently labeled cells, individual cells can be sorted on the basis of size, volume, intracellular structures, cytoplasmic granularity, intensity of fluorescence and light scattering properties. The cell soring characteristics of the flow cytometer are similar to the process of cell sorting by fluorescence activated cell sorters (FACs). The flow cytometer measures light scattered by each cell in a population of thousands to millions of cells. Light scattered in the forward direction of the laser light beam provides information about the size of the cell. Side scattered light perpendicular to the laser light beam provides information about the cytoplasmic granularity and intracellular membranous structures (Fig. 42.1). Granulocytes, monocytes and lymphocytes can be sorted and distinguished based on size, granularity and cytoplasmic contents. The granulocyte population can be gated and analyzed (Fig. 42.2a, b). The method employed for detecting cell surface antigens on leukocytes and identifying phenotypic differences in subpopulations of cells is known as immunophenotyping. Cell lineages, progenitor cells, differentiation stage and maturation of cells can be identified. Immunophenotyping can identify phenotypic changes in neoplastic cells, thereby aiding diagnosis, identifying malignant cells, also quantitating hematopoietic cell progenitors. Lymphocyte populations can also be identified and quantitated. For example antibodies against CD3 identify T lymphocytes. The use of antibodies against CD4 and CD8 will identify helper T cells and cytotoxic T cells,

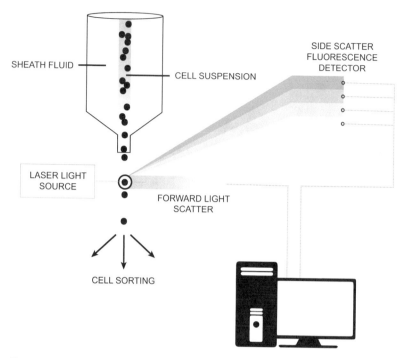

Fig. 42.1 Flow cytometry. Cells in suspension are passed through laser light source. Forward and side scattered light is detected. Fluorescent light is also detected as cells are sorted

respectively. The molecules CD19 and CD20 identify B lymphocytes and CD16 and CD56 identify natural killer (NK) cells. The lymphocyte population can be separated from other leukocytes with the use of antibodies against CD14 and CD45 and hematopoietic cells can be identified using antibodies against CD34. The **first objective** of this exercise is to perform flow cytometry for the identification of B and T cells in a lymphoid cell suspension. The **second objective** is to identify T helper and cytotoxic T cells from the T cell population.

Materials and Reagents (Per Pair)

Flow cytometer
Flow cytometry tubes (round bottom tubes)
Flow cytometry staining buffer
Blood cells
Red blood cell lysing buffer
Flow cytometry diluent and washing buffer
Centrifuge
Vortexer

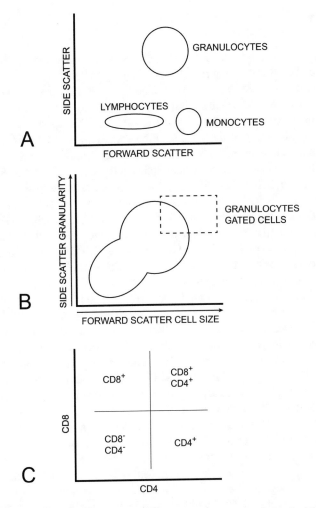

Fig. 42.2 (**a**) Illustration of side scatter and forward scatter plot of peripheral white blood cells (WBCs). (**b**) Different WBCs can be gated for further analysis. (**c**) The distribution of CD4$^+$ and CD8$^+$ T lymphocytes can be investigated using specific antibodies labeled with different colored fluorophores

Pipet squeezers
Pipets (P20, P200, P1000)
Pipet tips
Serological pipets (10 ml)

Procedure

1. Obtain mouse blood cell suspension as in Exercise 4 (see Chap. 28).
2. Lyse red blood cells using red blood cell lysing buffer.
3. Wash cells with PBS wash buffer containing 1% bovine serum albumin (BSA) and 1% sodium azide. (Flow cytometry buffer, FCB)
4. Perform cell count to obtain cells at 1×10^6–1×10^7 cells/mL.
5. Add 2 mL Fc receptor blocking solution containing anti-CD64 (other anti-Fc receptors include anti-CD16, CD32) or 1 μg IgG per 1×10^6 cells. This will block Fc receptors on macrophages and B cells. The origin of Fc receptor specific antibodies should be different from origin of primary antibodies.
6. Centrifuge cells for 5 min at 1300–1500 rpm and discard supernatant.
7. Add FCB and adjust cell count to 1×10^6 cells/100 μL volume for each tube.
8. Transfer 100 μL cells to each of five flow cytometry tubes. Label tubes. Unstained cells (tube 1), isotype control (tube 2), PBS control (tube 3), anti-CD4 (tube 4) and anti-CD8 (tube 5). The PBS control tube will be incubated with one of the conjugate antibodies.
9. Add diluted conjugated antibodies specific to membrane proteins on cell surface (for example, antibodies against CD3, CD4, CD8, CD19, CD20) of B and T lymphocytes. In this exercise antibodies against mouse CD4 and CD8 conjugated with two different fluorochromes will be used. Anti-mouse CD4 conjugated to Alexa Fluor 488 (or FITC) and anti-mouse CD8 conjugated to Alexa Fluor 647 (or phycoerythrin, PE) will be added at dilutions of 1:500–1:1000. Anti-mouse IgG to an irrelevant protein will be used for isotype control.
10. Incubate the cells for 45 min at 4 °C.
11. Centrifuge cells for 5 min at 1300–1500 rpm and remove unbound antibody
12. Wash cells twice with cold 2 mL FCB by centrifugation.
13. After the last wash, resuspend cells in 200–400 μL FCB.
14. Analyze cells using a Flow cytometer within 24 h. From the lymphocyte population, cells negative for both CD4 and CD8 will be in the lower left quadrant, cells positive for both CD4 and CD8 will be in the upper right quadrant, single positive cells for CD4 will be in the lower right quadrant and single positive cells for CD8 will be in the upper right quadrant.

NOTE: If unconjugated primary antibodies are used in step #9, secondary antibodies conjugated to fluorochromes will be added after the wash step in #12. Cells plus secondary antibodies will be incubated at 4 °C for 45 min, then centrifuged and washed as in steps #11–13. Flow cytometry analysis will be performed as in #14.

Selected Reference

Punt S, Jones O (2019) Kuby immunology, 8th edn. W.H. Freeman and Company, New York. "Antigen-antibody interactions" Ch 20

Chapter 43
Exercise 19: Complement Fixation Assays

Introduction

The complement system is composed of more than 50 proteins that function in three pathways: the classical, alternate and lectin pathways. Each pathway is composed of a series of steps. Some of these steps involve the activation of complement components that are proenzymes to enzymatically active forms, which use the next components in the sequence as substrates. Complement fixation (activation) is studied by measuring the degree of lysis of sheep red blood cells that occurs in the presence of specific antibody. Complement fixation is an extremely sensitive assay that detects the presence of IgM and IgG directed against a specific antigen. In order to detect the classical complement pathway, complement depletion is measured by the binding of antigen and antibody. An indicator system which indicates if complement remains unbound or bound, consists of sheep red blood cells (SRBCs) and anti-SRBC (i.e. hemolysin). If specific antibody is present in the test sample, complement will bind to the antigen-antibody complex and will not be available to lyse the SRBCs (positive test for complement). If no specific antibody is present, the complement is free to bind hemolysin, which is bound to SRBCs. This results in hemolysis of the SRBCs (negative test for complement). By titrating the unknown antibody or antigen a complement fixing titer can be obtained. This will yield a quantitative measure of the specific antibody in the system.

This method gives 100% lysis of SRBCs. The amount of complement in serum giving 50% lysis of sensitized SRBCs can also be measured spectrophotometrically. This gives a CH50 value. Complement-mediated lysis of sensitized SRBCs results in the release of hemoglobin, which is quantitated spectrophotometrically. The CH50 value is calculated as the inverse of the dilution which results in approximately 50% lysis of sensitized SRBCs. This is expressed in CH50 units/mL of serum.

The **objective** of this exercise is to learn the complement fixation assay and to compare the sensitivity of the assay to the agglutination assay. Sensitivity of an

© Springer Nature Switzerland AG 2021

T. Y. Sam-Yellowe, *Immunology: Overview and Laboratory Manual*,
https://doi.org/10.1007/978-3-030-64686-8_43

assay is a measure of how much antibody is required to produce a positive reaction. The more sensitive a test, the less antibody required to produce a positive reaction.

Materials and Reagents (Per Pair)

Two U-bottom microtiter plates
56 °C water
One 0.05 mL microdiluter
Beakers containing 70% ethanol
1 Gilson pipetman (0–200 μL)
Saline
Bench cover
Hemolysin
Gloves
Anti-BSA antiserum
Ice bucket
Normal Rabbit Serum
5 mL of 20% SRBC-BSA
5 mL of 20% SRBCs
Fresh guinea pig complement (1:20) 6 mL
37 °C incubator and water bath
Bench top centrifuge

Procedure

Part A

Negative system in microtiter plates

1. Divide fresh guinea pig complement into two aliquots. Place aliquot on ice, place the other aliquot in 56 °C water bath for 30 min.
2. Using the Gilson pipetman, add 0.05 mL saline diluent to wells #2–23. (Use two rows of the microtiter plate). Repeat with rows 3 and 4.
3. Using a pipetman, add 0.05 mL of normal rabbit serum to well #24 of rows 2 and 4.
4. Using a pipetman, add 0.05 mL hemolysin to wells 1 and 2 of rows 1 and 3.
5. Using the 50 μL microdiluter, make serial twofold dilutions of hemolysin starting in well #2 and ending in well #22. Rinse the microdiluter and repeat dilutions in rows 3–4.
6. Using a pipetman, add 0.05 mL of SRBCs to all wells. Mix well.
7. Using pipetman, add 0.05 mL of fresh guinea pig complement (from ice bucket) to all wells in rows 1 and 2. To all wells in rows 3 and 4, add 0.05 mL guinea pig complement (from 56 °C water bath).

8. Place microtiter plates at 37 °C for 30 min and observe for hemolysis or agglutination.

We will also use tanned SRBCs with absorbed BSA for complement fixation assay so that we can compare the sensitivity of this assay to that of passive agglutination.

Part B

The complement fixation test can also be performed in tubes. The indicator system can be performed by mixing sheep red blood cells, anti-sheep red blood cell antibody and Guinea pig complement. Anti-sheep red cell antibody binds to SRBC followed by complement fixation

Patient serum can be screened for antibodies specific to antigens of an infecting pathogen. The pathogen or specific antigen can be mixed with patient serum and complement. Patient serum can be serially diluted to determine the titer of the antibody fixing complement. If the patient serum contains specific antibody for the antigen, the antibody will bind to the antigen and the antigen-antibody complex will bind complement activating the complement cascade depleting complement proteins. Add SRBC and anti-sheep red blood cells to the tube. If antibody in patient serum is not specific to the antigen, complement will not be fixed and will bind to the sheep red blood cell-anti-sheep red blood cell complex resulting in lysis of the sheep red blood cells. This is a negative complement fixation test.

If sheep red blood cells are not lysed, then the test is a positive test indicating that complement fixing antibodies are present in the patient serum.

Complement is heat labile and when incubated at 56 °C will become inactivated and in the presence of antibody-antigen complex will not be fixed. Inactivated complement can be used as a negative control in the complement fixation test.

Complement proteins can be detected by antibodies specific to individual complement components by ELISA, western blotting or by immunofluorescence.

Procedure

1. Label two tubes "A" and "B". Add 0.25 mL antigen and 0.25 mL Guinea pig complement to tubes A and B each containing human antiserum (one antiserum is specific to the antigen).
2. Incubate tubes A and B in a water bath set to 37 °C for 30 min.
3. Add 0.25 mL 1% sheep red blood cells (SRBC) and 0.25 mL anti-sheep red blood cell antibody (hemolysin) and incubate for 3 min at 37 °C.
4. Examine the tubes for hemolysis and record the color of the tube contents.
5. Centrifuge the tubes for 5 min at 3500 rpm. Do not remove supernatants.
6. Check the pellets and record the appearance of the pellets.

Questions

1. Which tube has a red color and a loose "fluffy" and pellet consisting of red cell membrane ghost and debris.
2. Which tube has a clear color and compact pellet?
3. From Fig. 43.1, which tube is negative for hemolysis and is a positive test indication that the human antiserum used was specific for the antigen? Which tube was positive for hemolysis and is a negative test indicating that the human antiserum used did not contain specific antibodies for the antigen?
4. Add tubes C and D to the experiment. In tube C, add 0.25 mL normal human serum plus 0.25 mL complement. In tube D add 0.25 mL 1× PBS plus 0.25 mL complement. Incubate the tubes as indicated in #2. Add 0.25 mL SRBC and 0.25 mL hemolysin and incubate as in #3. Examine the tubes after incubation and record the results. What results would you expect? Was there hemolysis in the tubes? Explain.

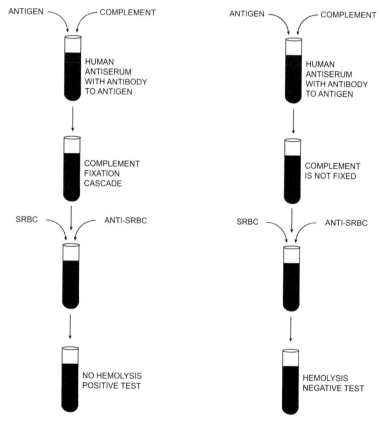

Fig. 43.1 Complement fixation. Indicator system determines the presence of specific antibody in patient serum. If specific antibody is absent in patient serum, complement will not be fixed and addition of SRBC and anti-SRBC will result in hemolysis of SRBC

NOTES:

Selected References

Barrett JT (1988) Textbook of Immunology. Mosby, St. Louis. Ch. 10, The complement system

Punt S, Jones O (2019) Kuby immunology, 8th edn. W. H. Freeman and Company, New York, Antigen-Antibody Interactions, Ch. 20

Sheehan C (1990) Principles and laboratory diagnosis: clinical immunology. J.B. Lippincott Company, Philadelphia. Ch. 13, Assays involving complement

Chapter 44
Tissue Culture Techniques: Introduction

Cell culture techniques were developed as a way to study animal cells in vitro. The behavior of single cells, organ culture and monolayer cells can be studied without the in vivo influences arising from physiological and environmental variations among experimental animals. Cell culture or tissue culture as the technique is widely known, was first described in 1907 (Freshney 1987) and through the decades has undergone extensive developments. These include the introduction of defined media, the development of continuous cell lines, cell fusion techniques and the extension of animal cell culture techniques to plant, insect and lower vertebrate cell culture.

The need to understand the growth mechanisms of tumor cells and animal viruses was a major stimulus in the development and standardization of tissue culture methods. Furthermore, the requirement for large scale production of cells to facilitate biochemical, genetic and in recent years molecular analysis, has led to the establishment of cell culture techniques as a major component of most biomedical and immunology laboratories.

Cell culture techniques rely heavily on sound aseptic techniques. In addition, most cells are fastidious in their growth requirements and efforts to maintain cell lines can become quite expensive. Tissue culture requires the availability of certain essential materials, namely; pure water (deionized, double distilled and sterile), a laminar flow hood or sterile cabinet, automatic pipetters, a CO_2 incubator, an oven/dryer, an autoclave for sterilizing glass ware, surgical equipment etc., microscopes (inverted and upright light microscopes equipped with phase optics), $-20\ °C$ and $-80\ °C$ freezers, liquid nitrogen storage tanks, refrigerators, centrifuges, cell counters, filtration devices and vacuum pumps. Other consumable sterile items essential for tissue culture work such as media, serum, tissue culture tubes, bottles, flasks, plates, and pipets etc. are also required.

The practice of aseptic technique cannot be overemphasized in cell culture work. This extends to the proper handling and manipulation of materials to prevent contamination of cultures (from the environment i.e. by bacteria, mold, yeast, prevention of cross contamination between cell lines, prevention of contamination

© Springer Nature Switzerland AG 2021
T. Y. Sam-Yellowe, *Immunology: Overview and Laboratory Manual*,
https://doi.org/10.1007/978-3-030-64686-8_44

by mycoplasma), proper organization and cleanliness of the work environment, and maintenance of personal hygiene i.e. hand washing, wearing of gloves, laboratory coats and face masks when necessary. These techniques including safety techniques, will be discussed in class.

Types of Cell Culture

1. **Organ culture:** Cell culture may be initiated directly from an organ e.g. liver, kidney etc. In organ culture the three dimensional architecture of the tissue is retained and the tissue is cultured in the liquid-gas interface on a raft, grid or gel. Differential properties of the cells are maintained and contact inhibitory properties of the cells are also maintained. Because the cells grow very slowly and propagation is not continuous, it is difficult to quantitate cells, or to obtain large numbers of cells. Primary explant cultures although not the same as organ culture, involve the culture of tissue fragments at the substrate-liquid interface to facilitate attachment, growth and migration of the cells. The substrate is solid and may be glass or plastic.

2. **Cell culture:** In cell culture, tissue from an organ or from a primary explant is either mechanically or enzymatically dispersed to give rise to single cells. These cells can then be cultured as single cell suspensions or as adherent cell monolayers. When cells reach a given cell density, they are subcultured, or diluted into fresh tissue culture flasks. Cells may be selected by cloning to retain uniform growth, morphologic, physiologic, genetic or biochemical characteristics. An increase in cell number over several generations in addition to the uniformity in cell culture characteristics results in the formation of a cell line after continuous passage of the daughter cells. Cell cultures can be maintained as **anchorage dependent,** or **anchorage independent** cultures. The former refers to cells that require attachment to a substrate and migration for growth and the later refers to cells (usually hematopoietic cells, malignant tumor cells, or transformed cells) that can proliferate in suspension **(suspension cultures),** without attachment. **Monolayer cultures** are for the most part anchorage dependent and are grown attached to a solid substrate. **Three-dimensional (3D) cell cultures** reviewed by Edmondson et al. (2014) are increasingly employed for investigating the expression of cell surface molecules participating in cell adhesion and in drug discovery. The use of 3D cultures in matrices such as hydrogel provides a more realistic tissue microenvironment like that found in vivo. Their wide spread use will depend on a better understanding of how to make the cultures more reflective of the in vivo environment to make their use more reproducible.

Use of Pipets (See Exercise 2)

Eppendorf micropipet should be manipulated correctly. Always adjust the pipet to the correct volume required. Never below or above the capacity indicated for the pipet. There are two positions on the pipetter for filling and dispensing liquids. To use the pipet, depress the plunger to the first position (you should feel a slight resistance at this point) to fill. Depress the plunger to the second position to dispense. At the second position the plunger will go no further. This is the final position. If you depress this far to fill the pipet, the volume obtained will be inaccurate.

Automatic pipeters (Pipet-aid) for 10, 5 and 1 mL pipets should also be manipulated correctly. The pipeter has two buttons for filling and dispensing liquids. The top button when depressed fills the pipet and the lower button right below, when depressed empties the pipet, dispensing the liquid. Care must be exercised when filling pipets such that the volume of liquid does not exceed the capacity of the pipet to wet the cotton plugs in the pipets.

Laboratory coats or gowns must be worn at all times. Hands must also be thoroughly washed before and after culturing procedures. Individuals with long hair need to have it tied back while working under the hood. No eating, drinking or smoking is permitted in the, laboratory and in the tissue culture area. When working under the hood with open containers, avoid carrying out lengthy conversations/discussions. Read and plan out the exercise before coming to the laboratory. (Refer to immunology laboratory policies)

Procedure for Using Tissue Culture Hood

1. Thoroughly wipe down the work surface under the hood with 70% ethanol before and after using the hood.
2. Organize pipets, flasks, pipeters, bottles, etc., neatly with enough space in front of you to perform your work. Only have in the hood the reagents and equipment that you need. Do not work directly over open bottles, tubes, or flasks. Be careful not to brush against open lids, pipet tips and open bottles. If you notice that you have done so, let the instructor know. The pipet or media may have to be discarded.
3. Every item to be used under the hood must be wiped with 70% ethanol including pens and pencils. If you have been outside the hood for more than 5 min handling nonsterile material, change your gloves before continuing with sterile work.
4. All waste media must be collected in a waste beaker/vessel under the hood and disposed of properly when culturing has been completed. If any spills occur, stop what you are doing, cover any open containers, clean up the spill with 70% ethanol before continuing.
5. Pipets, tubes, sterile squeezers, flasks and other disposable tissue culture ware must be disposed of in the biohazard bags provided for this purpose.
6. After using the inverted microscope, turn it off, rotate the nose piece and position the lowest objective above the condenser. Place the dust jacket over the microscope.

NOTES:

References

Edmondson R, Broglie JJ, Adcock A, Yang L (2014) Three-dimensional cell culture systems and their applications in drug discovery and cell-based biosensors. Assay Drug Dev Technol 12:207–218

Freshney RI (1987) Culture of animal cells. A manual of basic technique, 2nd edn. Wiley-Liss, New York. Chapter 1 and 2

Chapter 45
Exercise 20: Mitogen Induced Response of Lymphocytes. Detection of B and T Lymphocytes Using Immunofluorescence

Introduction

Mitogens are substances, which are capable of inducing mitosis in cells of the immune system. B and T lymphocytes are induced to proliferate when exposed to mitogens in the same way that proliferation is induced by exposure to antigen. The lymphocytes undergo the same cellular and chemical activation that occurs in antigen induced mitosis namely, blast transformation. In this mitotic state they are called lymphoblasts. Lymphoblasts can be found in lymphoid organs of animals responding to an antigenic challenge. When lymphoid cell suspensions are prepared from an animal immunized to a specific antigen, and then incubated with the antigen, blast formation occurs in response to the antigen. Several different mitogens can be used to demonstrate the same effect in culture. Many mitogens are plant lectins e.g. phytohemagglutinins (these will also agglutinate erythrocytes), and lipopolysaccharides (LPS) from the cell wall of gram negative bacteria. The mitogens bind to cell surface receptors on the lymphocytes.

LPS is highly mitogenic for murine B cells. It is not a potent mitogen of human B cells. Concanavalin A (Con A) is specifically mitogenic for T lymphocytes while pokeweed mitogen (PWM) and phytohemagglutinin (PHA) are mitogenic for B and T lymphocytes. In order to determine the degree of lymphocyte transformation, [^{3}H]-thymidine incorporation by the lymphocytes can be measured. Only the lymphocytes that are actively dividing incorporate the radiolabel into the newly synthesized DNA. The amount of radiolabel incorporated by the lymphocytes in a given period of time can be detected using a scintillation counter. The appearance of mitogen stimulated cells (2–7 days) can also be observed by light microscopy after staining the cells.

In this exercise, we will induce a mitotic response in mouse spleen cell suspensions enriched for lymphocytes by density gradient centrifugation on Histopaque-1077 (Sigma). We will incubate the cells with Con A, LPS, and Wheat germ agglutinin (WGA). The **first objective** of the exercise is to learn how to

© Springer Nature Switzerland AG 2021
T. Y. Sam-Yellowe, *Immunology: Overview and Laboratory Manual*,
https://doi.org/10.1007/978-3-030-64686-8_45

separate mononuclear cells using density gradient centrifugation. The **second objective** is to induce a mitogenic response in Band T lymphocytes, and to characterize cell surface markers by performing immunofluorescence assays using cell specific antibodies. Culture supernatants from cultures can also be examined for specific cytokine production.

Materials and Reagents (Per Group)

Three mouse spleens (Swiss mice)
Two sterile plastic petri dishes (one containing 10 mL RPMI plus sterile wire mesh)
One 10 mL plastic syringe
Two pr scissors and forceps
Pipetman 20 µL, 200 µL
Eppendorf tubes
70% alcohol in squeeze bottle and in 200 mL beaker
Glass slides and coverslips
3 mL of histopaque in 15 mL centrifuge tube
Two coplin jars
Pipet tips-yellow
One empty 200 mL beaker
Giemsa stain
Methanol
0.2% Trypan blue
Four 25 cm^2 tissue culture flasks
Four 15 mL centrifuge tubes
10 and 5 mL individually wrapped glass pipet (eight each)
Individually wrapped sterile squeezers (5)
RPMI 1640 medium with 5% fetal calf serum or human AB serum plus Gentamycin
Mitogens (Con A 1 mg/mL, LPS 2 mg/mL, WGA 1 mg/mL in RPMI). **Depending on the availability of mitogens or the activity of the mitogens, substitutions may be made for the exercise.**
Centrifuge
Microscope
Hemocytometers
Tally counters
Bench mats and plastic disposable bags
Gloves
Kimwipes and paper towels
Rabbit anti-mouse lgM-FITC
1× PBS and 50% glycerol in 1× PBS

Procedure

1. Prepare spleen cell suspensions as in Exercise #4. Be sure the mouse fur is completely soaked with 70% alcohol before performing splenectomy. Since the cells are to be incubated in culture for several days, sterile techniques have to be observed.
2. After first centrifugation, pool pellets into 4 mL of RPMI and resuspend the spleen cells. Remove a 0.1 mL aliquot for dilution (1:100) and determination of viability and 0.1 mL for Giemsa staining. Save the remaining cells on ice. Count and obtain # of cells. Pay attention to the size and morphology of the cells.
3. Very carefully layer 3 mL of spleen cells over 3 mL of histopaque in a 15 mL tube. Centrifuge at 400 × g for 10 min at room temperature. There will be four bands in the tube after centrifugation. The top band is the RPMI buffer, the second band is the mononuclear cell layer, the third band is histopaque, and the fourth band (pellet) is the red cell and granulocyte band (Fig. 45.1).
4. Very carefully, aspirate with a sterile squeezer the top layer i.e. RPMI buffer layer to within 0.5 cm of the mononuclear fraction and discard.
5. Carefully transfer the mononuclear fraction to a fresh centrifuge tube and add 10 mL of RPMI supplemented with 5% fetal calf serum. Resuspend gently (Fig. 45.1).
6. Centrifuge at 250 × g for 10 min, aspirate the supernatant and discard. Add 10 mL RPMI + 5% FCS and repeat centrifugation once more i.e. two centrifugation steps.
7. Resuspend the final pellet in 20 mL of RPMI/FCS. Transfer 5 mL into tissue culture flask, label #1. Transfer 5 mL into flask #2, #3, and #4. Adjust the volumes in each flask to 10 mL by adding an additional 5 mL of RPMI/FCS to the flasks.
8. Add Con A (1 μg Con A/1 × 10^6 cells, i. e. 10 μg/flask = #1), add 2–25 μg/mL LPS final concentration in culture-#2. Add the same concentration of WGA as Con A in flask #3. Add no mitogen in flask #4. This is your control flask.
9. Close the flasks and shake very gently from side to side. With caps slightly unscrewed to allow free passage of air through the flasks, incubate the flasks on their sides in a 37 °C, 5% CO_2 incubator for 2–7 days. After 2 days in culture, aliquot a sample from each flask and stain with trypan blue for viability. Also, take out an aliquot and centrifuge in an Eppendorf tube for Giemsa staining. Observe color changes in the stimulated and unstimulated control flasks. Record your observations and results. Do you notice any visible differences in cell size between the stimulated and unstimulated cells? How do the cells look when compared to cells from the day of preparation? **Note:** If vented caps are used for the flasks then the caps can be screwed on tight.

Procedure for Examination of Mitogen Stimulated Cells (Days 2 and 7)

1. Examine the T-flasks visually for any change in the color of the media. A yellow color may indicate increased or confluent cell growth or possible contamination (if culture is very turbid).

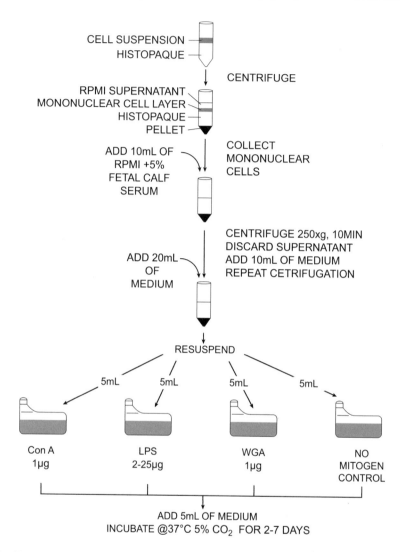

Fig. 45.1 Mitogen induced response of B and T lymphocytes. Mononuclear cells obtained from spleen cell suspension is treated with mitogens to induce cell proliferation. The lectins concanavalin A (Con A), wheat germ agglutinin (WGA) and the molecule lipopolysaccharide (LPS)

2. Examine the T-flask under an inverted microscope (in the presence of your TA or laboratory instructor) to confirm cell growth or contamination.

3. Under a laminar flow hood, remove 1.5 mL of culture from each flask into four Eppendorf tubes and centrifuge at 14,000 rpm for 2 min.

4. Remove supernatant to the 100 μL graduated mark on the tube and discard. Add an additional 1.5 mL of the cultures from the flasks and repeat centrifugation as in #3. Remove the supernatant to 100 μL mark.

5. Resuspend the cell pellet very gently in the remaining 100 μL media and use the cell suspension for (a) viability determination and (b) Giemsa staining-add a drop of the cell suspension to a clean glass slide and let the drop air dry. Do not use the blood smear technique. Fix the smear in absolute methanol, air dry and stain for 10 min with Giemsa stain.

6. Record your results very carefully and illustrate where necessary. Save your Giemsa slides.

7. On day 7, collect cells as in step #3. After centrifugation, collect supernatants, leaving 100 μL media above the pellets. Save the supernatants in fresh Eppendorf tubes. Label tubes. Resuspend the pellets in the remaining supernatant and prepare slides from each tube. Allow the slides to air dry, then fix the slides in absolute methanol for Giemsa stain and for IFA using anti-mouse CD19 (for B cells), anti-CD3, anti-CD4 and anti-CD8 antibodies (for T cells). Use the four antibodies to incubate with cells from each culture. Perform cell counts for viability to determine cell numbers in lectin treated cultures compared to the control (no mitogen control). Perform a capture ELISA assay using the supernatants from each culture to determine secretion of IL-2, IL-4 and IFNγ by the cells. Examine Giemsa stained cells for appearance of cell morphology in each culture.

Questions

1. Is there a difference in the distribution of anti-CD3 reactive cells in the LPS and Con A treated cultures?

2. How is the distribution of B cells similar or different from the cultures treated with Con A and LPS compared to cells treated with WGA?

3. Is there any antibody reactivity with cells in the control (no mitogen) culture?

4. In which of the culture would you expect to observe IL-2 secretion?

5. What other methods are used to enumerate and analyze B and T cell subsets?

NOTES:

NOTES:

NOTES:

NOTES:

NOTES AND QUIZZES:

Selected References

Barrett JT (1988) Textbook of Immunology, 5th edn. Mosby, St. Louis. Ch. 2 "Antigens, mitogens, haptens, and adjuvants"

DeToma FJ, MacDonald AB (1987) Experimental immunology. A guide book. Macmillan, New York. Ch. 12 "Blast transformation"

Goldsby RA, Kindy TJ, Osborne BA (2000) Kuby immunology. W.H. Freeman and Company, New York

Roitt IM, Brostoff J, Male DK (1989) Immunology. J.B. Lippincott Company, Philadelphia. Ch. 25 "Immunological Techniques"

Sheehan C (1990) Principles and laboratory diagnosis: clinical immunology. J.B. Lippincott Company, Philadelphia. Ch. 17 "Cellular Assays"

Chapter 46
Exercise 21: Induction of IL-2 Secretion from Mouse Lymphoma Cells (EL4.IL-2)

Introduction

Cytokines are low molecular weight proteins that possess regulatory functions for the immune system. They are antigenically nonspecific and are produced by a variety of cell types. T cells produce a number of cytokines that act synergistically or antagonistically to effect specific cell function. Cell lines have been described that produce specific cytokines or possess receptors to interact with specific cytokines. T helper cells are subdivided into THI or TH2 cells. Each subtype can be distinguished by the profile of cytokines produced. For example, TH1 cells produce IL-2, and IFNγ gamma, while TH2 cells produce IL-4, and IL-5. The particular profile will determine if the immune response generated will be humoral or cellular. In this exercise we will examine the mouse lymphoma cell line EL4.IL-2 (ATCC), an IL-2 secreting cell line. The **objective** of the exercise is to culture EL4.IL-2 cells and screen the cultures for IL-2 using ELISA with anti-IL-2 antibodies.

Materials and Reagents (Per Group)

EL4.IL-2 lymphoma cell line (from C57BL/6 mice) (ATCC)
3 C57BL/6 mice
70% ethanol in squeeze bottle
One empty 200 mL beaker
3 mL of Histopaque in 15 mL tube
Hank's balanced salt solution
Penicillin-Streptomycin
Two sterile plastic dishes with screens three pairs sterile scissors and forceps
Three coplin jars (1 empty, 1 containing ice cold acetone, 1 containing ice cold methanol) Giemsa stain, methanol

© Springer Nature Switzerland AG 2021
T.Y. Sam-Yellowe, *Immunology: Overview and Laboratory Manual*,
https://doi.org/10.1007/978-3-030-64686-8_46

Trypan blue
Four glass slides and cover slips
Sterile squeezers
Hemocytometer, tally counter
Bench mats
Dissection trays
Gloves
Kimwipes and paper towel
Plastic disposable bags
CO_2 incubator
Inverted microscope
Light microscope
Six 15 mL centrifuge tubes
Three 50 mL centrifuge tubes
Four 25 cm^2 tissue culture flasks
Clinical centrifuge
37 °C water baths
Dulbecco's modified Eagle's medium with 4.5 g/L glucose (DMEM)
Horse serum (HRS)
Fetal bovine serum (FBS)
Concanavalin-A (Con A) 1 mg stock solution
Lipopolysaccharide (LPS) 1 mg stock solution
Ionomycin
Phorbol-12-myristate-13-acetate (10 μg stock solution) (PMA)
Two 96-well plates with lids
ELISA coating buffer
Rabbit anti-IL-2
Anti-mouse CD4
Anti-mouse CD8
Goat anti-mouse ALEXA 488
Goat anti-rabbit-HRP (Horseradish peroxidase)
ELISA blocking buffer
1-step turbo TMB substrate solution (Pierce) 1 M H_2SO_4

Procedure

1. Follow procedures for preparing single cell suspension of mouse lymphoid tissue (spleen cell) in Exercise 4 (see Chap. 28) and for mitogen induction in Exercise 20 (see Chap. 45) using spleens from 3 C57BL/6 mice. Determine the cell count and cell viability from the spleen suspension and from the lymphoma cell culture provided in 25 cm^2 tissue culture flasks.
2. Resuspend the final pellet from the histopaque in 15 mL of 5% fetal bovine serum in RPMI = RPMI/FCS. Transfer 5 mL into tissue culture flask labeled #1, #2 and #3 (Fig. 46.1). Adjust the volumes in each flask to 10 mL by adding an

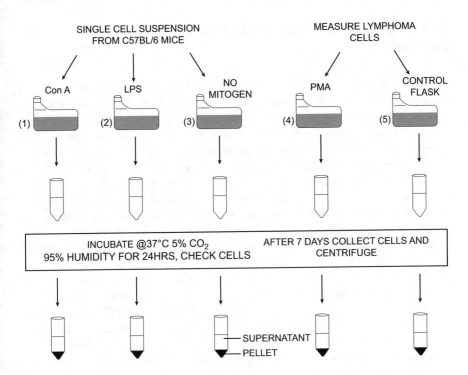

SINGLE CELL SUSPENSION
FROM C57BL/6 MICE

MEASURE LYMPHOMA
CELLS

Con A

LPS

NO
MITOGEN

PMA

CONTROL
FLASK

(1)   (2)   (3)   (4)   (5)

INCUBATE @37°C 5% CO_2
95% HUMIDITY FOR 24HRS, CHECK CELLS

AFTER 7 DAYS COLLECT CELLS AND
CENTRIFUGE

SUPERNATANT
PELLET

COLLECT SUPERNATANT AND ANALYZE USING ELISA TO DETECT CYTOKINES

COLLECT PELLET, RESUSPEND AND PREPARE SMEARS. FIX SMEARS AND ANALYZE BY IFA

Fig. 46.1 Induction of IL-2 secretion from mouse spleen cells and lymphoma cells. Spleen cells were incubated with concanavalin A (Con A) and lipopolysaccharide (LPS) and lymphoma cells were incubated with phorbol-12-myristate-13-acetate (PMA). Culture supernatants are tested for the secretion of the cytokine IL-2

additional 5 mL of RPMI/FCS to each flask. Add Con A (1 μg Con A/1 × 10^6 cells, i.e. 10 μg/flask for #1), add 2–25 μg/mL LPS final concentration in culture #2. Flask #3 is your control flask and will receive no mitogen. Cap flasks and shake gently from side to side. With the caps-slightly unscrewed, incubate the flasks on their flat sides and incubate at 37 °C, 5% CO_2 and 95% humidity.

The cultures will be examined periodically on the inverted microscope for 6 days. On day 6 viability determination, cell counts and Giemsa staining will be performed. Fresh media (5 mL) containing mitogens will also be added to flasks.

3. Mouse lymphoma cells obtained from the instructor will be maintained in 10% horse serum in DMEM = DMEM/HRS for 6 days. The cultures will be split, centrifuged and resuspended in 1% FBS/DMEM on day 6. Flasks will be labeled #4 and #5. Flask #4 will receive 20 ng/mL PMA (in some experiments PMA will be incubated with 1 μM ionomycin and PMA concentration will be varied up to 50 ng/mL) and flask #5 will be a no treatment control flask (Fig. 46.1). Cells will be cultured for 24 h at 37 °C, 5% CO_2, 95% humidity.

Screening for IL-2 Production by Elisa Using Anti-IL-2 Antisera

4. On day 7, collect all cultures into properly labeled, clean 15 mL tubes and centrifuge for 10 min at 1500 rpm. Collect supernatants into clean 15 mL centrifuge tubes. Prepare smears using the pellets, air-dry and fix in ice-cold acetone for direct and indirect immunofluorescence assays (IFAs) using rabbit α-mouse lgM-FITC, rabbit α-mouse IL-2 (secondary antibody, goat α-rabbit FITC) and mouse monoclonal antibody to Thy 1.2-TRITC (lgM). Monocolnal antibodies against CD4 and CD8 will also be used for IFA. Follow IFA procedure in Exercise 17 (see Chap. 41). Sign up to use the UV microscope following procedures in your department. Depending on the location of the microscope, you may only use the microscope accompanied by your instructor. Examine the morphology of Giemsa stained smears and record the appearance of the cells.

5. Use the supernatants collected to coat wells of an ELISA plate (2 plates). Follow the instructions from class and the procedures for the ELISA from Exercise16 (see Chap. 40). Prepare serial 1:2 dilutions of each supernatant using 2 rows of a 96 well plate (well #1 for each supernatant will be undiluted culture supernatant, well #2 will be 1:2, well #3 will be 1:4, etc.). Incubate plates for 24 h and in the next 2 days complete the assay. The antisera for IL-2 detection will be rabbit anti-IL-2. Control wells will contain either normal rabbit serum, no serum or no culture supernatant.

NOTES:

NOTES:

Selected Reference

Punt S, Jones O (2019) Kuby immunology, 8th edn. W.H. Freeman and Company, New York

Chapter 47
Exercise 22: Adoptive Transfer of Lymphocytes: B and T Lymphocyte Cooperation for Antibody Production

Introduction

In this exercise, we will demonstrate that combinations of B and T lymphocytes are required to efficiently produce antibodies against antigen. We will be using sheep red blood cells (SRBC) as the antigen. Irradiated CBA mice will serve as recipients for lymphoid cell suspensions from the spleen and thymus of a syngeneic donor. Mice exposed to whole body ionizing irradiation of 650–750 rads become immunologically suppressed. In addition, various biochemical and functional properties of the lymphocytes become impaired. Lymphocytes are highly sensitive to radiation and so animals whose lymphocytes have been inactivated can be reconstituted with various cell populations to study the functions of the different cells.

Hematopoietic cell transfer or transfer of sensitized lymphoid cells is referred to as adoptive transfer. Animals reconstituted with a combination of thymus and spleen cells will be challenged with antigen and the antibody response will be measured and compared to control animals reconstituted with spleen cells alone, thymus cells alone or saline as control. The **first objective** of this exercise is to learn procedures for adoptive transfer using i. v. injections. **The second objective** is to learn about B and T cell cooperation and the hemolytic plaque assay for enumerating antibody secreting plasma cells.

Materials and Reagents (Per Pair)

X-irradiation source
5 CBA mice (1 donor mouse, 4 irradiated mice)
Dissection trays and pins
Halothane chamber
Two sterile petri dishes containing wire meshes

© Springer Nature Switzerland AG 2021
T. Y. Sam-Yellowe, *Immunology: Overview and Laboratory Manual*,
https://doi.org/10.1007/978-3-030-64686-8_47

Hanks balanced salt solution
Centrifuge
Microscope
Six 15 mL centrifuge tubes
10% SRBC suspension
Sterile saline
1 and 10 mL pipets
Sterile 1 mL squeezers
Sterile Eppendorf tubes
Four pairs of sterile scissors and forceps
Mouse holders
Four 1 mL syringes and four 27 G needles
Sterile alcohol pads
Hemocytometers, cover slips and tally counters
Trypan blue
Ammonium chloride solution-Lysis buffer
Ice
Heparin
70% ethanol in squeeze bottle
200 mL waste beaker, Biohazard bags
Gloves
Capillary tubes
30 Sterile 13 × 100 mm tubes
Three empty cages with clean bedding and clean water
Materials from Exercise 6 (see Chap. 30) for hemolytic plaque assay

Procedure

1. Irradiate four CBA mice (600–800 rads) and keep in warm clean cages. Save fifth mouse for donating lymphoid cells. This will be done by your TA or instructor (*see* Fig. 47.1).

2. After 24 h prepare spleen and thymus cell suspension in Hank's balanced salt solution containing 25 units of heparin, following the procedure outlined in Exercise 2 (See Chap. 26). **USE THE NON-IRRADIATED MOUSE FOR OBTAINING LYMPHOID CELLS**. After the last wash count the cells, determine cell viability and resuspend the spleen cells to a final concentration of 5×10^6 cells/mL and the thymus cells to a final concentration of 3×10^8 cells/mL. Place the cells on ice until required for reconstitution.

3. Using 1 mL syringes and 27 G needles reconstitute irradiated mice with the lymphoid cell suspensions. Place the mice in a mouse holder and inject cells i.v. into the lateral tail vein.

   (a) Inject 0.2 mL of the spleen cell suspension into first mouse
   (b) Inject 0.2 mL of the thymus cell suspension into second mouse.

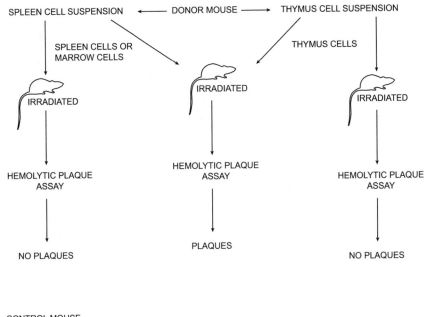

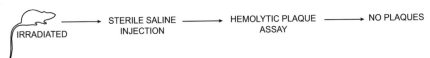

Fig. 47.1 Immune system reconstitution of irradiated mouse to demonstrate the requirement of B and T lymphocyte cooperation in immune response to antigen

(c) Inject 0.2 mL of mixture of 0.1 spleen and 0.1 mL thymus cell suspension into third mouse

(d) Inject 0.2 mL of sterile saline into fourth mouse.

4. After 24 h inject 0.2 mL of 10% SRBC into each of the four mice i.p.

5. After 5–6 days kill mice, obtain spleen cells and mix with SRBC and complement to perform the hemolytic plaque assay. Collect blood by cardiac puncture from the four mice into separate Eppendorf tubes for anti-serum. Your instructor will demonstrate. We will use the antiserum for direct agglutination reactions using SRBCs. Refer to Exercise #6 (see Chap. 30) for the hemolytic plaque assay procedure. Count and compare the number of plaques obtained from each mouse to determine the number of hemolysin (anti-SRBC antibody) secreting plasma cells. Are there any differences in the number of plaque forming units (PFUs) obtained from the four mice?

NOTES AND ILLUSTRATIONS:

NOTES:

NOTES:

Chapter 48
Exercise 23: Macrophage Migration Inhibition Test

Introduction

Migration inhibitory factor (MIF) is a pro-inflammatory, immunoregulatory cytokine with chemokine-like function. MIF has pleotropic effects on cells such as recruitment and also promoting cell arrest. Several cells, including B and T lymphocytes, macrophages, endothelial and epithelial cells secrete MIF. The MIF test is the in vitro correlate of delayed type hypersensitivity (DTH). In vivo, the DTH reaction is associated with the formation of granulomas and the recruitment of cells responding to chemokines in inflamm. The assay detects the secretion of MIF from T cells activated by antigen, which results in inhibition of macrophage migration. Peritoneal macrophages placed in a capillary tube in the presence of supernatant from activated T cells will remain in the capillary tube and not migrate. Control supernatant from unstimulated T cells, without MIF results in migration of macrophages when incubated with macrophages placed in a capillary tube. MIF can also be detected using ELISA and western blotting. However, with ELISA and western blotting, macrophages cannot be observed, since only the cytokine can be detected. Polymerase chain reaction (PCR) can also be used to amplify the gene encoding MIF. For quantitation of MIF expression, real-time-PCR (RT-PCR) may also be performed using cDNA template and primers targeting MIF. As with ELISA and western blotting, the macrophages cannot be detected when PCR is performed. Antibodies against MIF can detect MIF secreted by T cells. The levels of MIF secreted can be quantitated to determine the activation of T cells. MIF binds to CD74 and results in activation of the MAP kinase pathway and translocation of AP1. The **objective** of this exercise is to learn how to perform the MIF test.

© Springer Nature Switzerland AG 2021
T. Y. Sam-Yellowe, *Immunology: Overview and Laboratory Manual*,
https://doi.org/10.1007/978-3-030-64686-8_48

Materials and Reagents (Per Group)

Three ovalbumin sensitive Balb/c mice
Three 10 mL syringe with 18 G needle
6 mL incomplete Freund's adjuvant
Three 1 mL syringes with 25 G needle
Three 10 mL syringes with 20 G needle
100 mL cold DMEM with 10 units heparin (or 10% EDTA)/mL
Three 50 mL centrifuge tubes
Seven 15 mL centrifuge tubes
Six 1 and 10 mL pipets DMEM without heparin
DMEM with 5% Fetal bovine serum
12 sterile capillary tubes
Two pair of small forceps and clay block
Four sterile Sykes-Moore chambers with silicon grease and wrench assembly
    Diamond pencil
DMEM with 15% FBS
DMEM with 25 ug/mL ovalbumin
Two 1 mL syringes with four 26 G needles
White bond paper, pencil and pair of small scissors
Photographic enlarger
Centrifuge
Balance

Procedure

1. Inject ovalbumin sensitive Balb/c mice with 1 mL of incomplete Freund/s adjuvant i.p.

2. Approximately 72 h later, inject 5 mL of cold sterile DMEM containing 10 units heparin/mL into the peritoneal cavity using a 10 mL syringe attached to a 20 G needle. Gently massage the abdomen and carefully withdraw peritoneal fluid from the base of the peritoneum using a 20 G needle attached to a 10 mL syringe.

3. Place the peritoneal fluid in a sterile 50 mL centrifuge tube. Centrifuge the fluid for 10 min at 1000 rpm. Discard the supernatant. Resuspend and pool the cells, transfer to a 15 mL centrifuge tube and wash the cells twice with 10 mL of cold DMEM without heparin. Discard the supematants.

4. After the last wash, resuspend the cells to 10% concentration (e.g. if you have a 100 uL pellet, resuspend in 1 mL) in DMEM containing 15% FBS.

5. Fill eight sterile capillary tubes 2/3 full with the cell suspension and seal one end with clay to approximately 5 mm. Place the capillary tubes with sealed ends down in sterile test tube containing a plug of cotton and centrifuge in

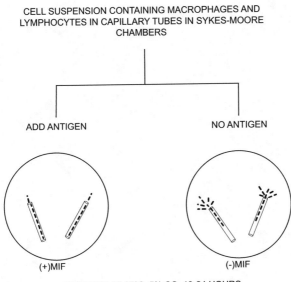

Fig. 48.1 Macrophage inhibitory factor (MIF) assay to demonstrate macrophage migration in response in absence of MIF and inhibition of macrophage migration in the presence of MIF

swing-bucket rotor at 500 rpm for 10 min. You may prepare several tubes in case some break.

6. Using the diamond knife cut the capillary tubes at the cell supernatant interface and place the ends containing the cells into sterile Sykes-Moore chambers. Secure the cut tubes with small amounts of silicone grease. Be sure the capillary tubes are resting on the glass cover slips. Use two capillary tubes per chamber and set tubes at an angle of about 40–450° to one another (Fig. 48.1).

7. Insert a 26 G needle into chamber through rubber gasket to vent the chamber after sealing, then fill them with DMEM containing 15% FBS with or without 25 µg of specific antigen. Prepare two chambers (four tubes) with antigen and two chambers without antigen.

8. Incubate the chambers at 37 °C, 5% CO_2 for 18–24 h. Observe and record your results by using a photographic enlarger or an overhead projector to enlarge the migration pattern. Make scale drawings of the migration patterns. Handle the chambers carefully, making sure that cells are not disturbed.

9. Using a small pair of scissors cut out migration patterns and determine the mean weight for each group.

10. Determine the % migration inhibition using the formula shown:

$$1 - \left(\text{mean weight of experimental cells}\right) \times 100 = \%\text{inhibition mean weight of control cells}$$

11. Show your results in a tabular form.

NOTES:

NOTES:

NOTES AND ILLUSTRATIONS:

Selected References

DeToma FJ, MacDonald AB (1987) Experimental immunology. A guidebook. Macmillan Publishing Company, New York. Chapter 13, An assay for leukocyte inhibitory factor

Kimball JW (1990) Introduction to immunology, 3rd edn. Macmillan Publishing Company, New York. Chapter 5, Cell-mediated immunity

Ortiz-Garcia YM, Garcia-Iglesias T, Morales-Velazquez G et al (2019) Macrophage migration inhibitory factor levelsin gingival crevicular fluid, saliva, and serum of chronic periodontitis patients. BioMed Res Int. https://doi.org/10.1155/2019/7850392

Punt S, Jones O (2019) Kuby immunology, 8th edn. W.H. Freeman and Company, New York

Chapter 49
Exercise 24: Monoclonal Antibody Production

Introduction

Monoclonal antibodies recognize and react with a single epitope on an antigen. Monoclonal antibodies are produced by a single B cell lineage i.e. a single clone of B cells propagated in culture. This is in contrast to polyclonal antibodies that recognize several different epitopes on a single antigen. The ability to prepare monoclonal antibodies has revolutionized biology and medicine. The unique specificity of the individual antibodies makes them particularly useful for mapping antigen epitopes. Monoclonal antibodies are routinely prepared by the fusion of immune Balb/c mouse spleen cells with non-Ig secreting **myeloma** cells of Balb/c origin, using polyethylene glycol. The antigen used for mouse immunizations does not have to be pure. The resulting hybrids, i.e. **hybridomas** are cultured in selective media consisting of HAT (**Hypoxanthine, Aminopterin and Thymidine**). The myeloma cells are deficient in hypoxanthine guanine phosphoribosyl transferase (HGPRT) or thymidine kinase (TK) and preferably non antibody producing (Ig) The spleen cells are HGPRT, TK+, Ig+. The components of the HAT medium suppress the growth of the parental myeloma cells and the spleen cells cannot survive indefinitely in culture. However, the hybridomas can grow in the presence of HAT and grow indefinitely. Hypoxanthine and thymidine are used in the salvage pathway, while aminopterin blocks DNA synthesis by the denovo pathway so that cells have to use the salvage pathway for DNA synthesis. The spent culture supernatants from the growing hybrids are screened for antibody production using ELISA assays or IFA. Antibody producing hybridomas are diluted and cloned to obtain single antibody producing cells. The clones are propagated and expanded in culture or grown as ascites in pristane-primed Balb/c mice for monoclonal antibody production. Mammalian expression host cells such as Chinese hamster ovary (CHO) cells are used to express recombinant monoclonal antibodies for therapeutic use. Recombinant DNA encoding immunoglobulin heavy and light chain genes is transfected into CHO cells through electroporation or the use of lipofectin.

© Springer Nature Switzerland AG 2021
T. Y. Sam-Yellowe, *Immunology: Overview and Laboratory Manual*,
https://doi.org/10.1007/978-3-030-64686-8_49

Monoclonal antibodies are used for a variety of procedures requiring exquisite specificity for antigen:

- protein purification by affinity purification
- mapping of antigen or antibody epitopes
- isolation of lymphocyte subpopulations
- identification of tumor associated antigens
- diagnostic ELISA, immunoblotting, immunoprecipitation and IFA assays
- tumor directed killing (therapeutic antibodies)

The objective of this exercise is to produce monoclonal antibodies against membrane proteins of *Plasmodium sp.* Antibody producing cells will be screened using ELISA and IFA.

Materials and Reagents (Per Pair)

Immunized Balb/c mice
Unimmunized Balb/c mice for feeder layers
Myeloma cells (P3/NS1/1/Ag4-1, Sp2/OAgl4, etc.) (ATCC)
Microscopes (Inverted and upright)
Laminar Flow Hood
Hemocytometers
Water bath (37 and 56 °C)
Centrifuge
CO_2 incubator
Timer
Fetal bovine serum
Dulbecco's Modified Eagle's Medium (DMEM) or RPMI
100× HAT solution
35% Polyethylene glycol (PEG) in PBS pH 8.3 (PEG 4000)
0.4% Trypan blue
Sterile lysing buffer (0.83% Ammonium chloride in 0.01 M Tris–HCl, pH 7.5)
15 and 50 mL centrifuge tubes
Sterile petri dishes
Sterile wire mesh screens
1 and 10 mL syringes, 26G needles and clean microfuge tubes
Sterile 1 mL squeezers
70% ethanol and waste beaker
24 and 96 well microtiter plates
1 and 10 mL pipets
Automatic pipeter (Pipet-aid)
Gilson pipetman 200, 20 µL
Sterile pipet tips
Sterile scissors and forceps
Sterile distilled water

Hybridomas can be grown in the presence of NCTC 109 (ThermoFisher), glutamine and OPI (Cisoxaloacetic acid, pyruvate and insulin) to enhance cell growth.

Procedure

1. Immunize 8–12 week old Balb/c mice with desired immunogen (50–100 μg) in complete Freund's adjuvant (CFA) i.p., or s.c. (or any other adjuvant of choice e.g. TiterMax Gold, Ribi adjuvant etc. Spleen cells may also be obtained from mice vaccinated with whole killed organisms (or infected with the replicating infectious organisms), followed by booster injections of the immunogen at 2–3 week intervals mixed in incomplete Freund's adjuvant (IFA). Three days before cell fusion, the mice are boosted with the immunogen in IFA i.p. or the soluble antigen is administered i.v. in the lateral tail vein.
2. Maintain myeloma cells in 10% FBS-DMEM-Gentamycin at approximately 1×10^6 cells/mL. 1–2 days before fusion split cultures, feed cells with fresh medium and check cell viability. Viability should be approximately 70–80%.

Day of Fusion

Prepare feeder cells (see protocol on next page) (Fusion can be successfully carried out without feeder layers). See Fig. 49.1 for fusion protocol.

3. Harvest myeloma cells by collecting cultures into 50 mL centrifuge tubes and centrifuging at 1500 rpms for 10 min. Collect supernatant into sterile bottles and store at 4 °C. This will be used as conditioned medium. Pool cell pellets and wash two times in DMEM without serum.
4. Resuspend the cells in 40 mL of DMEM without serum, dilute cells 1:20, count cells and determine viability. E.g. pipet 250 μL of cell suspension into centrifuge tube, add 250 μL of 0.4% Trypan blue and 4.5 mL of DMEM. Incubate cells for 1–2 min and count cells using a hemocytometer.
5. Kill immunized mouse by placing mouse in container with halothane soaked cotton, disinfect mouse with 70% ethanol by completely wetting mouse with 70% ethanol. Perform splenectomy-aseptically under hood- and collect immunized spleen into petri dish containing wire mesh and 10 mL DMEM without serum. Collect blood from the mouse into a clean eppendorf tube for hyperimmune anti-serum. "Ring" blood clot and incubate at 4 °C for antiserum collection 24 h later.
6. Gently tease spleen through wire mesh using the plunger from a 10 mL syringe. Transfer spleen cells into a 15 mL centrifuge tube. Let the large pieces settle, approximately 30 s then transfer cell suspension into fresh tubes and centrifuge cells for 10 min at 1500 rpms. Lyse erythrocytes by adding 1 mL of lysing

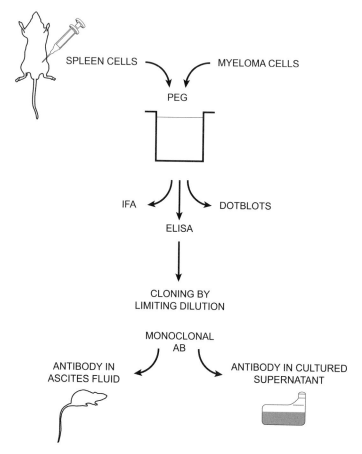

Fig. 49.1 Illustration of procedure for producing monoclonal antibodies. Spleen cells obtained from immunized mouse are fused with myeloma cells using polyethylene glycol (PEG). Hybridoma supernatants are screened for antibody production by ELISA, IFA or dot blots. Antibody positive hybridomas are cloned by limiting dilution for injection into mice to collect ascites fluid or grown in culture flasks to collect antibody in culture supernatant

solution (ammonium chloride) to spleen cell pellet, resuspend pellet for 1 min. Add DMEM to 10 mL and centrifuge 5 min at 1500 rpm. Wash the cells twice each time resuspending in 10 mL DMEM without serum. After last wash, resuspend cells in 10 mL DMEM without serum, prepare a 1:100 dilution of the cells into a separate tube count cells and determine the viability.

7. Transfer spleen cells to a 50 mL tube, add the myeloma cell suspension to the spleen cells, gently resuspend the cell mixture and centrifuge for 5 min at 1500 rpm.

8. Discard the supernatant and add 2 mL 35% PEG to pellet and very gently resuspend pellet for 3 min. Start the timer as soon as PEG is added. (Total time for PEG addition and centrifugation is 8 min.) Centrifuge cell mixture at 2000 rpm

for 2 min, add DMEM directly to cells plus supernatant to 50 mL resuspend gently and centrifuge for 3 min at 1500 rpm. Discard supernatant.

9. Add 25 mL of 15% FBS-DMEM-Gentamycin (50 mg/mL) to pellet, resuspend gently and distribute 1 mL aliquots to individual wells of a 24 well microtiter plate or 100 µL into 96 well plates with or without feeder cells.

10. After 18–24 h, add 1 mL of 2× HAT medium to cells in 24 well plates (100 µL of 2× HAT in 96 well). Feed cells 1× HAT media every 2–3 days by removing 1 mL media and replacing with 1 mL of fresh media. Around day 4–5 start checking for hybrids. By day 10 start screening for antibody production using ELISA, IFA or Dot blotting. **MAKE SURE YOU HAVE A RELIABLE SCREENING ASSAY BEFORE INITIATING CELL FUSION.**

11. When antibody production has been confirmed, clone the positive hybridomas by limiting dilution. Screen the supernatants from the clones, select positive clones and transfer cells to 24 well plates.

12. Repeat screening procedure using supernatants from 24 well plates and expand positive clones into tissue culture flasks. Slowly wean the cultures from 1x HAT by feeding the cultures 1× HT media and changing the media gradually to 15% FBS-DMEM-Gentamycin without additional additives. Determine the isotype and subisotype of the antibodies being secreted. It may be necessary to repeat the cloning procedure if a culture is suspected of having more than one clone.

13. Clones secreting antibody may be expanded in tissue culture flasks and the spent media collected as the source of antibody or clones ($1–3 \times 10^6$ cells/mL) may be injected into pristane primed Balb/c mice for ascites fluid production. The ascites fluid contains concentrated monoclonal antibodies approximately 1–10 mg/mL and once clarified by centrifugation followed by ammonium sulfate precipitation, can be used as the source of monoclonal antibodies. The antibodies may be purified and further characterizations performed to determine the specificity of the antibody.

Cloning by Limiting Dilution

Preparation of Feeder Cells

1. Kill an unimmunized Balb/c mouse by placing mouse in halothane chamber. Wet mouse thoroughly with 70% ethanol and aseptically splenectomize the mouse, placing the spleen on a sterile wire mesh in a sterile petri dish containing 10 mL of DMEM without serum.

2. Tease apart spleen cells using a plunger from a 10 mL syringe. Collect cells into a 15 mL centrifuge tube, allow large clumps to settle, approximately 30 s., transfer the spleen cell suspension into a fresh 15 ml centrifuge tube without disturbing clumps, and centrifuge the cells for 5 min at 1500 rpm.

3. Lyse erythrocytes using ammonium chloride lysing solution, add DMEM to 10 mL and centrifuge cells for 5 min at 1500 rpm. Wash spleen cells twice using

10 mL DMEM each wash. After last wash, resuspend the cells in 10 mL DMEM, prepare dilution, count cells and determine viability using trypan blue.

4. Adjust the cells to 1×10^7 cell/mL in I× HT or I× HAT depending on what the hybridoma cells are growing in. If the feeder cells are being prepared for use in cell fusion, resuspend the cells in 15% FBS-DMEM-Gentamycin. Add 100 µL of the cell suspension to each well of a 96 well plate.

Hybridoma Cells

1. Aspirate 1/2 the media from the wells to be cloned and save for screening.
2. Resuspend the cells in the well gently and transfer to a sterile 15 mL centrifuge tube. Count cells and determine viability using trypan blue as above. Adjust the cells to 1×10^4–1×10^5 cells/mL in media (same as the cells are growing in).
3. Prepare stock solution of cells i.e. bring cell volume up to 1–3 mL.
4. Arrange six sets of tubes and label A–F

(A) 0.5 mL of stock from #3 plus 4.5 mL of media
(B) 1 mL of A plus 2 mL of media
(C) 1 mL of B plus 2 mL of media
(D) 1 mL of C plus 2 mL of media
(E) 1 mL of D plus 2 mL of media
(F) 1 mL of E plus 2 mL of media

Add 100 µL of cell suspension from tubes A–F to feeder cells in 96 well plate. Freeze down the remaining cells in 10% DMSO. Incubate plates for 5–7 days without disturbing. Check plates occasionally for contamination and also check for growth of clones using an inverted microscope. When clones begin to grow, repeat screening procedure to detect antibody positive clones. Continue procedure as indicated above.

Selected References

Caldwell HD Monoclonal antibody production (modified), Rocky Mountain Laboratories, Hamilton, MT

Li F, Vijayasankaran N, Shen AY, Kiss R, Amanullah A (2010) Cell culture processes for monoclonal antibody production. mAbs 2:466–477

Murphy K, Weaver C (2017) Janeway's immunobiology, 9th edn. Garland Press, New York

Punt J, Stranford SA, Jones PP, Owen JA (2019) Kuby immunology, 8th edn. W.H. Freeman and Company, New York. Chapter 20, Antigen-antibody interactions.

Sam-Yellowe TY, Fujioka H, Aikawa M, Hall T, Drazba JA (2001) A *Plasmodium falciparum* protein located in Maurer's clefts underneath knobs and protein localization in association with Rhop-3 and SERA in the intracellular network infected erythrocytes. Parasitol Res 87:173–185

Tabll A, Abbas AT, El-Kafrawy S, Wahid A (2015) Monoclonal antibodies: principles and applications of immunodiagnosis and immunotherapy for hepatitis C virus. World J Hepatol 7:2369–2383

Chapter 50
Exercise 25: Immunization of Mice with a Recombinant Protein

Introduction

Following expression of a recombinant protein from *E. coli* and purification of the protein using a Nickel (Ni^{++}-NTA resin) column, the protein can be used to immunize mice for antibody production and as a vaccine for determining protection against a pathogen (*Plasmodium yoelii*). Using protocols approved by the institutional animal care and use committee (IACUC), mice can be immunized to investigate the immunogenicity of the recombinant protein, and antibodies generated can be used to investigate the characteristics of the protein. Eukaryotic proteins expressed in *E. coli* may be misfolded and lack post-translational modifications. In addition proteins may be found in aggregates or in inclusion bodies leading to the use of purification methods that may denature the proteins. Immunization with the recombinant proteins, generation of antisera and evaluation of the antisera using immunoassays can determine if the antibodies can be used in functional studies and in investigations to characterize the protein. Besides determining the titer of the antibodies, proteins that are part of large complexes such as those found in signaling pathways, can be co-precipitated using the antibody. The recombinant protein can be used in immunization challenge experiments to determine the effectiveness of antibodies produced against the recombinant protein in inhibiting parasite growth in vitro or preventing the establishment of infection in vivo. The **first objective** of this exercise is to learn how to immunize mice with a recombinant protein. The **second objective** is to learn how to screen the antisera using immunoassays to determine the titer of the antisera.

© Springer Nature Switzerland AG 2021
T. Y. Sam-Yellowe, *Immunology: Overview and Laboratory Manual*,
https://doi.org/10.1007/978-3-030-64686-8_50

Materials (Per Group)

Swiss Webster mice
Purified recombinant protein
TiterMax Gold adjuvant
Freund's complete adjuvant
Freund's incomplete adjuvant
Eppendorf tubes
1 mL syringes with 26 G needles
50 mL centrifuge tubes
15 mL centrifuge tubes
1× PBS
Sterile gauze
70% ethanol
Kimwipes

Procedure

Immunization of Mice for Antibody Production

Each mouse will receive 50 µL of protein (about 15 µg) plus 50 µL of adjuvant.

Four groups of five mice each will be used for immunizations. We will examine the effectiveness of two adjuvants; TiterMax Gold and Freund' adjuvant. The time interval between booster injections will also be tested. Mice will be immunized intraperitoneally (i. p.).

1. Divide mice into five groups:

   (a) Group 1: Titermax Gold adjuvant with boosts at one week intervals
   (b) Group 2: Titermax Gold adjuvant with boosts at two week intervals
   (c) Group 3: Freund's complete adjuvant with boosts at 1 week intervals with Freund's incomplete adjuvant
   (d) Group 4: Freund's complete adjuvant with boosts at 2 week intervals with Freund's incomplete adjuvant
   (e) Group 5: Unimmunized mice. Blood will be collected for normal mouse serum

2. Immunize mice i. p. using 100 µL of immunogen (50 µL protein plus 50 µL of adjuvant).

3. After the initial immunization, boost the mice after one week (for those mice receiving boosts at 1 week intervals) or 2 weeks (for those mice receiving boosts at 2 week intervals). Mice will receive a total of two boosts. Mice that were

immunized with Complete Freund's adjuvant for the initial immunization will receive boosters in incomplete Freund's adjuvant.

4. Two weeks after the second boost, blood will be obtained from each mouse for serum collection.

5. Centrifuge clotted mouse blood obtained from individual mice in each group. Label each tube. Pipet the antiserum from each tube into fresh Eppendorf tubes making sure that each tube is labeled.

6. For each group, pipet 50 µL of antiserum representing each mouse and add it to a labeled tube for pooled antiserum. Use a different pipet tip for each tube. There should be 250 µL of pooled antiserum for each of the five groups of mice.

7. The individual and pooled antisera from groups 1 to 4 will be analyzed using western blot, IFA, immunoprecipitation, and IEM to determine the specificity of the antibodies for the recombinant protein and to determine the titer of the antibodies for each immunoassay. Normal mouse serum will be used as a negative control for immunoassays. For western blotting and immunoprecipitation, cell extracts will also be analyzed for antibody reactivity to the native protein.

Immunization of Mice for Challenge Infection

1. Mice will be immunized as described above using the same antigen dosage. Mice will be arranged in seven groups.

   (a) Group 1: Freund's (boosts with Incomplete Freund's) alone (50 µL) as control

   (b) Group 2: Titermax Gold alone (50 µL)

   (c) Group 3: Freund's (50 µL) + 50 µL of protein (15 µg)

   (d) Group 4: Titermax Gold (50 µL) + 50 µL of protein (15 µg)

   (e) Group 5: PBS (50 µL) + protein (15 µg);

   (f) Group 6: PBS alone (100 µL);

   (g) Group 7: No treatment but only needle thrust (sham injection).

2. Immunize mice i.p. using 100 µL of immunogen (50 µL protein plus 50 µL of adjuvant) and controls.

3. Boost mice at two week interval.

4. Perform tail snips to collect small amounts of blood to detect antibody production using dot blots or double immunodiffusion.

5. Collect infected mouse blood in CPD from two infected mice and place in a 15 mL centrifuge tube. Wash the blood by centrifugation three times using RPMI medium.

6. After the last wash, remove the supernatant and save a volume of supernatant equal to the cell pellet. Prepare 2 smears for Giemsa staining and for determining the parasitemia of infection. Add RPMI to the pellet and bring the volume to 10 mL. Resuspend gently.

7. Pipet 10 µL of the cell suspension in #6 and add to 990 µL of RPMI to make a 1:100 diluition. Count the number of red cells in the 10 mL cell suspension by counting cells in 80 small square of a hemocytometer. Adjust the cells to 1×10^9, then make a 1:10 dilution to obtain 1×10^8 cells.

8. Inject each mouse with 100 µL of diluted cells which contains 1×10^7 cells for challenge injections.

9. The second day after challenge make blood smear from each mouse using tail snips for Giemsa staining.

10. Prepare blood smears daily for Giemsa staining to determine the level of parasitemia in the mice in each group. Check mice visually to determine if the mice appear well or moribund. Record the number of mice that survive the infection or die as compared to the controls. Analyze the results and perform statistics.

Selected References

Wang T, Fujioka H, Drazba JA, Sam-Yellowe TY (2006) Rhop-3 protein conservation among *Plasmodium* species and induced protection against lethal *P. yoelii* and *P. berghei* challenge. Parasitol Res 99:238–252

Chapter 51
Exercise 26: Polarization of T Helper Cells into TH1 Cells

Introduction

T helper cells undergo differentiation in response to cytokines released from antigen presenting dendritic cells (DCs) within the T cell zone of secondary lymphoid organs. IL-2 secretion and IL-2 receptor expression become upregulated following antigen contact. The nature of the antigen recognized by the naïve T helper cell and the cytokines received from the DC determines the TH subset that will be obtained and the type of effector function that cell will perform. In addition, the effect of the polarizing cytokines will also determine the activation of transcription factors that will drive the expression of effector cytokines. TH1 and TH2 helper subsets were initially described with TH1 cells characterized by IFNγ and TNFα secretion. TH2 cells are characterized by IL-4, IL-5 and IL-13 secretion. Intracellular infections by viruses, bacteria and parasites, aided by cytokines, polarize naïve T helper cells to THI as a result of IL-12 and IFNγ binding to receptors on naïve T helper cells.TH1 cells activate macrophages which along with TH1 cells are important for cytotoxity responses of CD8+ cytotoxic T cells. In response to IL-4, naïve T helper cells are polarized to TH2 cells in response to allergens from helminth parasites, leading to IgE secretion from B cells and activation of eosiniphils. The transcription factor (TF) T-bet drives expression of IFNγ and TH1 differentiation. The TF, GATA-3 is the master regulator for TH2 differentiation. Other subsets TH cells include TH17, TFH and TH9 which has effector characteristics similar to TH2 and also important for humoral immunity. TFH cell are important for germinal cell formation in the follicles of secondary and tertiary lymphoid organs. The **objective** of this exercise is to polarize T helper cells from a spleen suspension into TH1 cells.

© Springer Nature Switzerland AG 2021
T. Y. Sam-Yellowe, *Immunology: Overview and Laboratory Manual*,
https://doi.org/10.1007/978-3-030-64686-8_51

Materials (Per Pair)

Lamina flow hood
Swiss Webster mouse
70% ethanol
Sterile scissors and forceps
24 well and 6 well microtiter plates
Anti-mouse CD3 antibodies
Anti-mouse CD28 antibodies
Recombinant IL-2
Recombinant IL-12
Anti-mouse IL-4
Phorbol 12-myristate 13-acetate (PMA)
Ionomycin
Sterile 15 mL centrifuge tubes
DMEM
FBS
Penicillin/Streptomycin
RBC lysis buffer
DMEM containing 10% FBS and penicillin/streptomycin (complete medium)
PBS
Hemocytometer
Trypan blue
Sterile Petri dishes
10 mL serological pipets
P200
Yellow tips
Table top Centrifuge
Microfuge
37 °C incubator with 5% CO_2
Materials for capture ELISA

Procedure

1. Obtain spleen under a laminar flow hood from a Swiss Webster mouse killed and the fur sprayed with 70% ethanol (**as in Exercise 3**, see Chap. 27). Place the spleen in a petri dish containing sterile DMEM and a sterile wire mesh.
2. Prepare a cell suspension by gently teasing the spleen cells through the wire mesh using the plunger from a 10 mL syringe
3. Using a sterile 10 mL pipet, collect the cell suspension into a 15 mL sterile centrifuge tube. Cap the tube tightly and centrifuge for 10 min at 3500 rpm.

4. Using a sterile squeezer, discard the supernatant in the waste container provided. Resuspend the pellet in 1 mL of complete media and pipet 100 μL into an Eppendorf tube for cell counts.

5. Perform cell counts using a hemocytometer or automatic cell counter and adjust cells to 1×10^6 cells /ml.

6. Add additional 1 mL of complete media to the cells.

7. Add 500 μL of anti-mouse CD3 (1–3 μg/mL) and anti-mouse CD28 (1–3 μg/mL) antibodies to eight wells of a 24 well plate to coat the wells. Two sets of plates can be prepared. One set will be used for detecting IFNγ by ELISA and CD4 by IFA. The second set will be used for total RNA extraction from cells for T-bet expression by qPCR.

8. Incubate the plate at 37 °C for 2 h (the plates can be prepared before lab by coating the plates the day before and incubating the plate at 4 °C overnight)

9. Discard the unbound antibody from the wells by turning plate upside down over a waste container.

10. Wash the wells three times by adding 1 mL of PBS to the wells, gently shaking the plate from side to side and discarding the PBS as in step 9. Repeat the washes two more times.

11. Adjust cell count to 1×10^6 cells/mL and add 1 mL per well into 8 wells.

12. To wells 1 and 2 add IL-2 (5 ng/mL), IL-12 (10 ng/mL) and anti-mouse IL-4 (10 μg/mL), to wells 3 and 4 add IL-2 alone, to wells 5 and 6 add IL-12 alone and to wells 7 and 8 add IL-2 and IL-12 alone.

13. Incubate the plate at 37 °C, 5% CO_2

14. On day 3, check the plate for growth, by observing a change in color of the media from light orange to yellow.

15. Pool the duplicate wells for each treatment into the wells of 6-well plates. For example pool the contents of wells 1 and 2 from the 24 well plate into one well of a 6-well plate, contents of wells 3 and 4 from the 24 well plate into a well of the 6 well plate, contents of wells 5 and 6 from the 24 well plate into a well of the six well plate and contents of wells 7 and 8 from the 24 well plate to the 6 well plate. Add 2 mL of fresh complete media to each well containing cells in the 6 well plate and incubate cells at 37 °C, 5% CO_2

16. On day 5, add phorbol 12-myristate 13-acetate (50 ng/mL) and ionomycin (1 μg/mL) prepared in complete media, to cells in the 6 well plate.

17. Incubate plates at 37 °C, 5% CO_2 for 5 h

18. Using a sterile squeezer, collect supernatants into labeled 15 mL tubes. Supernatants will be used for capture ELISA to detect IFNγ secretion.

19. Add 1 mL of PBS to each well, resuspend the cells and transfer the cells to labelled Eppendorf tubes. Centrifuge the tube, discard the supernatants

20. Add 100 μL of PBS to the pellets, resuspend gently and prepare smears on glass slides. Prepare two slides per pellet. Air dry the smears and fix the cells in absolute methanol for immunofluorescence using anti-mouse CD4 antibodies.

21. For measuring the expression of the transcription factor T-bet, cells will be collected from plates processed from step 7 through step 19 into Eppendorf tubes for total RNA extraction using RNA-Bee (Tel-Test, Inc.)

22. RNA will be used to synthesize cDNA using SuperScript IV reverse transcriptase kit (ThermoFischer). cDNA can be stored at -20 °C until required for qPCR. Oligonucleotide primers targeting mouse T-bet will be used for qPCR and expression normalized to GAPDH.

Selected References

Flaherty S, Reynold JM (2015) Mouse naïve CD4+ T cell isolation and In vitro differentiation into T cell subsets. J Vis Exp (98):e52739. https://doi.org/10.3791/52739

Murphy K, Weaver C (2017) Janeway's immunobiology, 9th edn. Garland Press, New York

Punt J, Stranford SA, Jones PP, Owen JA (2019) Kuby immunology, 8th edn. W.H. Freeman and Company, New York. Chapter 20, Antigen-antibody interactions

Chapter 52
Exercise 27: Immunoprecipitation

Introduction

Antibodies or immunoglobulin binding proteins immobilized on sepharose or aga-rose beads can be used to bind immune complexes formed by antibody binding to antigen usually contained in an extract. The purified antigen is solubilized by boiling the beads in sample buffer. This process of pulling out a specific protein from a heterogeneous mixture of proteins from a cell extract is known as immunoprecipitation. The immunoglobulin binding proteins can be incubated with antibodies first, then incubated with the protein extract to pull out the specific protein from the extract. This is useful when antibody concentration is low. The antibody specific for the antigen is used to purify the protein out of the extract. Antibody may also be incubated with the cell extract to form the immune complex. Antibody or protein A immobilized beads may then be added to the antibody-antigen reaction, to pull out the immune complex. Proteins A, G and L are immunoglobulin binding proteins used for immunoprecipitation assays. Protein A is a 42 kDa surface protein produced by some strains of *Staphylococcus aureus*. Protein A binds to the Fc region of IgG. Protein G is produced by group C and G *Streptococcus* as a 58 and 65 kDa, protein respectively. Protein G also binds to the Fc region of IgG. Recombinant proteins containing protein A and G are also used for immunoprecipitation. Protein L is produced by *Peptostreptococcus magnus*, and is a 76 kDa protein that also bind immunoglobulin but binds to the light chain region of the molecule, specifically to kappa light chains. The immunoprecipitation assay is the basis for pull-down assays used to identify proteins in cell signaling pathways, identifying interacting protein partners in protein-protein interactions and in identifying DNA binding proteins in chromatin immunoprecipitation (ChIP). Immunoprecipitation assays are important in pulse chase experiments employing biosynthetically (^{35}S-methionine) labeled proteins. The **objective** of this exercise is to learn how to perform the immunoprecipitation assay.

© Springer Nature Switzerland AG 2021
T. Y. Sam-Yellowe, *Immunology: Overview and Laboratory Manual*,
https://doi.org/10.1007/978-3-030-64686-8_52

Materials (Per Group)

Protein A sepharose beads
Goat anti-mouse sepharose beads
Cell extracts
Rabbit and mouse antisera
End-over-end shaker
Microfuge
Table top IEC centrifuge
Balance
Parafilm
Markers
Pack of 1.5 mL Eppendorf tubes
1× PBS
15 mL centrifuge tubes
1 and 10 mL serological pipettes
Box of 1 mL plastic squeezers
Empty 500 mL beaker for waste/wash collection
Kimwipes
Buffers A, B, C and D
Materials for SDS-PAGE and western blotting

Procedure

1. Swell protein A-sepharose or goat anti-mouse IgG-sepharose beads by weighing 0.2 g beads and adding the beads to each of two 15 mL centrifuge tubes containing 10 mL 1× PBS. Goat anti-mouse IgG sepharose beads may also be supplied as a slurry. Protein A and goat anti-mouse IgG conjugated to agarose can also be used.
2. Resuspend the beads and incubate the tubes for 30 min at RT.
3. Centrifuge the tubes for 5 min at 1500 rpm. Discard the supernatant into a waste beaker, using a 1 mL plastic squeezer without disturbing the bead pellet.
4. Wash the beads three times by adding 5 mL of Buffer A to the beads, resuspending the beads gently and centrifuging each time for 5 min at 1500 rpm. The bead volume will be approximately 1 mL. Then add 5 mL of Buffer A to resuspend the beads. There will now be 200 μL of bead/mL.
5. Take 1.5 mL of resuspended beads into a 1.5 mL Eppendorf tube (about 250 μL of beads), centrifuge and discard supernatant.
6. Add 400 μL of primary antibody (1:10–1:50 of rabbit or mouse antiserum) into the tube, set the tube on an end-over-end shaker overnight in the cold room. If using monoclonal antibodies (Mabs) or anti-mouse IgG-sepharose beads, add

undiluted spent culture supernatant containing Mabs or ascites fluid diluted appropriately.

7. Centrifuge the tubes for 5 min in a microfuge at 13,000 rpm. Collect the supernatants containing unbound antibodies and save at −20 °C.

8. Wash the beads three times in cold Buffer A, each time centrifuging for 5 min in a microfuge at 13,000 rpm. Discard the wash supernatants and after the last wash, add 1 mL of buffer A to the bead pellet.

9. Distribute 200 μL bead suspension into Eppendorf tubes, each has 50 μL of beads, centrifuge as above and discard supernatant.

10. Add 200 μL of cell extract (0.1% Triton X-100 in PBS used for protein extraction) into the tube. Incubate 1 h at RT or overnight at 4 °C on an end-over-end shaker.

    (a) After incubation, centrifuge tubes, collect the supernatants into Eppendorf tube and save at −20 °C.

11. Wash the beads 2 times in Buffer A, 1 time in Buffer B, 1 time in Buffer C and 1 time in Buffer D. For each wash, discard the supernatant.

12. Add 100 μL of SDS-PAGE sample buffer plus DTT into the tubes, vortex and boil tubes for 3 min, vortex again and centrifuge the tubes for 5 min at 13,000 rpm.

13. Prepare SDS-PAGE gels and electrophoresis buffers for analysis of the precipitated proteins.

14. Load gel, each lane 20 μL and perform electrophoresis.

15. Assemble transfer sandwich and perform western transfer at 350–400 mA overnight at 4 °C.

16. After transfer, process the NCP for blocking and antibody incubation using the antibody used for precipitation, an unrelated antibody and a normal mouse or rabbit serum control.

17. Compare the results, record size of protein band detected on the NCP.

Make IP buffer A, B, C:
Buffer A: 1% BSA, 1% NP40, 1 mM EDTA in 1× PBS
Buffer B: 1% BSA, 1% NP40, 1 mM EDTA, 0.5 M NaCl in 1× PBS
Buffer C: 1% NP40, 1 mM EDTA in 1× PBS
Buffer D: 1 mM EDTA in 1× PBS

Chapter 53
Exercise 28: Induction of Apoptosis in T Lymphocytes and Detection of Apoptotic Markers

Introduction

Apoptosis is a programmed cell death process that occurs in response to extrinsic and intrinsic signals that leads to cell death. Binding of Fas (CD95) to Fas ligand (CD95L) on host cells such as cytotoxic T cells results in activation of the death pathway. Perforin and granzyme release from cytotoxic T cells into target cells leads to release of cytochrome c from mitochondria. Cysteine proteases that cleave after aspartic acid residues, known as caspases become activated and participate in the initiation and completion of the death process. Cells undergoing apoptosis display characteristic features that serve as markers for different stages of apoptosis. Proapoptotic molecules of the Bcl-2 family such as Bid, act on the mitochondria resulting in cytochrome c release. Procaspase 3 is cleaved and activated to caspase-3 which is required for apoptosis to occur. The **first objective** of this exercise is to induce apoptosis using staurosporine and anti-Fas antibody. The **second objective** is to detect apoptotic markers of different stages of apoptosis.

Materials (Per Pair)

Jurkat cells (ATCC)
RPMI 1640 medium
Fetal bovine serum (FBS)
Penicillin-streptomycin
Tissue culture flasks (T25 and T75)
Anti-Fas (CD95) antibody
Anti-caspase-3 antibody (specific for 17 kDa protein)
Staurosporine
Annexin V

© Springer Nature Switzerland AG 2021
T. Y. Sam-Yellowe, *Immunology: Overview and Laboratory Manual*,
https://doi.org/10.1007/978-3-030-64686-8_53

Propidium iodide
Bisbenzimidole Hoechst 33342
37 °C incubator
1× Dulbecco's PBS
Hemocytometer
Timer
Floating rack for microfuge tubes
Bench top centrifuge
15 and 50 mL centrifuge tubes
Serological pipets (1 and 10 mL)
Eppendorf pipettors 20 μL and 200 μL)
Microfuge tubes (1.5 mL)
Pipet tips (yellow tips)
Materials for SDS-PAGE and western blotting
Materials for flow cytometry
Materials for protein assay
Hot plate

Procedure

1. Grow Jurkat cells in tissue culture flasks (T75) containing RPMI medium supplemented with 10% FBS, 100 Units/mL penicillin, 100 μg/mL streptomycin (complete medium) in a 37 °C incubator with 5% CO_2 in humidified air.
2. Harvest cells by pipetting cells into 50 mL centrifuge tubes and centrifuging for 5 min at 300–350 × g. Discard supernatant and resuspend cells in complete medium.
3. Pipet 100 μL of the cell suspension, perform a cell count and adjust cells to 1 × 10^6 cells/mL in six T25 flasks. Label the flasks 1–6. In flask 1 add staurosporine to 0.5 μM, in flask 2 add staurosporine to 1 μM, in flask 3 add 2 mg/mL anti-Fas antibody, in flask 4 add 5 mg/mL anti-Fas antibody, in flask 5, add DMSO and in flask 6 will receive no treatment.
4. Incubate flasks as in step 1 for 4 h.
5. After incubation, collect the cells by pipetting cells into 50 mL centrifuge tubes and centrifuging as in step 2 and discard supernatant.
6. Wash the cells by resuspending the pellet in 1× dPBS and centrifuging as in step 2. Discard the supernatant and resuspend the pellet in 1× dPBS.
7. Label two sets of six microfuge tubes corresponding to each flask, then pipet 200 μL cells from each flask into the tubes.
8. To the first set of six tubes, add 1 μg/mL Bis-benzimidazole Hoechst and propidium iodide into each tube.
9. To the second set of six tubes, add annexin V-FITC to each tube and incubate cells in the dark.
10. Incubate tubes in the dark for 15 min at 37 °C.
11. Perform flow cytometry (Exercise 18, see Chap. 42).

12. Centrifuge the remaining cells in step 6, discard the supernatant and add 100 μL of electrophoresis sample buffer to the pellets.

13. Label six microfuge tubes corresponding to the flasks in step 3. Transfer the solubilized cells from step 11 into each tube. Place the tubes in a floating rack, transfer the rack to a 500 mL flask containing distilled water boiling on a hot plate. (Pellets can be extracted with1% Triton X-100 for protein determination. 40–50 μg total cell extract can be used to load each lane).

14. Boil the tubes for 2 min, remove the rack from the boiling water.

15. Assemble SDS-PAGE gel in gel chamber with running buffer. Load gels with samples and load pre-stained molecular weight markers in the first and last lanes of the gel.

16. While gel is running, prepare nitrocellulose and filter papers for western blotting. Label one NCP for antibody and the second NCP as control.

17. After electrophoresis, assemble sandwich for western transfer and place sandwich in transfer tank for protein transfer.

18. After protein transfer, block the nitrocellulose papers with 2% milk containing 0.05% Tween in blot buffer for 1 h at RT.

19. Prepare antibody dilution (1:500–1:1000 depending on supplier) for anti-caspase-3 antibody in 5 mL of 2% milk in a 15 mL centrifuge tube. Prepare control normal rabbit or mouse serum. Prepare plastic bags using a seal-a-meal device. Place NCPs in plastic bags and add the antibody mixture to one bag and label the bag. Seal the open end of the plastic bag and place sealed bag on a shaker. Add control serum to the second bag, label, seal and place the bag on the shaker. Incubate the NCPs overnight in a 4 °C cold room.

20. Cut one end of each plastic bag, collect the used antibody and control serum using a plastic squeezer pipet, place it into a 15 mL centrifuge tubes. Use a different squeezer for the antibody and control serum. The used antibody can be frozen and reused depending on the titer of the antibody. Remove the NCP and place it into a small Tupperware container containing 1× blot buffer. Wash the NCP four times, twice in 1× blot buffer, once in 1× blot buffer containing 0.5% Triton X-100 and once with 1× blot buffer.

21. Pour out the last wash and add species specific secondary antibody conjugated to HRP diluted 1:1000–1:5000 depending on vendor (Incubate the NCP 2 h at RT (or overnight at 4 °C).

22. Collect secondary antibody and wash NCP four times as in step 19.

23. Prepare developing solution: Solution A (30 mg tablet of powder of 4-chloro-1-naphtol to 10 mL of ice cold methanol in a 200 mL Erhlenmyer flask; Solution B (30 μL of 30% Hydrogen peroxide to 50 mls of ice-cold TBS in a 100 mL Erhlenmyer flask. Pour out wash buffer from NCP.

24. Swirl each flask to mix contents. Add solution B to A, mix and pour solution into container with NCP. Cover container and wrap with foil. Place the container on a shaker for 10 min. Observe the color development of the bands. If bands are faint, incubate for an additional 10 min. Pour out the developing solution and add distilled water to the NCP to stop the enzyme reaction. Record the results. Compare the NCP incubated with antibody to the control NCP incubated with normal rabbit or mouse serum.

Detecting Apoptosis

1. Which of the cells show features of apoptosis? Cells positive for annexin and PI staining or cells positive for PI but negative for annexin staining
2. What is the purpose of staining cells with Bis-benzimidazole Hoechst?

Selected References

Galluzi L, Zamzani N, de La Motte Rouge T, Lemaire C, Brenner C, Kroemer G (2007) Methods for the assessment of mitochondrial membrane permeabilization in apoptosis. Apoptosis 12:803–813

Chapter 54
Exercise 29: Cloning and Sequencing cDNAs of Mouse Variable Regions of H and L Chains of Monoclonal Antibodies

Introduction

Embryonic DNA contains multiple genes that encode the immunoglobulin (Ig) molecule. The Ig genes rearrange to form the variable region of the antibody molecule. Rearrangement takes place on the genes that encode both Heavy (H) and Light (L) chains. The variable regions on both chains form the antigen binding domain located in the Fab fragment of the antibody molecule. In L chains, variable (V) and joining (J) genes recombine to generate the V region. In H chains, V, J and diversity (D) genes recombine to generate the V region. RAG1 and RAG2 recombinases catalyze rearrangement by cleaving DNA at recombination signal sequences (RSSs) between the Ig coding junction and the RSS. Nonhomologous end joining events occur with use of repair enzymes, nucleotide addition by DNA polymerase and ligase activity to facilitate the rearrangement and formation of a contiguous coding sequence for the variable regions. Hybridomas secreting monoclonal antibodies contain a combination of rearranged V regions in H and L chains that encode different secreted antibodies. The type of VH and VL formed can be investigated by identifying the germline families of the V (D) J genes used. DNA isolated from hybridomas can be amplified using primers that target rearranged genes in hybridomas and compared to amplified DNA from embryonic cells. Sequencing of amplified product directly or cloned into a plasmid can be used to demonstrate the particular gene families utilized for rearrangement. Idiotypic homogeneity and cross-reactivity in the antibodies can also be investigated. The **first objective** of this exercise is to determine if monoclonal antibodies specific for the antigen contain different combinations of H and L chain region genes. The **second objective** is to determine the germ-line families of the genes. The **third objective** is to learn how to clone an insert into a plasmid and express the encoded recombinant protein.

© Springer Nature Switzerland AG 2021
T. Y. Sam-Yellowe, *Immunology: Overview and Laboratory Manual*,
https://doi.org/10.1007/978-3-030-64686-8_54

Materials (Per Pair)

Hybridomas
RNA extraction kit
Thermocycler
37 °C incubator and water bath
Ice bucket with ice
Bunsen burner
Cloning vector PUC19
Escherichia coli competent host cells DH5α and BL21 (DE3)
Restriction endonucleases EcoR1 and Bam H1
Ampicillin
X-Gal (5-bromo-4-chloro-3-indoyl-β-D-galacto-pyranoside)
IPTG
Nutrient agar
Luria Bertani (LB) broth and agar plates containing ampicillin
95% ethanol in 200 mL beaker for sterilizing bent glass rod spreaders
Protein L
Agarose
1× Tris acetate EDTA buffer
Ethidium bromide (Methylene blue can also be used)
Oligonucleotide primers targeting variable regions of heavy and light chains
Oligonucleotide primers (forward and reverse) for VLκ gene

Part A

Procedure:

1. Prepare hybridomas using spleen cells obtained from Balb/c mice immunized with antigen and myeloma cells (Exercise 24)
2. Screen for monoclonal antibody production and select clones secreting antibodies specific for the antigen.
3. Clone hybridomas by limiting dilution, propagate and screen to confirm antibody production and reactivity with antigen. Dilute cells to 1×10^9 cells/mL
4. Isolate total RNA from clones using RNA-Bee (Tel-Test, Inc.)
5. Reverse transcribe RNA to synthesize cDNA using SuperScript IV reverse transcriptase kit.
6. Use oligonucleotide primers targeting variable regions of heavy and light chains and primers targeting VLκ chain to perform PCR
7. Separate amplicons on 1% agarose containing ethidium bromide gels along with DNA standard markers.
8. Sequence PCR product from amplified VH, VL and VLκ genes
9. Compare DNA sequence of monoclonal antibodies with mouse Ig genes in GenBank by performing a BLAST search

Part B

1. Gel purify amplified DNA and perform restriction digest using EcoR1 and Bam H1
2. Clone VLκ DNA into PUC19 plasmid vector also restricted with EcoR1 and Bam H1 by ligating amplified DNA with plasmid DNA.
3. Transform competent *Escherichia coli* (strain DH5α) with recombinant plasmid and plate the cells on nutrient agar plates containing ampicillin and X-Gal (5-bromo-4-chloro-3-indoyl β-D-galacto-pyranoside) for blue/white colony selection.

   (a) To transform bacteria, add 5 μL of recombinant DNA to the tube of competent cells. Place the tube on ice for 15 min. Transfer the tube to 42 °C water bath for 1 min. Remove the tube from the water bath and set in a test tube rack at RT. Have the LB agar plates ready and labelled. Using a yellow pipet and P-200 pipetor, place 50 μL cell in one plate and 100 μL in the second plate. Remove the glass spreader from the alcohol, shake off the excess alcohol (carefully) and flame the spreader. Let the spreader cool for a few minutes then spread the cells on the surface of the plate. Repeat the process to spread the second plate. Incubate plates at 37 °C overnight (12–18 h)

4. Purify plasmid DNA from white colonies for use in sequencing
5. Transform competent *Escherichia coli* (strain BL21 (DE3)) with recombinant plasmid and plate the cells on nutrient agar for blue/white colony selection (see procedure above).
6. Select white colonies and inoculate in LB broth culture for induction of recombinant protein expression with IPTG induction.
7. Collect 1 mL cells at 30, 60 and 90 min following IPTG induction. Centrifuge cells, collect and save supernatant. Lyse bacterial pellets in 1% Triton X-100.
8. Incubate supernatants and bacterial lysates with Protein L-agarose for Kappa L chain binding using immunoprecipitation protocol in Exercise 27.
9. After elution of L chain from beads, perform SDS-PAGE and Coomassie blue staining to detect size of the protein band compared to molecular standards on the gel. A western blot can also be performed using HRP conjugated antibodies specific to Fab region or κL chain.

Questions:
1. What was the purpose of using agar plates containing ampicillin?
2. What is the cause of the white colonies on X-Gal plates? Why is the term insertional inactivation used when describing the recombinants in the white colonies?
3. How does the multiple cloning site in the plasmid help with cloning a DNA fragment into the plasmid?
4. What is the function of ligase in the cloning procedure?

NOTES:

Appendix

Vendors Where Supplies, Reagents, Equipment and Materials for Immunology Exercises Can Be Purchased

Abcam (www.abcam.com)
BioLegend (biolegend.com)
BioRad (www. Bio-rad.com)
Biotium (biotium.com)
BioVision, Inc. (www.biovision,com)
Cell Signaling (www.cellsignal.com)
Charles River Laboratories (www.criver.com)
Chromatek (www.chromatek.com)
Ebiosciences, Inc.
Invitrogen/ThermoFischer
Fischer Labs
Miltenyi Biotec (wwww.miltenyicbiotec.com)
Promega
SigmaAldrich
Sino Biologicals (www.sinbiologicals.com)
Southern Biotech (www.southernbiotech.com)
Taconic Biosciences (www.taconic.com)
Tel-test (www. Tel-testinc.com)
The Jackson Laboratory (www.jax.org)
ThermoFischer Scientific (www.thermofiscer.com)
VWR, Part of Avantor (www.vwr.com)

Helpful immunology websites and sites that have supply reagents useful for immunology experiments

www.cdc.gov/bam/diseases/immune/
https://www.cdc.gov
www.who.int
www.niaid.nih.gov/publichealth/PMH00725791
www.bio-alive.com/animations/anatomy.htm
www.miltenyibiotec.com/cytokines
www.abcam.com/pathways/chemokine-signaling-interactive-pathway
www.biolegend.com/basic_immunology
www.cellular-immunity.blogspot.com/2007/12/vdj-recombinant.html
www.rndsystems.com/resources/posters/t-cell-subsets
www.cellsignal.com
https://www.bio-rad-antibodies.com/mucosal-Immunology-minireview.html

www.jax.org
www.anatomybox.com
www.nature.com/subjects/cellsignalling/research
www.bio.davidson.edu/courses/movies.html
www.aaaai.org
https://www.immunotolerance.org
https://www.cancer.org
www.youtube.com
www.webmd.com/allergies

Buffers and Solutions

TRIS-TRICINE BUFFER pH 8.6

17.2 g Tricine
39.2 g Tris Base
0.8 g Sodium azide
0.4 g Calcium lactate

Mix with 800.0 mL dH_20, then bring up to 1.0 L. pH to 8.6 and then add 3.0 L
10× BLOT BUFFER

9.0 g NaCl
15.76 g Tris

Mix with 800.0 mL dH_20.then bring up to 1.0 L. pH to 7.4.
10× TRANSFER BUFFER

24.22 g Tris-Base
112.605 g Glycine

Mix with 800.0 mL dH_20.then bring up to 1.0 L.
10× PBS (Phosphate Buffered Saline)

2.0 g KCl
2.0 g KH_2PO_4
80.0 g NaCl
21.6 g Na_2HPO_4

Mix with 800.0 mL dH_20 then bring up to 1.0 L.
10× RUNNING BUFFER

30.3 g Tris-Base
144.2 g Glycine
10.0 g SDS (sodium dodecyl sulphate)

Mix with 800.0 mL dH$_2$0, then bring up to 1.0 L.

1.0 M TRIS BUFFER pH 8.8 and 6.8

121.0 g Tris-Base

Mix with 800.0 mL dH$_2$0, then bring up to 1.0 L. pH to 8.8 or 6.8 with cone. HCl.

10.0% SDS

10.0 g SDS

Mix with 80.0 mL dH$_2$0, then bring up to 100.0 mL.

Cell culture media:

RPMI
EBSS
HBSS
DMEM

NOTES:

Sample Practice Questions

I.

1. What is the final magnification of cells viewed under a light microscope using a 20× ocular lens and a high dry objective lens (40×)?
2. What is the magnification of a typical oil immersion lens on a light microscope?
3. How many grams of NaCl (Molecular weight 58.44) are required to prepare a 0.2 M solution in 500 mL of distilled water?
4. What is the molar concentration of physiological saline (NaCl)-0.85 % in 1 L of distilled water?
5. What is the clinical significance of the ABO blood antigen system?
6. If a woman is Rh (−) and the fetus that she is carrying is Rh (+), what is the potential danger to the fetus and to future pregnancies?
7. Name the primary and secondary lymphoid organs.
8. What are the major components of human blood?
9. Which of the following denotations is correct when it is used to indicate the hydrogen ion concentration of a solution?

   (a) PH
   (b) Ph
   (c) pH
   (d) ph

10. 1.5 milliliter (mL) equals _____ microliter (μL).
11. 28 milligrams (mg) equals _____ gram (g).
12. How much water must be added to 25.0 mL of 0.50 M KOH solution to produce a solution whose concentration is 0.35 M?
13. The serological technique for determining ABO and Rh blood types is known as _____
14. What blood group antigen is responsible for hemolytic disease of the new born?
15. John's blood group is AB+. What types of antibodies are present in his blood?

II.

1. From a mitogen stock solution of 1 mg/mL, what dilution is required to obtain a working solution of 2 μg/mL?
2. What two types of serial dilutions are routinely used in an immunology laboratory?
3. Kimberly prepared a working dilution of her new antibody by adding 0.05 mL of the antibody stock to 4.95 mL of PBS (1×). Calculate the following:

   (a) The dilution factor she prepared.
   (b) The antibody concentration in the diluent (PBS) expressed as a percentage.
   (c) The titer of the antibody after the dilution.
   (d) The volume of antibody she used expressed in microliters.

4. Kalada serially diluted a concentrated stock solution of ovalbumin (OVA) by diluting 5 mL of OVA in a tube containing 5 mL of distilled water. He then transferred 5 mL of the diluted OVA into a second tube containing 5 mL of water. Calculate the final dilution factor in the second tube. What type of serial dilution did Kalada perform?

5. If you perform the following dilutions: 1:2, 1:4, 1:8, 1:64 and 1:50 from a 25% solution of methylene blue, what will be the final concentration of dye in the final tube?

6. Illustrate the dilution scheme shown above, indicating the volumes of the diluent and dye stock required to achieve the correct dilutions.

III.

1. Identify the following lymphoid organs as primary or secondary

   (a) Thymus
   (b) Spleen
   (c) Gut-associated lymphoid tissue (GALT)
   (d) Bone marrow
   (e) Lymph nodes

2. What is the total cell number and percent cell viability (Trypan blue) from the following spleen cell count performed using a hemocytometer? Square I, 50 unstained, 8 stained; square II, 75 unstained, 10 stained; square III, 60 unstained, 9 stained; square IV, 65 unstained, 8 stained. The cells were counted from a 1:50 dilution prepared in a total volume of 5 mL.

3. Which instrument is used to determine the cell viability in a cell suspension?

4. If Trypan blue is used to stain a lymphoid cell suspension, how can you differentiate the live cells from the dead cells?

5. Name two other methods for determining cell viability besides Trypan blue staining.

6. If after diluting a cell suspension to perform a cell count, you only observe one or two cells in each large square, what might you do differently to obtain acceptable counts on the hemocytometer?

7. Name a subclass of lymphocytes, which mature in the thymus.

8. Name the lymphoid organ where hematopoiesis takes place.

9. You are going to dilute 12 μL of a cell suspension (the dilution factor is 1:10) with 0.2% trypan blue and HBSS, and let the final concentration of trypan blue become 0.01%. How many μL of 0.2% trypan blue and how many μl of HBSS will be used?

IV.

1. What is the RES or MPS system?
2. What are the major cells of the RES system?
3. What are the clinical terms for the following conditions:

   (a) Enlarged spleen
   (b) Enlarged liver
   (c) Enlarged lymph nodes

4. What does adoptive transfer mean?
5. What is a mitogen? Name a specific B cell mitogen and a specific T cell mitogen.
6. Name four precautions that must be observed to maintain aseptic conditions in tissue culture work.
7. John diluted 0.01 mL of blood cells with 990 μL of sterile saline.

   (a) Calculate the dilution factor of the cell suspension.
   (b) What is the percentage of blood cells if the resulting cell suspension was further diluted with saline at 1:2?

V.

1. Name a cell which actively participates in the RES system to remove blood borne particles.
2. Kamere injected 1×10^6 bacterial cells i.v. into a mouse. After 30 min he recovered only 1×10^2 cells. What is the clearance rate of the bacterial cells by the mouse?
3. What type of cells are (a) Langerhans cells; (b) Kupffer cells; (c) dendritic cells?
4. Are bacterial cells eukaryotic or prokaryotic cells?
5. From the following dilution scheme: Five tubes containing saline blanks of 4.5 mLs with 0.5 transferred between each tube followed by two tubes, each containing 9.9 mL of saline with 0.1 and transferred from the last 4.5 mL blank through the last 9.9 mL tube. What is the dilution in each tube? What is the final dilution factor of the series? What type of dilution series was performed?
6. If a cell suspension containing 3×10^{10} bacterial cells/mL was diluted using the dilution scheme in #5, calculate the cell number in each tube. If 100 μL of the cell suspension from each tube was plated on nutrient agar, how would this change the final dilution in each plate? If the 250 colony forming units (CFU) are counted in tube #4, calculate the number of cells/ml in tube # 4.
7. From a culture containing 5×10^8 cells/mL, calculate the dilution required to obtain 100 CFU on a nutirent agar plate.

VI.

1. The direct hemoly-tic plaque assay measures only cells secreting IgG antibodies. (a) True or (b) False.
2. What is the purpose of using Guinea pig complement in the hemolytic plaque assay? What is the purpose of using the sheep red blood cells?

   (a) Antigen
   (b) Immune complex
   (c) Agglutination
   (d) Precipitation
   (e) Titer
   (f) Tanning

3. In general why are agglutination reactions more sensitive than precipitation reactions?
4. What is the difference between direct hemagglutination and passive hemagglutination?
5. When soluble antigens react with their respective antisera _____ will form.
6. In general, _____ are less sensitive in detecting the presence of specific antibodies than agglutination reactions

   (a) complement fixation
   (b) precipitation reactions
   (c) none of the above

7. When particulate antigens react with their respective antisera _____ will form.

   (a) precipitation
   (b) agglutination
   (c) none of the above

8. Maximum precipitation occurs when the antigen and antibody concentration are in _____.
9. Name the individual who developed the Ouchterlony gel immunodiffusion technique.
10. In immunoelectrophoresis technique _____ diffuse

    (a) antigen
    (b) antibody
    (c) both antigen and antibody
    (d) none of the above

VII.

1. The dye-binding protein assay is based on the principle of _____.
2. Why would you want to know the protein concentration in an unknown sample before performing SDS-PAGE or other protocols?
3. If the OD of an unknown sample is much higher than the OD of the protein standard used to generate the standard curve, how will you go about determining the protein concentration in your unknown sample? Why is necessary to prepare a standard curve?
4. Briefly describe how you would collect and process blood collected from a rabbit.
5. What does SDS-PAGE stand for?
6. What is the difference between reducing and non-reducing SDS-PAGE? What is the function of SDS?
7. What difference will be observed when purified IgG is separated under reducing conditions or nonreducing conditions?
8. You have been handed notes from your lab partner detailing the preparation of buffers. One of the solutions, a 10 mL 0.5% ovalbumin solution was prepared from a 20% stock solution. The notes show that 500 µL of the stock solution was diluted in 10 mL to give 0.5% concentration. What is the problem with the calculation?
9. What do you understand by the following terms: (illustrate an example of each system). **simple diffusion system, double diffusion system, identity precipitation, partial identity precipitation, non-identity precipitation,** and **rocket immunoelectrophoresis**
10. What three factors can affect or influence the rate of protein diffusion through a gel matrix?

VIII.

1. Why is 2% non-fat milk used in the western blotting procedure?
2. What will be the appearance of the NCP at the end of a Western Blot procedure if the blocking step is omitted?
3. Name an assay that can be used to detect single antibody or cytokine secreting cells. Name one major advantage of this assay over an ELISA assay.
4. How can you detect proteins separated on an SDS-PAGE gel? What method can be used to identify a single protein from the complex mixture of proteins separated on the gel?
5. Name two matrices which may be used for protein separation.
6. Briefly and clearly describe the immunoblotting and immunofluorescence techniques.
7. Tissue culture techniques were developed to study animal cells in vivo. (a) True or (b) False.
8. What specific technique allows one to enrich for mononuclear cells?

9. Cell culture can be maintained as anchorage dependent or anchorage independent. How do these two techniques differ?
10. What does aseptic technique mean?
11. What organism serves as the source for Protein A? What cells respond mitogenically to Protein A, lipopolysaccharide or concanavalin A?
12. What are superantigens?
13. Name two procedures where having a high lymphocyte viability (80–90%) is advantageous.
14. After performing a serial 1:2 dilution of antiserum, eleven times using PBS, calculate the final dilution factor of the antiserum.

IX.

1. What are cytokines?
2. What are the sources and the functions of the following cytokines?

   (a) IL-1
   (b) IL-2
   (b) IL-4
   (c) IL-5
   (d) IL-8
   (e) IL-10
   (f) IL-12
   (g) GM-CSF

3. Define immunity.
4. List advantages of primary binding assays.
5. If you have 2 rabbit antisera specific for CD4 antigens and IgD, design an IFA experiment which will allow you to differentiate B and T cell subpopulations from a spleen cell and a thymus cell suspension. Would the ratio of T and B cells differ in the two cell suspensions?
6. Describe (a) direct ELISA; (b) indirect ELISA; (c) competitive ELISA
7. What do the following assays detect:

   (a) Northern blotting
   (b) Southern blotting
   (c) Western blotting

8. What is bacterial transformation? Why are the bacterial cells made competent before transformation?
9. Briefly describe how DNA is engineered to generate a recombinant DNA molecule.
10. What is the difference between genomic DNA and complementary DNA?
11. Briefly describe the process of gene cloning into a plasmid and expression in an E. coli host cell.

12. Define the following terms:

  (a) Purines
  (b) Pyrimidines
  (c) Transcription
  (d) Replication
  (e) Operon
  (f) Origin of Replication
  (g) Restriction Endonuclease
  (h) Restriction Site
  (i) Deoxynucleotide Triphosphates (dNTPs)
  (j) Polymerase Chain Reaction (PCR)
  (k) Cathode
  (l) Anode
  (m) Buffer
  (n) Ph
  (o) Hybridization
  (p) Absorbance
  (q) Antibiotic
  (r) Selectable Marker
  (s) Clone
  (t) Colony
  (u) Log phase
  (v) Complimentarity
  (w) Plasmid
  (x) Phage
  (y) Sterilization
  (z) Blue/White Colony Selection

Selected References

Corradini P, Boccadoro M, Voena C, Pileri A (1993) Evidence for a bone marrow B cell transcribing malignant plasma cell VDJ joined to Cμ sequence in immunoglobulin (IGG)- and IgA-secreting multiple myeloma. J Exp Med 178:1091–1096

Kotloff DB, Bosma MJ, Ruetsch NR (1993) V(D)J recombination in peritoneal B cells of leaky scid mice. J Exp Med 178:1981–1994

Sollbach AE, Wu GE (1995) Inversions produced during V(D)J rearrangement at IgH, the immunoglobulin Heavy-chain locus. Mol Cell Biol 15:671–681

Index

Printed in the United States
by Baker & Taylor Publisher Services